Aromadermatology

Aromatherapy in the treatment and care of common skin conditions

Janetta Bensouilah
Private Practitioner of Acupuncture and Aromatherapy, Surrey
Registered Principal Tutor, International Federation of
Professional Aromatherapists

and

Philippa Buck
Aromatherapy Practitioner in Private Practice, Surrey
Registered Tutor, International Federation of
Professional Aromatherapists

Forewords by

Robert Tisserand

and

Angela Avis

Radcliffe Publishing
Oxford • Seattle

Radcliffe Publishing Ltd
18 Marcham Road
Abingdon
Oxon OX14 1AA
United Kingdom

www.radcliffe-oxford.com
Electronic catalogue and worldwide online ordering facility.

Every effort has been made in the preparation of this publication to provide
accurate and up-to-date information at the time of publication. However,
aromatherapy is a rapidly changing field as clinical standards and practices are
constantly broadened through research and adapted in line with regulation.
Readers are strongly advised to check the product information provided by the
manufacturer of any product or preparation that they plan to use. Neither the
publisher nor authors assume any liability for direct or consequential damages
arising from the use of material in this publication.

British Library Cataloguing in Publication Data

A catalogue record for this book is available from the British Library.

ISBN-10: 1 85775 775 0
ISBN-13: 978 1 85775 775 0

Typeset by Anne Joshua & Associates, Oxford
Printed and bound by TJ International Ltd, Padstow, Cornwall

Contents

Foreword

There are very few evidence-based texts dealing with the therapeutic application of essential oils and, until now, there were none that covered the skin. This paucity of coverage is surprising, considering that dermal application of essential oils is the most frequent mode of use. Perhaps because this subject area is only lightly touched on in most aromatherapy books, it has remained a source of debate and confusion.

Bensouilah and Buck have gone a long way to dispelling this confusion through their detailed discussion of, for example, transdermal permeation and skin barrier issues, excipients, and dosages and concentrations, as well as therapeutic effects. These discussions are woven into a foundation covering the basics of skin structure and function, essential oil chemistry and safety issues.

The risk of skin sensitisation from preservatives, both natural and synthetic, could perhaps have been more fully considered, but generally there is a good awareness and understanding of dermatological safety. This is a particularly difficult area, since allergic skin reactions to essential oils are not easy to anticipate, and the pre-emptive use of patch testing remains controversial. It is good to see the subject of essential oil oxidation being discussed in the context of skin reactions, since its important safety implications are often not appreciated by those who use the oils.

The reader is frequently reminded to weigh risk against benefit (such as in the case of tea tree oil) and this may help to counter the largely negative view of essential oils held by some dermatologists. The *Skin and psyche* chapter is particularly interesting, and is a potent reminder that the therapeutic effects of essential oils can take place through a number of mechanisms, some purely physical and some not.

This well-illustrated, thorough and authoritative text is written in a language and style that is clear and accessible to a variety of healthcare practitioners, without talking down to anyone – an accomplishment in itself. A thorough understanding of dermatology underpins the book, and both current research and clinical knowledge are elegantly applied to the skin conditions discussed. Because of these factors, the few unsupported statements that are made can be forgiven, and the cohesion and structure of the book hold together well, considering the diversity of subjects covered.

Robert Tisserand
Ojai, California
August 2006

Foreword

With the growing interest in aromatherapy, it is important that therapists and healthcare professionals are able to offer a valid rationale when integrating essential oils into clinical care. Sound knowledge of bio-chemical principles and the ability to critically appraise and apply relevant research are fundamental requirements. This book offers a comprehensive, in-depth view of current knowledge. The authors have skilfully woven research and clinical application. A range of therapeutic possibilities is explored and offers practitioners alternative approaches to the management of skin conditions. These include detailed discussions on different methods of application. I hope that this book will become a standard text on both pre-qualifying and CPD courses in aromatherapy.

Angela Avis MBE

RGN, DNCert, PGDip Ed, PGDip Advanced Healthcare Practice, MA

Senior Lecturer, Oxford Brookes University

Formerly, Chair, RCN Complementary Therapies Forum

August 2006

Preface

In recent years there has been a considerable increase in the expectation that advocates of traditional approaches to healthcare will be able to provide sound scientific evidence to support their integration into conventional medicine. To meet these expectations, modern aromatherapy – with its origins set firmly in a folkloric, empirical tradition and drawing upon a rich diversity of styles and approaches – faces significant challenges. One main challenge is the urgent need to reconcile conflicts that exist between different approaches to the theoretical basis of aromatherapy. By actively engaging with the science behind the therapy, although this may challenge much of the established dogma, this will encourage scientifically sound and person-centred holistic styles of practice to emerge which are fully able to integrate with mainstream medicine.

This book is an attempt to meet some of the challenges by exploring the evidence for one area of aromatherapy practice where the science assuredly supports an integrated approach to care. We attempt to accurately extrapolate from scientific studies information that can be used to develop a host of effective treatment strategies for common dermatological conditions. Through the course of our work, we have encountered individuals seeking relief from the symptoms of many skin disorders and aromadermatology is as much about offering an integrated, complementary approach as it is about providing alternatives in cases where mainstream approaches have little to offer.

Although large-scale clinical trials are lacking, we have used evidence from a variety of sources and have concentrated on common conditions seen in clinical practice. By bringing a degree of clarity to this area of aromatherapy practice, it is our aim to encourage the adoption of approaches that make full use of the proven benefits of essential oils and other natural products. It may also be that by seeking to present an approach that represents a harmony between research, theory and practice, avenues for future studies in this field are pursued.

The aim throughout the book is to keep speculative ideas to a minimum, while at the same time identifying scope for originality, enabling a flexible approach to aromatic formulations to emerge. It was never our intention to write a book of definitive recipes or formulations, and it is very far from our wish that the formulations we provide be slavishly adopted. They are given merely to illustrate the direction with which we as practitioners might approach a topic where we feel it adds something to the matter under discussion. Our expectation is that any practitioner referring to this book will always apply their professional judgement in any given case, using the information herein for further exploration.

We have assumed the reader is familiar with the basic concepts of aromatherapy. The first three chapters provide an overview of essential oil sciences and safety that are directly relevant to aromadermatology, without going over ground that is covered in other texts. For a refresher in essential oil chemistry, readers may like to consult *The Chemistry of Aromatherapeutic Oils* by E Joy Bowles (2003, Allen & Unwin), as it is one of the best books currently available on this topic. The remaining chapters span a range of common conditions where aromatherapy has something valuable to offer in clinical practice. There may be overlaps between topics and chapters (we are after all focused here on a single body-system) and, although we have tried to cluster together, in a logical order, conditions and appropriate treatment strategies, the reader will find it helpful to move flexibly around the book when looking for information on a particular condition. This is especially the case with the inflammatory disorder dermatitis, a condition that comes up in several contexts throughout the book.

Finally, we hope that in the intellectual rigours of sifting and sorting the huge volume of research papers in the preparation of this book, we have managed to retain here the essence of what is a wonderful, remarkably eclectic, person-centred rather than symptom-centred therapy with masses of potential yet to be fully exploited.

Janetta Bensouilah
Philippa Buck
August 2006

About the authors

Janetta Bensouilah MBAcC, LicAc, MIFPA, CertEd

Janetta holds professional qualifications in clinical and holistic aromatherapy, reflexology and acupuncture. Her clinical experience includes the setting up and running of a multidisciplinary complementary therapy clinic in a council-funded day-care centre for the elderly and she currently maintains a private practice where she provides multidisciplinary treatments to patients.

Over the years Janetta has developed and written a range of professional level courses in aromatherapy and holds Principal Tutor status with the International Federation of Professional Aromatherapists (IFPA).

Philippa Buck BPharm, MRPharmS, PGCert MedToxicol, MIFPA

Philippa qualified and registered as a Pharmaceutical Chemist in 1986. In 1991, after having worked as a hospital and community pharmacist, she worked as a Clinical Research Associate for a multinational company involved in dermatological clinical trials. Philippa holds professional qualifications in clinical and holistic aromatherapy and has studied Medical Toxicology at the University of Wales College of Medicine which allowed her to develop a fuller understanding of the safety of essential oils.

She currently teaches pathophysiology, pharmacology, essential oil sciences and aromatherapy on IFPA accredited courses. She runs a private aromatherapy practice, specialising in aromadermatology and paediatrics.

Acknowledgements

We are very grateful to so many people who have helped us in the completion of this book and it is with a small degree of anxiety that we attempt to recognise individuals for fear of missing anyone out. However, we would like to first thank many of our colleagues for giving us much needed support and encouragement: in particular Vivienne Parker for her unfailing understanding when we were absent from the office for longer than we probably ought to have been; Wendy Allen for her refreshing humour and Rhiannon Harris who gave valuable advice and insightful suggestions; Lisa Cadman for providing the drawings; and Lynn Bertram for getting us started. Finally, very special and heartfelt thanks to our friends and families, especially Michel, Lois, David and Jonathon, for their endless patience and loving support.

Botanical terminology

We have adopted the convention of using botanical names, followed by English common names, when referring to plant extracts in this book. With botanical names we have attempted to ensure that the most globally relevant and up to date are used and given in the usual botanical format with italicised generic names starting with an upper-case letter, followed by the species in lower case. Chemotypes and plant parts are given where of particular note but naming botanists are not; these can be found in the Appendix, along with the botanical families and a range of synonyms.

List of abbreviations

ACD	allergic contact dermatitis
ACTH	adrenocorticotrophic hormone
AD	atopic dermatitis
AGM	absorbent gelling material
AHA	alpha-hydroxy acid
BP	balsam of Peru
CAM	complementary and alternative medicine
CNS	central nervous system
CPD	continuing professional development
CRF	corticotrophin releasing factor
CSF	colony stimulating factor
DGLA	dihomogammalinolenic acid
DMAPP	dimethylallyl diphosphate
DMMB	dimethoxymethylbenzene
DNA	deoxyribonucleic acid
EFA	essential fatty acid
EP	European Pharmacopoeia
ESR	erythrocyte sedimentation rate
EU	European Union
FM	fragrance mix
GAG	glycosaminoglycan
GLA	gamma-linolenic acid
GSE	grapefruit seed extract
HIV	human immunodeficiency virus
HPA	hypothalamic pituitary axis
HPV	human papilloma virus
HSV	herpes simplex virus
HT	hepatotoxic
IAPT	International Association for Plant Taxonomy
ICD	irritant contact dermatitis
IFRA	International Fragrance Association
IL	interleukin
IPP	isopentyl pyrophosphate
MBC	minimum bactericidal concentration
MBP	methyl-p-hydroxybenzoate
MCV	molluscum contagiosum virus
MHC	major histocompatibility complex
MIC	minimum inhibitory concentration
MRSA	methicillin resistant *Staphylococcus aureus*
NMF	natural moisturising factors
NK	Natural Killer (cells)
NT	neurotoxic

OCD	obsessive-compulsive disorder
O/W	oil-in-water
PEA	phenylethyl alcohol
PG	prostaglandin
PNI	psychoneuroimmunology
PPM	parts per million
RIFM	Research Institute for Fragrance Materials
RNA	ribonucleic acid
SCCNFP	Scientific Committee on Cosmetics and Non-Food Products
SCCP	Scientific Committee on Consumer Products
SLS	sodium lauryl sulphate
SPF	sun protection factor
TEWL	transepidermal water loss
TNF	tumour necrosis factor
UV	ultraviolet
UVR	ultraviolet radiation
V/V	volume-volume percentage
VZV	varicella-zoster virus
W/O	water-in-oil

Chapter 1

Skin structure and function

Introduction

The integument or skin is the largest organ of the body, making up 16% of body weight, with a surface area of 1.8 m². It has several functions, the most important being to form a physical barrier to the environment, allowing and limiting the inward and outward passage of water, electrolytes and various substances while providing protection against micro-organisms, ultraviolet radiation, toxic agents and mechanical insults. There are three structural layers to the skin: the epidermis, the dermis and subcutis. Hair, nails, sebaceous, sweat and apocrine glands are regarded as derivatives of skin (*see* Figure 1.1). Skin is a dynamic organ in a constant state of change, as cells of the outer layers are continuously shed and replaced by inner cells moving up to the surface. Although structurally

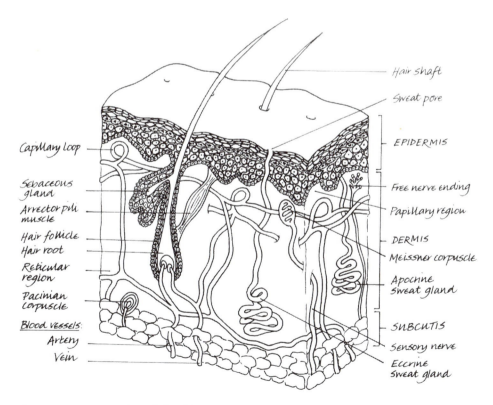

Figure 1.1 Cross-section of the skin.

Table 1.1 Layers of the skin.

Skin layer	Description
Epidermis	The external layer mainly composed of layers of keratinocytes but also containing melanocytes, Langerhans cells and Merkel cells.
Basement membrane	The multilayered structure forming the dermoepidermal junction.
Dermis	The area of supportive connective tissue between the epidermis and the underlying subcutis: contains sweat glands, hair roots, nervous cells and fibres, blood and lymph vessels.
Subcutis	The layer of loose connective tissue and fat beneath the dermis.

consistent throughout the body, skin varies in thickness according to anatomical site and age of the individual.

Skin anatomy

The epidermis is the outer layer, serving as the physical and chemical barrier between the interior body and exterior environment; the dermis is the deeper layer providing the structural support of the skin, below which is a loose connective tissue layer, the subcutis or hypodermis which is an important depot of fat (*see* Table 1.1).

Epidermis

The epidermis is stratified squamous epithelium. The main cells of the epidermis are the keratinocytes, which synthesise the protein keratin. Protein bridges called desmosomes connect the keratinocytes, which are in a constant state of transition from the deeper layers to the superficial (*see* Figure 1.2). The four separate layers of the epidermis are formed by the differing stages of keratin maturation. The epidermis varies in thickness from 0.05 mm on the eyelids to 0.8–1.5 mm on the soles of the feet and palms of the hand. Moving from the lower layers upwards to the surface, the four layers of the epidermis are:

- stratum basale (basal or germinativum cell layer)
- stratum spinosum (spinous or prickle cell layer)
- stratum granulosum (granular cell layer)
- stratum corneum (horny layer).

In addition, the stratum lucidum is a thin layer of translucent cells seen in thick epidermis. It represents a transition from the stratum granulosum and stratum corneum and is not usually seen in thin epidermis. Together, the stratum spinosum and stratum granulosum are sometimes referred to as the Malphigian layer.

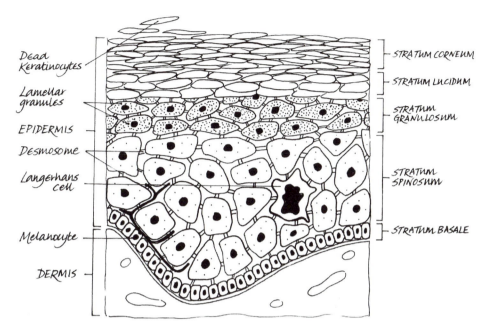

Figure 1.2 Layers of the epidermis.

Stratum basale

The innermost layer of the epidermis which lies adjacent to the dermis comprises mainly dividing and non-dividing keratinocytes, which are attached to the basement membrane by hemidesmosomes. As keratinocytes divide and differentiate, they move from this deeper layer to the surface. Making up a small proportion of the basal cell population is the pigment (melanin) producing melanocytes. These cells are characterised by dendritric processes, which stretch between relatively large numbers of neighbouring keratinocytes. Melanin accumulates in melanosomes that are transferred to the adjacent keratinocytes where they remain as granules. Melanin pigment provides protection against ultraviolet (UV) radiation; chronic exposure to light increases the ratio of melanocytes to keratinocytes, so more are found in facial skin compared to the lower back and a greater number on the outer arm compared to the inner arm. The number of melanocytes is the same in equivalent body sites in white and black skin but the distribution and rate of production of melanin is different. Intrinsic ageing diminishes the melanocyte population.

Merkel cells are also found in the basal layer with large numbers in touch-sensitive sites such as the fingertips and lips. They are closely associated with cutaneous nerves and seem to be involved in light touch sensation.

Stratum spinosum

As basal cells reproduce and mature, they move towards the outer layer of skin, initially forming the stratum spinosum. Intercellular bridges, the desmosomes, which appear as 'prickles' at a microscopic level, connect the cells. Langerhans cells are dendritic, immunologically active cells derived from the bone marrow, and are found on all epidermal surfaces but are mainly located in the middle of this layer. They play a significant role in immune reactions of the skin, acting as antigen-presenting cells.

Stratum granulosum

Continuing their transition to the surface the cells continue to flatten, lose their nuclei and their cytoplasm appears granular at this level.

Stratum corneum

The final outcome of keratinocyte maturation is found in the stratum corneum, which is made up of layers of hexagonal-shaped, non-viable cornified cells known as corneocytes. In most areas of the skin, there are 10–30 layers of stacked corneocytes with the palms and soles having the most. Each corneocyte is surrounded by a protein envelope and is filled with water-retaining keratin proteins. The cellular shape and orientation of the keratin proteins add strength to the stratum corneum. Surrounding the cells in the extracellular space are stacked layers of lipid bilayers (*see* Figure 1.3).

The resulting structure provides the natural physical and water-retaining barrier of the skin. The corneocyte layer can absorb three times its weight in water but if its water content drops below 10% it no longer remains pliable and cracks. The movement of epidermal cells to this layer usually takes about 28 days and is known as the epidermal transit time.

Dermoepidermal junction/basement membrane

This is a complex structure composed of two layers. Abnormalities here result in the expression of rare skin diseases such as bullous pemphigoid and epidermolysis bullosa. The structure is highly irregular, with dermal papillae from the papillary dermis projecting perpendicular to the skin surface. It is via diffusion at this junction that the epidermis obtains nutrients and disposes of waste. The dermoepidermal junction flattens during ageing which accounts in part for some of the visual signs of ageing.

Dermis

The dermis varies in thickness, ranging from 0.6 mm on the eyelids to 3 mm on the back, palms and soles. It is found below the epidermis and is composed of a tough, supportive cell matrix. Two layers comprise the dermis:

- a thin papillary layer
- a thicker reticular layer.

The papillary dermis lies below and connects with the epidermis. It contains thin loosely arranged collagen fibres. Thicker bundles of collagen run parallel to the skin surface in the deeper reticular layer, which extends from the base of the papillary layer to the subcutis tissue. The dermis is made up of fibroblasts, which produce collagen, elastin and structural proteoglycans, together with immunocompetent mast cells and macrophages. Collagen fibres make up 70% of the dermis, giving it strength and toughness. Elastin maintains normal elasticity and flexibility while proteoglycans provide viscosity and hydration. Embedded

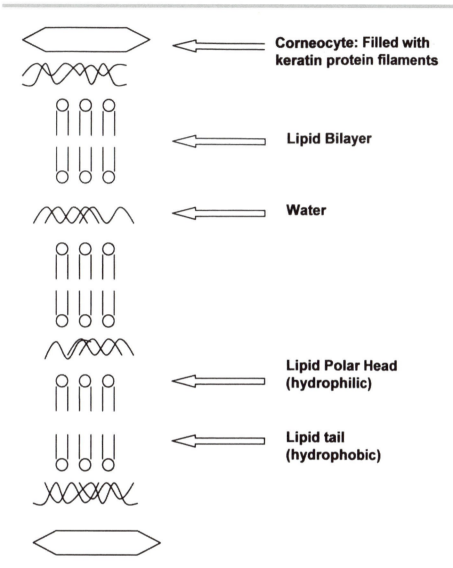

Figure 1.3 Corneocyte lipid bilayers.

within the fibrous tissue of the dermis are the dermal vasculature, lymphatics, nervous cells and fibres, sweat glands, hair roots and small quantities of striated muscle.

Subcutis

This is made up of loose connective tissue and fat, which can be up to 3 cm thick on the abdomen.

Blood and lymphatic vessels

The dermis receives a rich blood supply. A superficial artery plexus is formed at the papillary and reticular dermal boundary by branches of the subcutis artery.

Branches from this plexus form capillary loops in the papillae of the dermis, each with a single loop of capillary vessels, one arterial and one venous. The veins drain into mid-dermal and subcutaneous venous networks. Dilatation or constriction of these capillary loops plays a direct role in thermoregulation of the skin. Lymphatic drainage of the skin occurs through abundant lymphatic meshes that originate in the papillae and feed into larger lymphatic vessels that drain into regional lymph nodes.

Nerve supply

The skin has a rich innervation with the hands, face and genitalia having the highest density of nerves. All cutaneous nerves have their cell bodies in the dorsal root ganglia and both myelinated and non-myelinated fibres are found. Free sensory nerve endings lie in the dermis where they detect pain, itch and temperature. Specialised corpuscular receptors also lie in the dermis allowing sensations of touch to be received by Meissner's corpuscles and pressure and vibration by Pacinian corpuscles. The autonomic nervous system supplies the motor innervation of the skin: adrenergic fibres innervate blood vessels, hair erector muscles and apocrine glands while cholinergic fibres innervate eccrine sweat glands. The endocrine system regulates the sebaceous glands, which are not innervated by autonomic fibres.

Derivative structures of the skin

Hair

Hair can be found in varying densities of growth over the entire surface of the body, exceptions being on the palms, soles and glans penis. Follicles are most dense on the scalp and face and are derived from the epidermis and the dermis. Each hair follicle is lined by germinative cells, which produce keratin and melanocytes, which synthesise pigment. The hair shaft consists of an outer cuticle, a cortex of keratinocytes and an inner medulla. The root sheath, which surrounds the hair bulb, is composed of an outer and inner layer. An erector pili muscle is associated with the hair shaft and contracts with cold, fear and emotion to pull the hair erect, giving the skin 'goose bumps'.

Nails

Nails consist of a dense plate of hardened keratin between 0.3 and 0.5 mm thick. Fingernails function to protect the tip of the fingers and to aid grasping. The nail is made up of a nail bed, nail matrix and a nail plate. The nail matrix is composed of dividing keratinocytes, which mature and keratinise into the nail plate. Underneath the nail plate lies the nail bed. The nail plate appears pink due to adjacent dermal capillaries and the white lunula at the base of the plate is the distal, visible part of the matrix. The thickened epidermis which underlies the free margin of the nail at the proximal end is called the hyponychium. Fingernails grow at 0.1 mm per day; the toenails more slowly (*see* Figure 1.4).

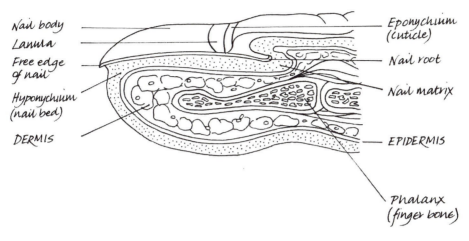

Figure 1.4 Nail structure.

Sebaceous glands

These glands are derived from epidermal cells and are closely associated with hair follicles especially those of the scalp, face, chest and back; they are not found in hairless areas. They are small in children, enlarging and becoming active at puberty, being sensitive to androgens. They produce an oily sebum by holocrine secretion in which the cells break down and release their lipid cytoplasm. The full function of sebum is unknown at present but it does play a role in the following:[1]

- maintaining the epidermal permeability barrier, structure and differentiation
- skin-specific hormonal signalling
- transporting antioxidants to the skin surface
- protection from UV radiation.

Sweat glands

There are thought to be over 2.5 million on the skin surface and they are present over the majority of the body. They are located within the dermis and are composed of coiled tubes, which secrete a watery substance. They are classified into two different types: eccrine and apocrine.

- Eccrine glands are found all over the skin especially on the palms, soles, axillae and forehead. They are under psychological and thermal control. Sympathetic (cholinergic) nerve fibres innervate eccrine glands. The watery fluid they secrete contains chloride, lactic acid, fatty acids, urea, glycoproteins and mucopolysaccharides.
- Apocrine glands are larger, the ducts of which empty out into the hair follicles. They are present in the axillae, anogenital region and areolae and are under thermal control. They become active at puberty, producing an odourless protein-rich secretion which when acted upon by skin bacteria gives out a characteristic odour. These glands are under the control of sympathetic (adrenergic) nerve fibres.

Table 1.2 Functions of the skin.

- Provides a protective barrier against mechanical, thermal and physical injury and noxious agents.
- Prevents loss of moisture.
- Reduces the harmful effects of UV radiation.
- Acts as a sensory organ.
- Helps regulate temperature control.
- Plays a role in immunological surveillance.
- Synthesises vitamin D_3 (cholecalciferol).
- Has cosmetic, social and sexual associations.

Skin functions

The skin is a complex metabolically active organ, which performs important physiological functions that are summarised in Table 1.2.

Barrier function and skin desquamation

As the viable cells move towards the stratum corneum they begin to clump proteins into granules in the granular layer (*see* Figure 1.5). The granules are filled with the protein fillagrin, which becomes complexed with keratin to prevent the breakdown of fillagrin by proteolytic enzymes. As the degenerating cells move towards the outer layer, enzymes break down the keratin-fillagrin complex. Fillagrin forms on the outside of the corneocytes while the water-retaining keratin remains inside.

When the moisture content of the skin reduces, fillagrin is further broken down into free amino acids by specific proteolytic enzymes in the stratum corneum. The breakdown of fillagrin only occurs when the skin is dry in order to control the osmotic pressure and the amount of water it holds: in healthy skin the water content of the stratum corneum is normally around 30%. The free amino acids, along with other components such as lactic acid, urea and salts, are known as 'natural moisturising factors' (NMF) and are responsible for keeping the skin moist and pliable due to their ability to attract and hold water.

Lipids

The major factor in the maintenance of a moist, pliable skin barrier is the presence of intercellular lipids. These form stacked bilayers that surround the corneocytes and incorporate water into the stratum corneum. The lipids are derived from lamellar granules, which are released into extracellular spaces of degrading cells in the granular layer; the membranes of these cells also release lipids. Lipids include cholesterol, free fatty acids and sphingolipids.

Ceramide, a type of sphingolipid, is mainly responsible for generating the stacked lipid structures that trap water molecules in their hydrophilic region. These stacked lipids surround the corneocytes and provide an impermeable barrier by preventing the movement of water and NMF out of the surface layers of the skin. After the age of 40 there is a sharp decline in skin lipids thus increasing our susceptibility to dry skin conditions.

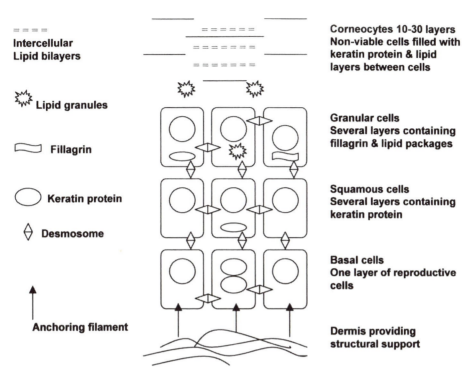

Figure 1.5 Barrier function of the epidermis.

Shedding (desquamation) of skin cells

Shedding the cells of the stratum corneum is an important factor in maintaining skin integrity and smoothness. Desquamation involves the enzymatic process of dissolving the protein bridges, the desmosomes, between the corneocytes, and the eventual shedding of these cells (*see* Figure 1.2). The proteolytic enzymes responsible for desquamation are located intracellularly and function in the presence of a well-hydrated stratum corneum. In the absence of water the cells do not desquamate normally and the skin becomes roughened, dry, thickened and scaly. In normal healthy skin there is a balance in the production and shedding of corneocytes. In diseases such as psoriasis, which involve increased corneocyte production, and where decreases in shedding occur, the result is dry, rough skin as the cells accumulate on the skin.

Remaining functions

UV protection

Melanocytes, located in the basal layer, and melanin have important roles in the skin's barrier function by preventing damage by UV radiation. In the inner layers of the epidermis, melanin granules form a protective shield over the nuclei of the keratinocytes; in the outer layers, they are more evenly distributed. Melanin

Table 1.3 Immune components of the skin.

Defence type	Component	Immune action
Structural	Skin	Impenetrable physical barrier to most external organisms.
	Blood and lymphatic vessels	Provision of transport network for cellular defence.
Cellular	Langerhans cells	Antigen presentation.
	T lymphocytes	Facilitate immune reactions. Self-regulating through the action of T suppressor cells.
	Mast cells	Facilitate inflammatory skin reactions.
	Keratinocytes	Secrete inflammatory cytokines; have ability to express surface immune reactive molecules.
Systemic	Cytokines and eicosanoids	Cytokines: cell mediation chemicals produced by components of the cellular defence system.
		Eicosanoids: non-specific inflammatory mediators produced by mast cells, macrophages and keratinocytes.
	Adhesion molecules	Increase the number of cellular defence facilitators in an area by binding to T cells.
	Complement cascade	Activation of this initiates a host of destructive mechanisms, including opsonisation, lysis, chemotaxis and mast cell degranulation.
Immunogenetic	Major histocompatibility complex (MHC)	Enables immunological recognition of antigens.

absorbs UV radiation, thus protecting the cell's nuclei from DNA (deoxyribonucleic acid) damage. UV radiation induces keratinocyte proliferation, leading to thickening of the epidermis.

Thermoregulation

The skin plays an important role in maintaining a constant body temperature through changes in blood flow in the cutaneous vascular system and evaporation of sweat from the surface.

Immunological surveillance

As well acting as a physical barrier, skin also plays an important immunological role. It normally contains all the elements of cellular immunity, with the exception of B cells.[2] Immune components of the skin are given in Table 1.3.

References

1 Ro BI, Dawson TL. The role of sebaceous gland activity and scalp microfloral metabolism in the etiology of seborrheic dermatitis and dandruff. *J Investigative Dermatol SP.* 2005; **10**(3): 194–7.
2 Gawkrodger DJ. *Dermatology, An Illustrated Colour Text.* 3rd ed. Edinburgh: Churchill Livingstone; 2002.

Chapter 2

Essential oil sciences in context

Introduction

For centuries, skin treatments were entirely of natural origin and were derived from herbs, animal products and inorganic materials, with herbs forming the largest proportion of remedies. The science of pharmacognosy, which grew from these traditional approaches, demonstrates that plants provide a vast and complex source of phytochemicals which not only calm, restore and heal the epidermal barrier but are also capable of surviving the scrutiny of clinical trial and pharmacological testing.[1] Volatile essential oils, fixed oils and hydrosols are extracted from a wide variety of plants and form the main tools used in aromatherapy practice today. This chapter will focus on the science underlying the dermo-therapeutic use of essential oils; a more detailed discussion of fixed oils and hydrosols can be found in Chapter 4. In line with the remit of this book, the chemistry presented here will largely focus on that most relevant to aromadermatology. A comprehensive account of essential oil chemistry can be found elsewhere.

Essential oils

An essential oil is the volatile odoriferous oil extracted from aromatic vegetable plant material by physical means. The physical methods used are distillation (steam, steam/water and water) or expression, which refers to the mechanical cold-pressing of the citrus fruit pericarp. An essential oil is not a solvent-extracted product. These are classified differently; using solvents such as benzene, acetone, ethanol and hexane produces absolutes and resinoids. Solvent extraction is used for fragrant flowers and other plant material that cannot be steam distilled either because the yield is extremely low or the odoriferous components are thermo-labile. The use of absolutes is not advocated by all aromatherapists since not all solvent molecules can be removed from the concrete or absolute, which could pose chronic toxicity problems or cause skin reactions.

Carbon dioxide (CO_2) extracts are relatively new introductions to aromatherapy practice and are briefly included in this chapter, if only to highlight future avenues for research. They contain interesting therapeutically active compounds that are either thermo-labile or not sufficiently volatile to be extracted by steam distillation. *Calendula officinalis* (calendula) CO_2 extract is of keen interest for its pronounced anti-inflammatory activity and research to date indicates little concern with safety.[2] However, depending upon operational procedures the composition and hence toxicological profile of CO_2 extracts will vary. Therefore until greater standardisation of their composition and detailed toxicological data can be provided, caution is needed before they can be more widely accepted into aromatherapy practice.

Botanical origins of essential oils

Botanical nomenclature

As essential oils arise from plant material, in professional practice the convention is to refer to them (and hydrosols and vegetable oils) by their botanical names rather than the ambiguous and sometimes misleading common names. For example, 'lavender' essential oil might refer to that from any species of the genus Lavandula (*Lavandula angustifolia, Lavandula latifolia, Lavandula stoechas, etc.*) with each having a particular chemical profile. The rules of botanical naming can be found in the International Code of Botanical Nomenclature and International Code of Nomenclature for Cultivated Plants, published by the International Association for Plant Taxonomy (IAPT).[3]

In aromatherapy, it is ideal (but not always possible for a host of reasons) to have available the following information when identifying essential oils:

- botanical family
- botanical name, including the name (most usually the abbreviation) of the naming botanist, and the variety or subspecies
- the part of the plant from which the oil is obtained
- country of origin
- chemotype.

In this text, the convention we have followed is to give the botanical name, followed by one of the main synonyms. As there are often several different synonyms that might be used, we have strenuously attempted to remain consistent in those given. On occasion, published papers may not have provided botanical names and, in such circumstances, we have by necessity omitted them. A detailed listing of the essential oils, hydrosols and vegetable oils referred to in the book along with their botanical families and synonyms and common botanical abbreviations can be found in the Appendix.

Genesis and classification of aromatic compounds

Essential oils are present in the plant within distinctive oil cells or secretory glands either on the surface of the plant or within plant tissue. These secretory glands, which are an important characteristic of many plant families, are generally found to predominate in one particular part of the plant such as the leaves, flowers, pericarp, wood, bark, roots, rhizomes or seeds. Abbreviations for these are usually included when one plant species produces distinctly different oils from different structures. For example, *Cinnamomum zeylanicum* fol. refers to the leaf oil of cinnamon, whereas *Cinnamomum zeylanicum* cort. refers to that of the bark.

Essential oils are produced by 'secondary metabolism', which describes the production of any compound not essential to the growth and basic needs of the plant. It has been estimated that 50,000 to 100,000 secondary compounds exist in the plant kingdom with only a tiny proportion of these having been identified.[4] Essential oils are highly complex chemical substances produced in nature to serve ecological and evolutionary roles.

An overview of essential oil chemistry

An understanding of essential oil composition is vital for everyone intending to work with these chemically complex substances in order to:

* identify oils with appropriate activity for the treatment of a given condition
* identify the toxicological profile of individual oils and formulations, which in turn will influence dosage and exposure duration
* predict reactivity of oils with oxygen, which affects shelf life.

Essential oils are oxidised over time by contact with air, producing resinous products and artefacts that can cause sensitivity and detract from the original odour profile. Exposure to heat, sunlight and moisture accelerates decomposition of oils. Table 2.1 provides storage guidelines necessary to minimise their degradation.

Essential oils are primarily complex mixtures of mono (C_{10}) and sesquiterpene hydrocarbons (C_{15}), and oxygenated compounds derived from these hydrocarbons, which include alcohols, aldehydes, esters, ketones, phenols, acids and oxides. These terpenoid compounds are formed from biochemically active isoprene units, isopentyl pyrophosphate (IPP) and dimethylallyl diphosphate (DMAPP) via the mevalonate biosynthetic pathway. Other commonly occurring compounds include phenylpropanoids, from the shikimate pathway and their biotransformation products. In addition to these major groups, specific compounds containing sulphur and nitrogen can be found and the metabolism of fatty acids and amino acids produces further constituents (*see* Table 2.2).

Terpenoid compounds

The isoprene unit is the starting point for the manufacture of terpenoid compounds. The number of isoprene units (*see* Figure 2.1) dictates the size of

Table 2.1 Storage conditions for essential oils.

* Containers should not interact physically or chemically with the oil. Small quantities can be stored satisfactorily in small dark glass bottles. Metal containers provide complete protection against light and are used by suppliers.
* Plastic containers are avoided as they can adsorb or bind essential oil molecules to their surface and leach components of the plastic into the essential oil.
* Bottles need to be kept cool, ideally refrigerated (+2 to +8°C refrigerator air temperature) to retard chemical reactions.
* Closures or bottle caps must prevent the penetration of air or water vapour into the bottle and the escape of volatile components.
* Bottles used in aromatherapy practice should be fitted with a screw cap with dropper dispensers.
* Childproof caps should be considered when working in an environment with young children.

Table 2.2 Commonly occurring chemical constituents of steam-distilled and expressed essential oils.

Terpenes
Monoterpenes (C10) – cyclic, acyclic or bicyclic

Hydrocarbons

Addition of oxygen-containing functional groups provides further classification

C10 – alcohols
C10 – phenols
C10 – aldehydes
C10 – esters
C10 – oxides
C10 – ketones
C10 – lactones

Sesquiterpenes (C15) – bicyclic and open chain

Hydrocarbons

C15 – alcohols
C15 – aldehydes
C15 – ketones
C15 – lactones

Diterpenes (C20)

Hydrocarbons

C20 – alcohols

Phenylpropanoids
Phenyl methyl ethers
Aromatic aldehydes

Coumarins
Furanocoumarins

---

the compounds, which are broadly divided into two classes: the monoterpenoids (10C) or sesquiterpenoids (15C). Small amounts of diterpenoids (20C) are found in some oils but steam distillation limits their extraction.

Hydrocarbon terpenes

Monoterpenes

These are unsaturated hydrocarbons, which have 10 carbon atoms and at least one double bond between carbon atoms and are among the most volatile of essential oil compounds. Monoterpenes can either be acyclic (e.g. myrcene) or contain one ring (e.g. limonene) or two ring structures such as α-pinene and δ-3-carene (*see* Figure 2.2). The closed rings of the cyclic structures add complexity to the molecules, which may increase their specificity for different chemical reactions in the body.[5]

Monoterpene hydrocarbons such as α- and β-pinenes, limonene, δ-3-carene, α-phellandrene and myrcene are found as complex mixtures in most essential oils, particularly plant leaf oils, while seed and flower oils contain more specialised monoterpenes.[6] Therapeutic effects in the context of skin treatments include:

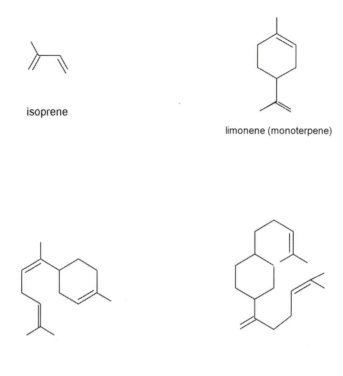

isoprene

limonene (monoterpene)

alpha-bisabolene
(sesquiterpene)

camphorene (diterpene)

Figure 2.1 Examples of a monoterpene (C10), sesquiterpene (C15) and diterpene (C20).

- bactericidal and antiviral activity[7,8]
- prevention of initiation, promotion and progression of cancerous cells[9,10]
- skin penetration enhancing activity.[11]

Monoterpenes are frequently cited as causing skin irritation. In the main, pure monoterpenes are not skin irritants but their oxidation products, peroxides, epoxides and endoperoxides formed during storage are sensitising agents, a topic further discussed in Chapter 3.[5,6,12] Inhalation of pinene-rich oils can produce a concentration-dependent throat irritation and increased airway resistance in some individuals.[13] The administration method and concentration of pinene-rich oils requires evaluation when treating clients with asthma and other airway hypersensitivity disorders.

Sesquiterpenes
Sesquiterpenes are hydrocarbons with 15 carbon atoms. They are less volatile and more viscous than monoterpenes. Many woody oils contain high percentages of sesquiterpenes and sesquiterpenols. Sesquiterpenes also oxidise on storage, forming epoxides and alcohols and eventually polymerise to form long chain resins. Unlike the monoterpenes their oxidation products have not been

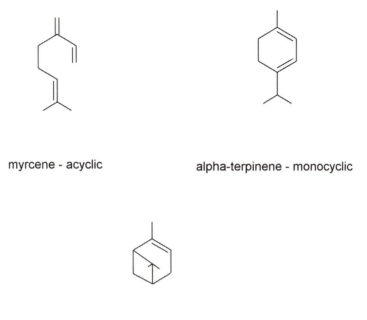

myrcene - acyclic   alpha-terpinene - monocyclic

alpha-pinene - bicyclic

Figure 2.2 Examples of commonly occurring acyclic, monocyclic and bicyclic mono-terpenes.

shown to be skin irritants, but shelf life and storage conditions are still important considerations for the preservation of their therapeutic activity.

Demonstrated anti-inflammatory activity of some sesquiterpenes (*see* Figure 2.3) found in oils widely used in skin care has been shown, including:

- β-caryophyllene found in *Pogostemon cablin* (patchouli).[14,15] Other oils containing appreciable levels of β-caryophyllene include *Helichrysum italicum* subsp. *italicum*[16] and *Achillea millefolium* (yarrow);[17] these both demonstrate notable anti-inflammatory activity in practice
- guaiazulene found in *Callitris intratropica* (blue cypress)[18]
- chamazulene (C14), in *Matricaria recutita* (German chamomile).

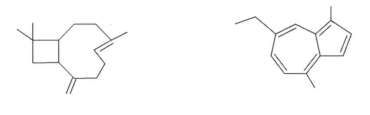

beta-caryophyllene   chamazulene (C14)

Figure 2.3 Isolates with demonstrated anti-inflammatory activity.

The anti-inflammatory effect of chamazulene is due to inhibition of the formation of leucotriene B4 in neutrophils.[19] It is likely this inhibition is responsible for the traditional use of *Matricaria recutita* in the suppression of allergic responses, since chamazulene has little influence on the degranulation of mast cells or granulocytes and hence the release of histamine.[20] *Achillea millefolium* (yarrow) essential oil is also traditionally valued in this realm, probably due to its chamazulene content, but the levels are highly variable and cannot be assumed for any single batch of oil.[21]

Chamazulene, although not strictly a sesquiterpene, is formed during steam distillation from the decomposition of matricin, a sesquiterpene lactone. Matricin, present in the CO_2 extract of *Matricaria recutita* (German chamomile), has significantly stronger anti-inflammatory properties than chamazulene or guaiazulene.[18,22]

Alcohols

Terpenoid alcohols have a hydroxyl group (OH) attached to one of the carbon atoms of the monoterpene, sesquiterpene or diterpene chain. The addition of the hydroxyl group can be added anywhere along the carbon chain forming either:

- primary alcohols, where the –OH group is attached to a carbon atom which in turn is attached to only one other carbon atom
- secondary alcohols where the carbon atom is attached to two others
- tertiary alcohols where the carbon atom is attached to three other carbon atoms (*see* Figure 2.4).

Monoterpenols

Primary monoterpenols such as geraniol are slowly oxidised in the presence of air and light to aldehydes or acids or to form resins.

Monoterpenols have demonstrated antibacterial and antifungal activity and are generally well tolerated on the skin and mucous membranes. Pattnaik *et al.*[23] investigated the antimicrobial activity of linalol, geraniol and menthol against 18 bacteria species and 12 fungi. Antibacterial activity was demonstrated in the order linalol > geraniol > menthol while antifungal activity was found to be geraniol > linalol > menthol. Virucidal activity against herpes simplex virus-1 (HSV-1), the cause of cold sores, has been demonstrated by the monoterpenols isoborneol,[24] borneol,[24] terpinen-4-ol[25–27] and α-terpineol.[25] Table 2.3 identifies monoterpenols with specific dermo-therapeutic activity.

Sesquiterpenols

Unlike monoterpenols, sesquiterpenols are often complex molecules possessing two or three closed rings (*see* Figure 2.5). Oils such as *Pogostemon cablin* (patchouli) and *Santalum album* (sandalwood) produce characteristic sesquiterpenols: patchoulol and the santalols. Penetration into the skin is slowed by their larger molecular size and irritation is unlikely to arise. Sesquiterpenol-rich oils are viscous which affects the size of drop that is delivered from a standard dropper-insert. This underlines the importance of using measuring cylinders for accuracy in essential oil formulations rather than relying on the somewhat arbitrary drop measurements.

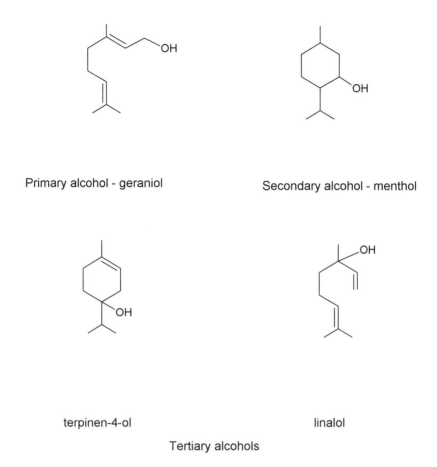

Primary alcohol - geraniol   Secondary alcohol - menthol

terpinen-4-ol   linalol

Tertiary alcohols

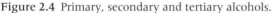

Figure 2.4 Primary, secondary and tertiary alcohols.

The sesquiterpenol α-bisabolol found in *Matricaria recutita* (German chamomile) is promoted for skin healing in the commercial preparations Camoderm® and Camillosan®. (–)-α-bisabolol is considered highly significant in the anti-inflammatory and skin-healing effect of *Matriciaria recutita*, possessing greater activity than chamazulene.[36,37] Animal studies demonstrate cicatrisant activity with the promotion of epithelialisation and granulation,[35,37] making this of particular value in wound care.

Santalum album (sandalwood) consisting largely of sesquiterpenes and the sesquiterpenols α- and β-santalol have demonstrated virucidal activity in vitro against the herpes simplex virus-1, a common cause of cold sores.[38]

Aromatic alcohols

2-phenylethyl alcohol (PEA) is the most commonly occurring aromatic alcohol, which is synthesised via the shikimate pathway. It is found in distilled rose oil but greater concentrations are present in the hydrosol due to its water solubility. It is used in the perfumery industry for its mild floral rose odour and is found in smaller quantities in *Jasminum grandiflorum* (jasmine absolute), *Citrus aurantium* flos. (neroli) and *Pelargonium graveolens* (geranium).[6]

Table 2.3 Examples of essential oils containing useful levels of monoterpenols with dermo-therapeutic activity.

Monoterpenol	Therapeutic activity	Essential oil
Geraniol	Antibacterial, antifungal[23]	Cymbopogon martini Cymbopogon nardus Pelargonium graveolens Rosa damascena
Linalol	Antimicrobial[23] Anti-inflammatory[28,29] Sedative[30,31] Anaesthetic/analgesic[32]	Aniba rosaeodora Cinnamomum camphora Coriandrum sativum Lavandula angustifolia Ocimum basilicum ct linalol Thymus vulgaris ct linalol
Menthol	Anaesthetic/analgesic[33] Antibacterial, antifungal[23]	Mentha arvensis Mentha piperita Mentha spicata
Terpinen-4-ol	Antibacterial, antifungal[34] Antiviral[25–27]	Melaleuca alternifolia Origanum majorana Pistacia lentiscus
α-terpineol	Cicatrisant[35] Antiviral[25] Antimicrobial[23]	Eucalyptus radiata Melaleuca quinquenervia Myrtus communis Ravensara aromatica

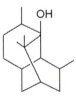

Figure 2.5 Patchoulol – a tricyclic, tertiary sesquiterpenol.

Phenols

Structurally, phenols occurring in essential oils have a hydroxyl (-OH) group connected to an aromatic benzene ring system, which distinguishes them from alcohols (*see* Figure 2.6). The term 'aromatic' is used to describe a six-membered ring where all the bonds in the ring are the same length and possess a special configuration of electrons. Phenols can arise from the terpenoid mevalonate pathway (thymol, carvacrol) or via the shikimate pathway (eugenol, chavicol). They behave like weak acids and readily form ions, which react with other polar or positively charged molecules including protein molecules in the skin. Consequently, despite demonstrating greater antimicrobial activity compared to alcohols, some phenols such as eugenol are dermal and mucous membrane irritants. Moreover, some, when regularly ingested in high concentrations, have the potential to induce liver damage by the depletion of liver glutathione.[5]

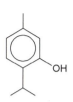

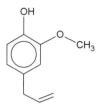

aromatic benzene ring
structure

Thymol - a terpenic phenol   Eugenol - a phenylpropanoid

Figure 2.6 Examples of phenols.

Table 2.4 Examples of antimicrobial phenol-rich
oils. Their judicious use may be indicated in some
skin conditions for limited periods. All oils in this list
have dermocaustic potential requiring dose
attenuation.

Phenol	Essential oil
Carvacrol	*Origanum vulgare* *Satureja hortensis* *Satureja montana* *Thymus capitatus* *Thymus vulgaris* ct carvacrol
Eugenol	*Cinnamomum zeylanicum* fol. *Syzygium aromaticum* gem./fol.
Thymol	*Origanum vulgare* *Satureja hortensis* *Satureja montana* *Thymus capitatus* *Thymus vulgaris* ct thymol

Phenols are highly effective anti-infectious agents, preventing growth and in many cases killing many types of micro-organisms including *Staphylococcus aureus* and *Pseudomonas aeruginosa*. The bactericidal mechanism of carvacrol and thymol is via disruption of membrane integrity, which affects bacterial pH homeostasis and equilibrium of inorganic ions such as potassium and hydrogen.[39]

Phenol-rich essential oils listed in Table 2.4 are first-line treatment for acute skin infections; however, their dermocaustic and hepatotoxic hazard limits dosage concentration and frequency of exposure. Careful blending with the well-tolerated alcohol and ester rich oils is required to balance skin tolerability of preparations.

The antiviral activity of phenols is less well established. The concomitant use of the pharmaceutical acyclovir and eugenol against herpes simplex virus (HSV-1) in vitro synergistically inhibits HSV-1 replication.[38] Thymol, carvacrol and eugenol rich oils are cited as being of therapeutic interest for the treatment of disease associated with the human papilloma virus (HPV).[40]

Aldehydes

Aldehydes characteristically possess the structure HC=O on a terminal carbon atom (*see* Figure 2.7). They are produced by the oxidation of a primary alcohol and are readily oxidised themselves to carboxylic acids. Aldehydes may be:

- non-terpenoid such as trans-2-hexenal, octanal, nonanal and decanal
- aromatic: benzaldehyde, phenylacetaldehyde
- monoterpenoid or sesquiterpenoid.

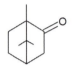

camphor - a ketone

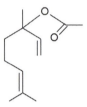

linalyl acetate - an ester

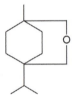

1,8 cineole - an oxide

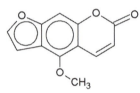

bergapten - a furanocoumarin

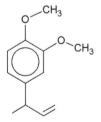

methyl eugenol - a phenyl methyl ether

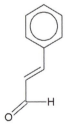

cinnamic aldehyde - an aromatic aldehyde

Figure 2.7 Examples of oxygenated compounds that occur in essential oils.

Table 2.5 Notable citral- and cinnamic aldehyde-containing essential oils that have specific and limited indications for use in aromadermatology.

Citral-rich oils	Cinnamic aldehyde-rich oils
Backhousia citriodora	Cinnamomum zeylanicum cort.
Cymbopogon flexuosus	
Cymbopogon citratus	
Litsea cubeba	
Melissa officinalis	

Citral, a monoterpene aldehyde, nearly always occurs as a mixture of two isomers, neral and geranial, and is a highly reactive and unstable substance.[41] It is associated with dermal sensitisation,[42] and the safety of this and cinnamic aldehyde is discussed fully in Chapter 3. Notable oils are listed in Table 2.5.

Therapeutically, certain aldehydes are anti-infectious, particularly with regard to fungi; however, with the exception of cinnamic aldehydes, antibacterial and antiviral activity is not found to be as consistent as that demonstrated by alcohols or phenols. The following aldehydes have demonstrated antimicrobial activity:

- antibacterial: citral,[43,44] citronellal,[44,45] cinnamic aldehyde[46]
- antifungal: citral,[47] cinnamic aldehyde[47]
- antiviral: citral.[48,49]

Melissa officinalis (lemon balm) and *Cymbopogon flexuosus* (lemongrass) are traditionally recognised for the treatment of anxiety, restlessness, excitability, stress and insomnia. These citral-rich oils have shown favourable results in the management of agitation associated with dementia and responsiveness in people with profound learning disabilities.[50,51] Although there is no research to date demonstrating this is due specifically to their aldehyde contents, there is a clear opportunity for using them in the psychosomatic management of skin disorders where strong psychogenic factors are implicated (*see* Chapter 6).

Ketones

Ketones have a carbonyl group (C=O) where the carbon atom is additionally connected to two other atoms, usually carbon, which renders them less reactive than aldehydes (*see* Figure 2.7). They are derived from the oxidation of secondary alcohols (monoterpenoid or sesquiterpenoid), which generally occurs in the plant. Many, particularly the more ubiquitous monoterpenoid ketones, have powerful odours, for example damascenone and ionone which make up less than 1% of *Rosa damascena* oil (rose) but contribute greatly to the aroma.

Ketones have long been cited for their wound-healing properties and for preventing the overproduction of scar tissue and keloid formation.[52] Guba[53] included two ketone-rich essential oils, *Artemesia vulgaris* (mugwort) and *Salvia officinalis* (sage), each at a concentration of 10 mg/g in a wound-healing cream.

Table 2.6 Essential oils containing high percentages of ketones with direct relevance to skin care.

Ketone	Neurotoxic (NT) Hepatotoxic (HT)	Essential oil
Camphor	NT	*Achillea millefolium* *Rosmarinus officinalis* ct camphor *Salvia officinalis*
Carvone (+) (−)		*Carum carvi* *Mentha spicata*
Fenchone	?NT	*Foeniculum vulgare*
Iso-pinocamphone	NT	*Hyssopus officinalis*
cis jasmone		*Jasminum grandiflorum* (absolute)
Menthone (−)		*Mentha arvensis* *Mentha piperita*
Pulegone	NT/HT	*Mentha pulegium*
Thujone	NT	*Thuja occidentalis* *Salvia officinalis*
Tumerone		*Curcuma longa*
Verbenone		*Rosmarinus officinalis* ct verbenone *Eucalyptus globulus*

Wound Heal Formula was applied at a dose of 0.5–2.0 g daily and resolved a variety of wounds, presenting in nursing homes, on average 116% more quickly than untreated control wounds.

Anecdotal reports suggest that the diketones (containing two ketone groups), notably the italidiones found in *Helichrysum italicum* (immortelle), possess anti-haematomal properties. Thujone and cryptone are suggested by Baudoux *et al.* for the treatment of HPV infections.[40]

The high ketone concentration of certain oils poses potential toxicity risks. Single dermal doses are unlikely to be of any consequence but the high stability and resistance of ketones to metabolism by the liver could result in cumulative chronic toxicity with repeated daily doses over prolonged periods. Ketones considered to be neurotoxic and/or hepatotoxic are further reviewed in Chapter 3. Table 2.6 lists essential oils of relevance to skin care that contain high levels of ketones.

Carboxylic acids

The carboxylic acid group (-COOH) renders many of the essential oil acids too soluble in water to be found in anything but traces in the oils, but greater concentrations are found in the waters of distillation – the hydrosols. The plant extract of *Boswellia carterii* (frankincense) contains the anti-inflammatory tri-terpenoid boswellic acids. Although often found in commercial cosmetic preparations, they are not found in the steam-distilled oil.

Esters

In plants, acids and alcohols readily combine together to form esters (*see* Figure 2.7) with the elimination of water. This reaction is reversible being dependent on the right combination of water and acids. Esters are more resistant to oxidation than alcohols or aldehydes but are hydrolysed in the presence of heat and water. They are well tolerated on the skin but may induce sensitisation if used for prolonged periods.

The only esters with known toxicity are sabinyl acetate, a teratogen with demonstrated liver toxicity in mice,[54] and methyl salicylate, which can result in systemic toxicity when applied topically to damaged skin.[55] *Salvia lavandulifolia* (Spanish sage) is the only sabinyl acetate-containing oil likely to be used in aromatherapy. Methyl salicylate found in *Betula lenta* (sweet birch) and *Gaultheria procumbens* (wintergreen) is a counter-irritant indicated for rheumatic conditions. Neither of these oils is indicated for the treatment of skin disorders.

Therapeutic effects demonstrated by certain esters, which can be exploited in aromadermatology, include sedative and anti-inflammatory activity, which is particularly useful in the treatment of pruritic and painful skin conditions that cause disturbed sleep and restlessness. *Anthemis nobilis* (Roman chamomile) is rich in non-terpenoid esters (angelates, tiglates and butyrates) and has demonstrated anti-inflammatory and sedative activity.[56,57] The concentration of angelates has the greatest influence on sedation.[57]

Linalyl acetate and linalol are reported as being responsible for the sedative reputation of certain oils. A study by Buchbauer *et al.*[30] in mice found sedation achieved by these isolates to be mediated through direct activity with cell membrane lipids in the cortex, particularly depressing the motor cortex. Linalyl acetate has a major role in the overall anti-inflammatory activity of an essential oil.[29] When compared with linalol such as in *Lavandula angustifolia* (lavender), it produces a less pronounced effect but is highly significant in terms of synergy.

Oxides

These are formed where a hydroxyl (-OH) group is altered in such a manner that the H atoms are removed and the oxygen atom bonds to another carbon atom to form a closed ring (*see* Figure 2.7) The most commonly occurring oxide in essential oils is 1,8 cineole. Other less commonly encountered oxides include linalol oxide, caryophyllene oxide, α-bisabolol oxide and rose oxide. Little is known about their therapeutic effects apart from 1,8 cineole, which is mainly indicated in the treatment of respiratory tract disorders.

It is pertinent when using essential oils topically to be aware that 1,8 cineole has been shown to disrupt stratum corneum lipid bilayers;[11] this alters permeant diffusivity through the stratum corneum, including that of essential oil based preparations. We will return to this later in the chapter.

Neurological side effects in children associated with the oral ingestion of 1,8 cineole (from eucalyptus oil) are reported by Day *et al.*[58] and Tibbals.[59] Eucalyptus oil should not be applied to the face or noses of young children and infants.[60]

Chemical families of limited interest in aromadermatology

The chemical families described below offer little therapeutic interest for skin disorders, apart from the potent antimicrobial activity of the phenyl propanoids cinnamic aldehyde and eugenol. However, in order to provide reliable guidance for safe formulation it is useful to review them briefly.

Lactones

A lactone is an ester group incorporated into a carbon ring system and can be monoterpenoid (e.g. nepetalactone), sesquiterpenoid (e.g. alantolactone, helenaline) or non-terpenoid (e.g. jasmine lactone).

Lactones are recognised skin sensitisers, in particular the sesquiterpenoid lactones commonly occurring in plants from the Asteraceae family.[61] They do not occur as major constituents in any essential oils used in aromatherapy, with only traces ever being present in steam-distilled oils. However, greater concentrations are increasingly likely to occur in CO_2 extracts. Matricin, a sesquiterpenoid lactone found in the CO_2 extract of *Matricaria recutita*, is absent in the steam-distilled oil. Caution should be used before advocating the indiscriminate use of such extracts despite evidence that matricin is significantly more anti-inflammatory than chamzulene.[62]

Coumarins

Coumarins have a lactone ring adjoined to a benzene ring which itself may have several groups attached thereby making it difficult to predict which functional group properties will dominate. Due to their low volatility coumarins are more prevalent in absolutes and solvent extracts.

Furanocoumarins have a five-membered ring attached to the coumarin structure (*see* Figure 2.7). They are particularly abundant in the Apiaceae and Rutaceae families, which synthesise linear furanocoumarins (syn. psoralens) and angular furanocoumarins. The linear furanocoumarins, bergapten (5-methoxypsoralen) and xanthotoxin (8-methoxypsoralen), produce a clinically significant photosensitising reaction which is reviewed in Chapter 3.

Phenylpropanoids

These are phenolic compounds with an aromatic ring containing a three carbon (propyl) side chain. Phenylpropanoids such as cinnamic aldehyde (*see* Figure 2.7), eugenol, methyl eugenol, anethole, methyl chavicol, safrole and apiol are potentially hazardous and oils containing these in significant quantities are recommended for short-term, low-dose applications only.

Phenyl methyl ethers are derived from phenols and are the most common ethers in essential oils. Eugenol is both a phenol and a methyl ether (*see* Figure 2.6) and therefore unsurprisingly shares properties of both functional groups. Eugenol possesses strong anti-infectious properties, which may be utilised in the treatment of skin infections.

The phenyl methyl ethers safrole, methyl chavicol and methyl eugenol have been identified as carcinogens in rodent studies. The metabolic pathways necessary to produce reactive electrophiles from safrole, methyl chavicol and methyl eugenol are regulated by dose.[63–65] The large doses and lengthy exposure time needed to demonstrate carcinogenic potential of these compounds in rodent studies most likely overestimates the potential risk to humans.

Isomerism

Essential oil chemical complexity is further enhanced by the formation of isomers. Two molecules can have the same molecular formulae but have different structural ones, known as structural isomers. Linalol and geraniol posses the same molecular formula $C_{10}H_{17}OH$, but have a different arrangement of their atoms; this results in different aroma and antibacterial activity. The position of a double bond may result in much smaller differences in structure, denoted as *alpha-* (α) or *beta-* (β) isomers, an example being α- and β-pinene.

However, it is the existence of stereoisomers, geometric isomers and enantiomers that are of particular interest. Stereoisomers have the same structure and bond order but their atoms and groups of atoms are arranged differently in space resulting in their molecules being non-superimposable. Geometric isomerism involves a double bond, preventing the rotation of atoms about this bond, resulting in *cis-* and *trans-*isomers, which can have different chemical and therapeutic properties.

Many components possess one or more asymmetric carbon atoms that exhibit optical activity. Two molecules can be three-dimensional, non-superimposable mirror images of one another and are known as enantiomers (*see* Figure 2.8). Such molecules are dextrorotatory (+) or laevorotatory (–), which indicates their ability to rotate plane polarised light. Since these compounds evolved by biosynthetic processes that were enzymatically controlled, plants naturally produce only one enantiomer. Enantiomers often display different olfactory properties. Examples include the (+)- carvone, which is the main constituent of *Carum carvi* (caraway seed) oil, whereas its enantiomeric mirror image (–)-carvone is the main constituent of *Mentha spicata* (spearmint) oil,[66] both producing quite different aromas.

Different chiral isomers of the same component have been shown to have varying physiological effects and therefore the pharmacological action could be greatly affected by the proportion of enantiomers present in a preparation.[67] Inhalation of (+)-limonene has been demonstrated to increase systolic blood pressure and change alertness and restlessness in individuals, while (–)-limonene only affected blood pressure.[68]

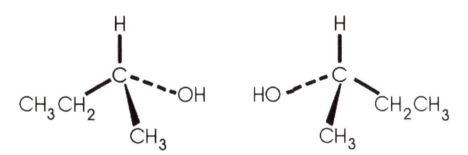

Figure 2.8 Enantiomers – three-dimensional, non-superimposable mirror images.

Essential oil synergy: enhancement and antagonism

Aromatherapists work with complete, pure and unrefined oils in the understanding that the whole oil or extract is more effective and has greater therapeutic activity than individual isolated compounds. There is abundant evidence that confirms this traditionally favoured view, with research identifying synergistic reactions between components within individual oils.[69,70]

Aromatic synergy is also the rationale for blending essential oils together to produce a product with greater therapeutic activity than the sum of the known and unknown chemical components.[71] It must be remembered that synergy is not always positive however, and within a blend there may be antagonism in addition to potentiation, depending upon the dose, application method and base into which the blend is mixed (*see* Table 2.7).[72,73]

As a general rule, there is no single chemical component that predominates in any essential oil, as seen in the oil of *Origanum majorana* (sweet marjoram), where individual chemicals each form no greater than 0.1–10% of total oil volume. In certain oils, however, one constituent may form the majority of the chemistry. For example, linalol can be found at concentrations of 80–90% in *Cinnamomum camphora* (ho leaf), 60–90% in *Aniba rosaeodora* (rosewood) and 60–80% in *Coriandrum sativum* (coriander seed) oil.[6] However, the presence of trace components can influence odour, flavour and biological activity of the oil.[69,70]

Variations in essential oil composition

Therapists working with essential oils recognise and accept that natural variations in essential oil chemistry are inherent in non-standardised natural materials. So long as they remain within defined boundaries and occur due to environmental or genetic influences and not from adulteration, this is an accepted part of aromatherapy practice. It does however underline the importance of obtaining batch-specific data from essential oil suppliers, as some of these variations significantly alter therapeutic and toxicological profiles.

Chemotypes

Morphologically identical plants can possess marked differences in essential oil composition from a specific part of the plant. Referred to as chemotypes or chemo

Table 2.7 Interactions resulting in synergy enhancement or antagonism.

Even before blending, interactions may occur between:
- individual components of the essential oil itself
- essential oils and pesticides.

In the final preparation interactions may occur between:
- essential oils in a blend
- essential oils and other plant extracts
- essential oils and other ingredients present.

When applied, interactions may occur between:
- essential oils and drugs.

varieties, these are distinguished by the differences in major components of the essential oil. They are thought to have evolved as a response to the environmental and living conditions of the plant, which has resulted in inheritable genetic biosynthetic changes necessary to secure the viability of the plant.

Chemotypes are a common occurrence in the Lamiaceae family, notably the *Thymus* and *Rosmarinus* genera. For example, *Thymus vulgaris* (thyme) is thought to have seven genetically distinct chemotypes, six of which can be found in the south of France: geraniol, α-terpineol, thujanol-4, linalol, carvacrol and thymol. In Spanish populations, 1,8 cineole is present but the geraniol chemotype has not yet been found.[74] The importance of knowing which chemotype is being used in practice is illustrated well with thyme oils. Phenol-rich chemotypes, containing carvacrol and thymol, require caution when applying to the skin due to their dermocaustic nature whereas those containing linalol and geraniol are safe to apply at greater concentrations. Antimicrobial activity also varies, with some research demonstrating greatest antifungal activity with the thymol chemotype.[75]

Environmental influences

Other reasons for natural chemical variations of essential oils include:

- time of harvest[76]
- plant maturity[77]
- geographical origin/climate[78]
- soil type[78]
- part of plant used and position of leaves on the stem
- extraction processes.[79]

Quality control issues

The addition of synthetic or natural components to standardise essential oils does occur and is a concern for aromatherapists. In 2001 Health Which identified gross adulteration of aromatherapy oils for retail sale.[80] Therefore it is imperative that steps are taken to determine whether an oil is natural and genuine before using it in aromatic medicine. The two main concerns of adulteration are:

- the interference of adulterants with components of the natural oil; this may affect synergy and the expected physiological and psychophysiological activities of the oil
- toxicity implications of the adulterants.

A more complete exploration of this and the detection methods used for spotting adulteration lie beyond the scope of this book. For in-depth discussion of what can be a highly contentious area of aromatherapy, the reader is directed elsewhere.

Transdermal permeation of essential oils

For the majority of aromatherapists, dermal application provides the principal route for essential oil administration and it is axiomatic that it is the primary

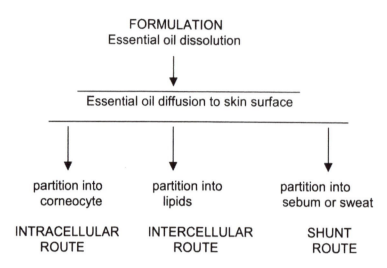

FORMULATION
Essential oil dissolution

Essential oil diffusion to skin surface

| partition into corneocyte | partition into lipids | partition into sebum or sweat |
| INTRACELLULAR ROUTE | INTERCELLULAR ROUTE | SHUNT ROUTE |

Figure 2.9 Routes through the stratum corneum.

route for dermatological care. Transdermal permeation of essential oil molecules is complex, involving many possible steps from initial application to their arrival in the systemic circulation. The clinical significance of the amount of essential oil absorbed into the systemic circulation is frequently disputed. However, they have been shown to penetrate into and through the skin,[81,82] where they exert local therapeutic effects.

The stratum corneum for most molecules is the rate-limiting barrier to further permeation. There are three ways (*see* Figure 2.9) that intact stratum corneum can be crossed:

1 intercellular – via lipid domains
2 intracellular – diffusion through the corneocyte
3 shunt routes – via hair follicles and sweat glands.

Intercellular permeation

There is an extremely large variability in rates of dermal absorption between different chemicals. In general, lipophilic substances such as essential oil components are absorbed more readily as the stratum corneum provides a formidable barrier for hydrophilic compounds, which penetrate more slowly.[83] Polar and non-polar molecules are thought to diffuse through the skin by different mechanisms. The lipid bilayers provide a continuous phase within the stratum corneum and the principal pathway by which small, uncharged molecules cross the stratum corneum.[84,85] The intercellular pathway for a molecule by this route is greater than the thickness of the stratum corneum (*see* Figure 2.10).

Intracellular permeation and 'shunt routes'

The intracellular route is usually regarded as a pathway for polar (hydrophilic) molecules, since cellular components are predominantly aqueous in nature.

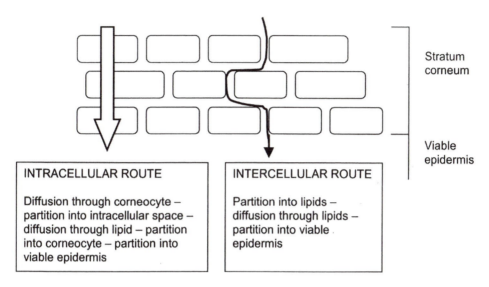

Figure 2.10 Intracellular and intercellular routes of essential oil absorption.

Here the pathway is directly across the stratum corneum, the rate-limiting barrier being the multiple bilayered lipids that must be crossed (*see* Figure 2.10).

The appendages, occupying around 0.1% of the total skin surface,[86] offer pores that bypass the barrier of the stratum corneum creating 'shunt routes'. Eccrine sweat glands are numerous on the palms and the soles of the feet, but their openings are very small and, beyond this, ducts are either evacuated or actively secreting sweat, which would diminish the inward diffusion of topically applied essential oils.

The opening of the follicular pore is much larger by comparison, although less numerous. The duct of the sebaceous gland is filled with sebum, which is lipoidal in nature and therefore more favourable for the dissolution of essential oil molecules compared to the aqueous nature of sweat. Consideration of the shunt routes is particularly useful when targeting essential oils to the pilosebaceous units in the treatment of acneform eruptions, boils and carbuncles. Recent work has indicated that the transfollicular route may be involved to a greater extent than previously recognised in topical drug applications; a finding that prompted researchers to look at maximising the follicular concentration of *Melaleuca alternifolia* (tea tree) oil in the development of acne vulgaris preparations.[87]

If appendages are modified by trauma such as burned skin, the short-cut diffusion of substances through these appendages may be impaired even after wound healing has occurred.[88] The three pathways are not mutually exclusive and most molecules will pass through the stratum corneum by a combination of these routes.[86] A generalised order of site permeability is:

genitals > head and neck > trunk > arm > leg

Although it is of practical value to consider site-specific variations, it is important to view any regional variations in context with all factors affecting permeation.[86]

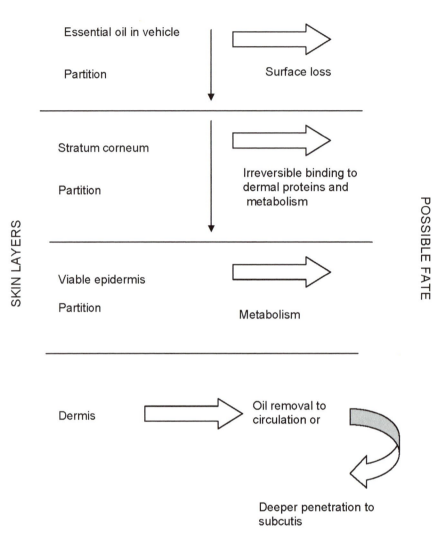

Figure 2.11 Potential fate of essential oil components when applied to skin.

The fate of essential oil molecules

At the stratum corneum/viable epidermis junction essential oil molecules must partition into the viable tissue before further diffusion to the dermoepidermal junction. Partitioning occurs once more at this site, followed by diffusion through the dermal tissue to the vascular capillaries (*see* Figure 2.11). In addition to these partitioning and diffusion processes there are other potential fates for essential oil molecules entering the skin which include:

- irreversible binding to cutaneous proteins such as keratin
- degradation or biotransformation by cutaneous enzymes
- partitioning into and forming a reservoir in the subcutis.

Essential oils as skin penetration enhancers

The pharmaceutical industry has studied the use of terpenoid compounds as penetration enhancers in a quest to deliver drugs topically or transdermally. Penetration enhancers partition into the stratum corneum and interact with tissue components to reduce the barrier properties of this membrane without causing damage to the underlying skin cells. d-limonene and 1,8 cineole have both been shown to disrupt stratum corneum lipid bilayers thereby modifying permeant diffusivity through the stratum corneum.[11]

Effects of mediums on essential oil permeation

Essential oils are rarely applied neat, but in a vehicle, which can either enhance or inhibit percutaneous absorption. In skin care, the vehicle is of equal therapeutic importance to the choice of essential oils and requires careful selection. Zatz[89] demonstrated the negation of the antiseptic effect of phenol when applied to the skin in a fatty formulation; Orafidiya *et al.* recorded similar findings.[73]

Due to their lipophilicity essential oil molecules will partition into the stratum corneum lipids from an aqueous formulation such as a lotion or cream more readily than from an oily vehicle or ointment. Only essential oil molecules adjacent to the skin can partition from the vehicle into the tissue, thus movement through the vehicle to the skin surface is important. Diffusion through the vehicle depends on the nature of the formulation such as its viscosity.

Other permeation variables

Transdermal essential oil permeation is influenced by many variables. Those that are accepted as enhancing permeation include:

- warmth of the skin
- increasing the dose applied
- extending the duration of contact
- humidity
- occlusion
- skin hydration.

The physiochemical properties of the complete preparation may either retard of enhance permeation. Interestingly, although skin hydration increases the bulk of the skin and therefore might plausibly be assumed to decrease absorption, an increased rate of percutaneous absorption of both hydrophilic and lipophilic components occurs.[90]

Effect of disease on essential oil transdermal permeation

Whether the skin is diseased by a transient infection or a chronic condition such as psoriasis or dermatitis, in general it is more permeable than healthy, normal skin. A notable exception occurs when the skin becomes thickened or lichenified. Pathological processes may influence skin barrier function by either directly influencing the protein or lipid composition of the stratum corneum through changes in structural or enzymatic proteins or cause improper formation of the stratum corneum by increasing keratinocyte proliferation.

The damage caused to the skin barrier integrity will vary depending on the severity and nature of the disorder. It is obvious that in severe infections, such as necrotising fasciitis, the skin barrier is seriously impaired. However, in the case of a wart, only a very small fraction of the skin's surface is involved and the effect of hyperkeratinisation on essential oil flux through the site is likely to be very small. What is apparent is that in most cases of infection the effect on skin barrier function will be to diminish its effectiveness. This is usually favourable for topical treatment using essential oils, but it must be remembered that the barrier is dynamic and will be restored as the condition improves, therefore essential oil flux across the repairing tissue will be expected to slow. It might therefore be necessary to either increase or decrease the essential oil concentration, depending on the clinical aims of treatment. Paradoxically when treating a fungal infection it might be necessary to increase the essential oil concentration as the condition improves and barrier function is restored to ensure full mycological cure.

References

1 Dweck AC. African fragranced plants. *Cosmetics Toiletries*. 1997; **112**: 47–54.
2 Quirin, K, Gerard, D. New aspects on calendula CO_2 extract as a cosmetic ingredient. *Cosmetics Toiletries*. 1999; **112**(4): 55–8.
3 www.bgbm.org/iapt/nomenclature/code/default.htm (accessed 21.01.06).
4 Stern KR, Jansky S, Bidlack JE. *Introductory Plant Biology*. 9th ed. Boston: McGraw Hill; 2003.
5 Bowles EJ. *The Chemistry of Aromatherapeutic Oils*. 3rd ed. Australia: Allen & Unwin; 2003.
6 Burfield T. *Natural Aromatic Materials – odours and origins*. Florida: The Atlantic Institute of Aromatherapy; 2000.
7 Raman A, Weir U, Bloomfield SF. Antimicrobial effects of tea tree oil, and its major components on *Staphylococcus aureus, Staphylococcus epidermidis* and *Propionibacterium acnes*. *Lett Appl Microbiol*. 1995; **21**(4): 242–5.
8 Dorman HJD, Deans SG. Antimicrobial agents from plants: antibacterial activity of plant volatile oils. *J Appl Microbiol*. 2000; **88**: 306–16.
9 Gould MN. Cancer chemoprevention and therapy by monoterpenes. *Environ Health Perspect*. 1997; **105**(4): 977–9.
10 Vigushin DM, Poon GK, Boddy A *et al*. Phase I and pharmacokinetic study of D-limonene in patients with advanced cancer. Cancer Research Campaign Phase I/II Clinical Trials Committee. *Cancer Chemother Pharmacol*. 1998; **42**(2): 111–17.
11 Cornwall PA, Barry BW, Bootstrap JA *et al*. Modes of action of terpene penetration enhancers in human skin: differential scanning calorimetric, small angle X-ray diffraction and enhancer uptake studies. *Ind J Pharm*. 1996; **127**: 9–26.
12 Hausen BM, Reichling J, Harkenthal M. Degradation products of monoterpenes and the sensitising agents in tea tree oil. *Am J Contact Dermat*. 1999; **10**(2): 68–77.
13 Filipsson AF. Short term inhalation exposure to turpentine: toxicokinetics and acute effects in men. *Occup Environ Med*. 1996; **53**(2): 100–5.
14 Martin S, Padilla E, Ocete MA *et al*. Anti-inflammatory activity of the essential oil of *Bupleurum fruticescens*. *Planta Med*. 1993; **59**: 533–6.
15 Tambe Y, Tsujiuchi H, Haonda G *et al*. Gastric cytoprotection of the non-steroidal anti-inflammatory sesquiterpene β-caryophyllene. *Planta Med*. 1996; **62**(5): 469–70.

16 Bianchini A, Tomi P, Bernardini AF *et al*. A comparative study of volatile constituents of two *Helichrysum italicum* (roth) Guss. Don Fil subspecies growing in Corsica (France), Tuscany and Sardinia (Italy). *Flav Fragr J*. 2003; **18**: 487–91.

17 Agnihotri VK, Lattoo SK, Thappa RK *et al*. Chemical variability in the essential oil components of *Achillea millefolium* Agg. from different Himalayan habitats (India). *Planta Med*. 2005; **71**: 280–3.

18 Jakovlev V, Flaskamp I, Flaskamp E. Pharmacological investigations with the compounds of chamomile. VI. Investigations on the antiphlogistic effects of chamazulene and matricine. *Planta Med*. 1986; **49**: 67–73.

19 Safayhi H, Sabieraj J, Sailer ER *et al*. Chamazulene: an anti-oxidant-type inhibitor of leukotriene B4 formation. *Planta Med*. 1994; **60**(5): 410–13.

20 Miller TM, Wittstock U, Lindequist U *et al*. Effects of the essential oil of chamomile, *Chamomilla recutita*, on histamine release from rat mast cells. *Planta Med*. 1996; **62**(1): 60–1.

21 Spinarova S, Petrikova K. Variability of the content and quality of some active substances within *Achillea millefolium* complex. *Hort Sc*. 2003; **30**(1): 7–13.

22 Guba R. The modern alchemy of carbon dioxide extraction. *Int J Aromatherapy*. 2002; **12**(3): 120–6.

23 Pattnaik S, Subramanyam VR, Bapaji M *et al*. Antibacterial and antifungal activity of aromatic constituents of essential oils. *Microbios*. 1997; **89**: 39–46.

24 Armaka M, Papanikolaou E, Sivropoulou A *et al*. Antiviral properties of isoborneol, a potent inhibitor of herpes simplex virus type 1. *Antiviral Res*. 1999; **43**: 79–92.

25 Schnitzler P, Schon K, Reichling J. Antiviral activity of Australian tea tree and eucalyptus oil against herpes simplex virus in cell culture. *Die Pharmazie*. 2001; **56**: 343–7.

26 Cox SD, Mann CM, Markham JL. Interactions between components of the essential oil of *Melaleuca alternifolia*. *J Appl Microbiol*. 2001; **91**: 492–7.

27 Farag RS, Shalaby AS, El-Baroty GA *et al*. Chemical and biological evaluation of the essential oils of different *Melaleuca* species. *Phytother Res*. 2004; **18**: 30–5.

28 Moretti MD, Peana AT, Satta M. A study on anti-inflammatory and peripheral analgesic action of *Salvia sclarea* oil and its main components. *JEOR*. 1997; **9**: 199–204.

29 Peana AT, D'Aquila PS, Panin F *et al*. Anti-inflammatory activity of linalol and linalyl acetate constituents of essential oils. *Phytomedicine*. 2002; **9**: 721–2.

30 Buchbauer G, Jirovetz L, Jager W. Fragrance compounds and essential oils with sedative effects upon inhalation. *J Pharmaceut Sci*. 1993; **82**(6): 660–4.

31 Elisabetsky E, Marschner J, Souza DO. Effects of linalool on glutamatergic system in the rat cerebral cortex. *Neurochem Res*. 1995; **10**(4): 461–5.

32 Ghelardini C, Galeotti N, Salvatore G *et al*. Local anaesthetic activity of the essential oil of *Lavandula angustifolia*. *Planta Med*. 1999; **65**: 700–3.

33 Galeotti N, Mannelli DC, Mazzanti A. Menthol: a natural analgesic compound. *Neurosci Lett*. 2002; **322**(3): 145–8.

34 Carson CF, Riley TV. Antimicrobial activity of the major components of the essential oil of *Melaleuca alternifolia*. *J Appl Bacteriol*. 1995; **78**(3): 264–9.

35 Villegas LF, Marcalo A, Martin J *et al*. (+)-epi-alpha-bisabolol is the wound healing principle of *Peperomia galioides*: investigation of the in vivo wound healing activity of related terpenoids. *J Nat Prod*. 2001; **64**: 1357–9.

36 Carle R, Gomaa K. The medicinal use of *Matricariae* flos. *Brit J Phytother*. 1992; **2**(4): 147–53.

37 Issac O. Pharmacological investigations with compounds of chamomile. On the pharmacology of (–)-α-bisabolol and bisabolol oxides (Review). *Planta Med*. 1979; **35**:118–24.

38 Benencia F, Courreges MC. In vitro and in vivo activity of eugenol on human herpes virus. *Phytother Res*. 2000; **14**: 495–500.

39 Lambert RJW, Skandamis PN, Coote PJ *et al*. A study of the minimum inhibitory concentration and mode of action of oregano essential oil, thymol and carvacrol. *J Appl Microbiol*. 2001; **91**(3): 453–62.

40 Baudoux D, Zhiri A. Aromatherapy alternatives for gynaecological pathologies: recurrent vaginal Candida and infection caused by the human papilloma virus (HPV). *Int J Clinical Aromather*. 2005; **2**: 34–9.

41 Burfield T. The adulteration of essential oils – and the consequences to aromatherapy and natural perfumery practice. Presented to IFA annual AGM; 2003 Oct 11; London.

42 Tisserand R, Balacs T. *Essential Oil Safety*. Edinburgh: Churchill Livingstone; 1995.

43 Hayes AJ, Markovic B. Toxicity of Australian essential oil *Backhousia citriodora* (Lemon myrtle). Part 1. Antimicrobial activity and in vitro cytotoxicity. *Food Chem Toxicol*. 2002; **40**: 535–43.

44 Dorman HJD, Deans SG. Antimicrobial agents from plants: antibacterial activity of plant volatile oils. *J Appl Microbiol*. 2000; **88**: 306–16.

45 Low D, Rawal BD, Griffin WJ. Antibacterial action of the essential oils of some Australian Myrtaceae with special reference to the activity of chromatographic fractions of *Eucalyptus citriodora*. *Planta Med*. 1974; **26**; 184–9.

46 Moleyar V, Narisiashimham P. Antibacterial activity of essential oil components. *Int J Food Microbiol*. 1992; **16**(4): 337–42.

47 Viollon C, Chaumont JP. Antifungal properties of essential oils and their main components upon Cryptococcus neoformans. *Mycopathologia*. 1994; **128**(3): 151–3.

48 Minami M, Kita M, Nakaya T *et al*. The inhibitory effect of essential oils on Herpes simplex virus type-1 replication *in vitro*. *Microbiol Immunol*. 2003; **47**(9): 681–4.

49 Allahverdiyev A, Duran N, Ozguven M *et al*. Antiviral activity of the volatile oils of *Melissa officinalis* L. against Herpes simplex virus type-2. *Phytomedicine*. 2004; **11**: 657–61.

50 Lindsay WR, Pitcaithly D, Geelen N *et al*. A comparison of the effects of four therapy procedures on concentration and responsiveness in people with profound learning disabilities. *Journal Intellect Disabil Res*. 1997; **42**(3): 201–7.

51 Ballard CG, O'Brien JT, Reichelt K *et al*. Aromatherapy as a safe and effective treatment for the management of agitation in severe dementia: the results of a double-blind placebo-controlled trial with melissa. *J Clin Psychiatr*. 2002; **63**(7): 553–8.

52 Franchomme P, Penoel D. *L'aromatherapie Exactement*. Limoges: Roger Jollois; 1990.

53 Guba R. Wound healing; a pilot study using an essential oil-based cream to heal dermal wounds and ulcers. *Int J Aromatherapy*. 1998/1999; **9**(2): 67–74.

54 Pages N, Fournier G, Chamorro M *et al*. Teratological evaluation of *Juniperus sabina* essential oil in mice. *Planta Med*. 1989; **55**(2): 144–6.

55 Heng MC. Local necrosis and interstitial nephritis due to topical methyl salicylate and menthol. *Cutis*. 1987; **39**(5): 442–4.

56 Wolfe A, Herzeberg J. Can aromatherapy oils promote sleep in severely demented patients? *Int J Geriatric Psychol*. 1996; **11**: 926–7.

57 Melegari M, Albasini A, Pecorari G *et al*. Chemical characteristics and pharmacological properties of the essential oils of *Anthemis nobilis*. *Fitoterapia*. 1989; **59**(6): 449–55.

58 Day LM, Ozanne-Smith J, Parsons BJ *et al*. Eucalyptus poisoning among young children: mechanisms of access and the potential for prevention. *Aust NZ Journal Public Health*. 1997; **21**(3): 297–302.

59 Tibbals J. Clinical effects and management of Eucalyptus oil ingestion in infants and young children. *Med J Australia*. 1995; **163**(4): 177–80.

60 Blumenthal M, editor. *The Complete German Commission E Monographs*. Austin, Texas: American Botanical Council; 1998.

61 Paulsen E. Contact sensitization from Compositae-containing herbal remedies and cosmetics. *Contact Derm*. 2002; **47**: 189–98.

62 Della Loggia R, Tubaro A, Sosa S *et al*. The role of triterpenoids in the topical anti-

inflammatory activity of Calendula officinalis flowers. *Planta Med.* 1994; **60**(6): 516–20.

63 Chan VSW, Caldwell J. Comparitive induction of unscheduled DNA synthesis in cultured rat hepatocytes by allylbenzenes and their 1'-hydroxy metabolites. *Food Chem Toxicol.* 1992; **30**: 831–6.

64 Benedetti MS, Malnoe A, Broillet AL. Absorption, metabolism and excretion of safrole in the rat and man. *Toxicology.* 1977; **7**(1): 69–83.

65 Anthony A, Caldwell J, Hutt AJ *et al.* Metabolism of estragole in rat and mouse and the influence of dose size on excretion of the proximate carcinogen 1'-hydroxyestragole. *Food Chem Toxicol.* 1987; **25**: 799–806.

66 Boelens MH, Boelens H, van Gemert LJ. Sensory properties of optical isomers. *Perfumer Flavorist.* 1993; **18**(6): 2–16.

67 Balchin LM, Onchoka RJ, Deans SG *et al.* Bioactivity of the enantiomers of limonene. *Med Sci Res.* 1996; **24**: 309–10.

68 Huenberger E, Hongratanaworakit T, Bohm C *et al.* Effects of chiral fragrances on human autonomic nervous system parameters and self-evaluation. *Chem Senses.* 2001; **26**(3): 281–92.

69 Nostro A, Blanco AR, Cannatelli MA *et al.* Susceptibility of methicillin-resistant staphylococci to oregano essential oil, carvacrol and thymol. *FEMS Microbiol Lett.* 2004; **230**: 191–5.

70 Cox SD, Mann CM, Markham JL. Interactions between components of the essential oil of *Melaleuca alternifolia*. *J Appl Microbiol.* 2001; **91**: 492–7.

71 Cassella S, Cassella J, Smith I. Synergistic antifungal activity of tea tree (*Melaleuca alternifolia*) and lavender (*Lavandula angustifolia*) essential oils against dermatophytes infection. *Int J Aromatherapy.* 2002; **12**(1): 2–15.

72 Harris R. Synergism in the essential oil world. *Int J Aromatherapy.* 2002; **12**(4): 179–86.

73 Orafidiya LO, Oyedele AO, Shittu AO *et al.* The formulation of an effective topical antibacterial product containing *Ocimum gratissimum* leaf essential oil. *Int J Aromatherapy.* 2002; **12**(1): 16–21.

74 Linhart YB, Thompson JD. Thyme is of the essence: biochemical polymorphism and multi-species deterrence. *Evol Ecol Res.* 1999; **1**: 151–71.

75 Giordani R, Regli P, Kaloustian J *et al.* Antifungal effect of various essential oils against *Candida albicans*. Potentiation of antifungal action of amphotericin B by essential oil from *Thymus vulgaris*. *Phytother Res.* 2005; **18**(12): 990–5.

76 Basker D, Putievsky E. Seasonal variation in the yields of leaf and essential oil in some Labiatae species. *J Hort Sci.* 1978; **53**(3): 179–83.

77 Porter NG, Smale PE, Nelson MA *et al.* Variability in essential oil chemistry and plant morphology within a *Leptospernum scoparium* population. *NZ J Botany.* 1998; **36**: 125–33.

78 Simon J, Chadwick AF, Craker LE. *Herbs: an indexed biography 1971–1980: the scientific literature on selected herbs, and aromatic and medicinal plants of the temperate zone.* Connecticut: Archon Books; 1984.

79 Lawrence B. Essential oils: from agriculture to chemistry. *Int J Aromatherapy.* 2000; **10**(3/4): 82–96.

80 *Health Which.* Feb 2001; 18–20.

81 Jager W. Percutaneous absorption of lavender oil from a massage oil. *J Soc Cosmet Chem.* 1992; **43**: 49–54.

82 Fuchs N, Jager W, Lenhardt A *et al.* Systemic absorption of topically applied carvone: influence of massage. *J Soc Cosmet Chem.* 1977; **48**: 277–82.

83 Wester RC, Maibach HI. Understanding percutaneous absorption for occupational health and safety. *Int J Occup Environ Health.* 2000; **6**: 86–92.

84 Abraham MH, Chanda HS, Mitchell RC. The factors that influence skin penetration of solutes. *J Pharm Pharmacol.* 1995; **47**: 8–16.

85 Roberts MS, Pugh WJ, Hadgraft J. Epidermal permeability-penetrant structure relationships 3: the effect of H-bonding groups in penetrants on their diffusion through the stratum corneum. *Int J Pharm.* 1996; **132**: 23–32.

86 Williams AC. *Transdermal and Topical Drug Delivery: from theory to clinical practice.* London: Pharmaceutical Press; 2003.

87 Biju SS, Ahuja A, Khar RK. Tea tree oil concentration in follicular casts after topical delivery: determination by high-performance thin layer chromatography using a perfused bovine udder model. *J Pharm Sci.* 2005; **94**(2): 240–5.

88 Illel B, Schaefer H. Transfollicular percutaneous absorption. *Acta Derm Venereol.* 1988; **68**: 427–30.

89 Zatz JL. Modification of skin permeation by solvents. *Cosmetics Toiletries. 1991;* **106**(7): 89–94.

90 Behl CR, Flynn GL, Kurihara T. Hydration and percutaneous absorption. I. Influence of hydration on alkanol permeation through hairless mouse skin. *J Invest Dermatol.* 1980; **75**: 346–52.

Chapter 3

Aromadermatology and safety issues

Introduction

Essential oils, absolutes, plant extracts and vegetable oils are all capable of producing adverse reactions or undesirable effects. This is despite the popular misconception among some that natural products are less likely to be toxic and will be dealt with more effectively by the body. Aromatic materials are potentially hazardous but their informed use determines the exposure dose and therefore the degree of safety or hazard involved. Paracelsus (1491–1541), regarded as the 'father of pharmacology', comprehensively used natural compounds in the treatment of disease. He understood the importance of dose titration of medicines and wrote:

> All substances are poisons. There is none that is not a poison. The right
> dose differentiates a poison from a remedy.

The implication of this concept directly applies to the modern practice of aromatherapy. The safety of essential oil use is a topic that generates much debate and is on occasion subjected to inaccurate use of data. In this chapter, we give special attention to the conditions where the topical application of aromatherapy formulations may be harmful.

Specifically, the review provided here is in line with the focus of the book, namely we engage with safety issues of direct importance to the topical use of preparations in the care of common skin conditions. Therefore subjects that are not closely related to this are not covered, including the safety of essential oils that have little relevance in dermal care. Instead detailed attention is given to skin safety and reactions. For a discussion of the wider remit of aromatherapy safety the reader is directed to other specialised texts.

In general, effective aromatherapy massage for routine use favours low dosage formulations (usually between 1 and 3% essential oil concentration). Throughout this book comparatively higher dosage formulations are advocated to achieve desired therapeutic effects in certain clinical situations that demand specific interventions. Full and careful consideration of chemical and toxicological profiles of aromatic materials, alongside their proven and traditional effects, determine each recommendation made herein.

In the absence of a single monitoring body, recommendations for the safe use of essential oils are often derived from the work of the International Fragrance Association (IFRA). Established in 1973 primarily to assess the large amount of safety data generated by the Research Institute for Fragrance Materials (RIFM), guidelines issued by the IFRA either ban or restrict ingredients used in fragrance and cosmetic products. Many of the guidelines covering essential oils relate to skin sensitisation and phototoxicity and although they have certain implications for aromatherapy, they only cover the use of essential oils in perfumery and cosmetics. The safety implications are therefore not strictly comparable since aromatherapy formulations are generally unlikely to be applied on a daily basis over a number of years. Nevertheless, relevant IFRA data is included in this chapter to aid the reliability of the guidance provided.

Skin irritation

A skin irritant is any non-infectious agent, physical or chemical, capable of causing cell damage if applied to the skin for sufficient time and in sufficient concentration. Exposure to skin irritants is the major cause of non-immunological inflammation of the skin.[1] Irritation reaction patterns can be defined as follows.

- *Acute irritation* – a local, reversible non-immunological inflammatory response of normal living skin to direct injury caused by application of an irritant substance. Irritation can also describe subjective sensations such as burning or itching, which are non-inflammatory.
- *Irritant contact dermatitis* – this can be the result of an acute toxic insult to the skin (acute irritant dermatitis) such as acids or alkalis or repeated and cumulative damage from more marginal physical or chemical irritants (chronic irritant contact dermatitis).
- *Corrosion* – this arises from direct chemical action on normal living skin, resulting in its disintegration and irreversible alteration at the site of contact, healing with the formation of a scar.

Many essential oils have a dose-dependent ability to cause acute irritation or irritant contact dermatitis and some oils that are classed as moderate irritants, such as cinnamon and clove, when undiluted can cause corrosive burns and blistering.

The assessment and clinical presentation of irritation

Assessing acute skin irritation of essential oils by animal tests has been based on the method of Draize *et al.*[2] The significance of animal irritancy data to the human situation is questionable and recent reports suggest that animal tests can lead to the misclassification of chemicals.[3,4] Together with the ethical opposition to animal testing, this has led to alternative procedures such as in vitro methodology, human patch testing and structure-activity relationships being developed. Erythema and oedema are the main clinical manifestations of the dermal irritant response. Mild effects include skin dryness while more severe cases may lead to blistering.

With their greater exposure rates to essential oils, it is plausible that aromatherapists will display the greatest incidence of adverse effects. Therefore, it is no surprise that the incidence of self-reported hand dermatitis in aromatherapists is greater than found in the general population.[5] However, this may not entirely be due to their increased exposure to essential oils. In a study of massage therapists (ibid.) only 4% of those surveyed reported that the use of aromatherapy products aggravated their dermatitis, whereas frequent hand washing was cited as the most significant factor.

Water is a weak irritant and significant water exposure can cause the loss of soluble natural moisturising factors (NMF) and protective lipids resulting in an increase in transepidermal water loss (TEWL), the major cause of dry, scaly skin. Soap and cleansers are also mild irritants with repeated prolonged exposure causing the denaturation of skin proteins, disorganisation of lipid lamellae layers, removal of the protective intracellular lipids, loss of NMF and decreased cohesion between cells. Furthermore, the warmth of water can increase irritancy since it enhances absorption of the cleanser. For therapists, the implementation of hand-care practices such as judicious hand washing, avoidance of harsh soaps and use of emollient barrier products should be considered. These measures will help to minimise disruption of the skin barrier function thereby lessening penetration of irritants and sensitisers.

Factors influencing skin reactivity

Susceptibility to skin irritation varies widely among the general population and is frequently unpredictable. Possible population-based differences in skin reactivity include age, race, skin type and disease. Environmental conditions such as humidity and season have also been shown to have some influence. Intra-individual variations in skin irritation responses can also occur. Two chemicals with a similar overall irritant potential may show very different comparative responses; the susceptibility to one chemical cannot always predict that to another.[6]

Age

Lower reactivity and less severe reactions are reported in older (56–74 years) subjects than in younger age clusters.[6,7] However, the skin of women at the beginning of the menopause is more sensitive to various environmental threats since it becomes thinner at this stage resulting in higher percutaneous absorption.[8]

Race

Although it is clinically accepted that black skin is the least reactive and Asians are more reactive than Caucasians, many of the studies in this area do not reach statistical significance.[9] Arakami et al.[10] found no significant differences between Japanese and German women after sodium lauryl sulphate (SLS) testing but significant subjective sensory differences. The researchers concluded that Japanese women might complain about stronger sensations reflecting a different cultural behaviour rather than measurable differences in skin physiology.

Skin type and atopic dermatitis

Greater skin reactivity and subjective sensory irritation has been reported with skin type I (that is, skin that easily burns and never tans).[11,12] However, a study covering all six skin types, involving SLS under four-hour occlusion, demonstrated no significant dose-response differences between the groups.[13]

Sensitive skin is defined as a subjective cutaneous hyperactivity to environmental factors and approximately 40% of the population consider themselves to have the condition.[14] Increased permeability of the stratum corneum and acceleration of the nerve response are thought to be responsible for the hyper-sensitivity.[15] Individuals often show no sign of irritation but report itching, burning, stinging and a tight sensation after contact with substances that are not always considered irritants.[16] Elevated levels of nerve growth factor and sensitivity to electrical stimuli relative to non-sensitive skin suggest that the hyper-sensitive reaction is closely related to nerve fibres innervating the epidermis. Sensitive skin has been classified into three types, according to physiological parameters:

- type 1 – low barrier function
- type II – inflammation but normal barrier function
- type III – normal barrier function and no inflammatory changes.

In atopic dermatitis, heightened skin reactivity occurs because the compromised epidermal barrier allows greater penetration of irritants and sensitisers.[17,18]

Environmental factors

Skin irritability increases during winter with low ambient temperatures and absolute humidity causing disruption of the epidermal barrier. Weather-exposed skin will show visible changes such as dryness and scaling and may affect subjective feelings like itching, burning and tightness.[19] Some have found increased irritability even on skin not exposed to climate conditions during the winter season.[20,21]

Essential oils and skin irritation

Irritant essential oils can be divided into those with severe, strong, moderate or weak irritancy,[22] though in practice there is likely to be a continuous graduation in strength: a strong irritant by sufficient dilution can be converted to a weak one. Strong irritants are capable of provoking visible skin damage after just a single exposure, whereas weak irritants require frequent multiple exposures over months or even years to produce cumulative or chronic irritant contact dermatitis. Mucous membranes line various internal organs and body cavities that are exposed to the external environment and in several places are continuous with the skin: the nostrils, lips, ears, genital area and anus. These areas lack the keratinised cell layers of the skin (as do the eyes), making them more fragile and permeable, thus any essential oil is potentially irritant in these locations.

Essential oil chemistry

Phenols and aromatic aldehydes are the most irritant essential oil components and readily bind to skin proteins.[23] Table 3.1 lists oils rich in phenols or aromatic aldehydes used in aromatherapy dermatological practice that are classed as moderate irritants and Figure 3.1 outlines the general progress of irritation reactions.

Non-oxidised monoterpenes are mostly not considered as skin irritants.[ibid] However, their oxidation products such as peroxides, epoxides and endoperoxides can cause irritancy and, of greater concern, act as sensitising agents. Therefore, careful attention to correct storage conditions and expiry dates for oils

Table 3.1 Essential oils containing phenols or aromatic aldehydes used in aromatherapy dermatological practice that are classed as moderate irritants.

Phenol	Essential oil
Eugenol	*Cinnamomum zeylanicum* fol.
	Syzygium aromaticum gem./fol.
Thymol	*Ocimum gratissimum*
Carvacrol	*Origanum vulgare*
	Origanum vulgare ssp. hirtum
	Origanum onites
	Satureja hortensis
	Satureja montana
	Thymus vulgaris ct thymol
	Thymus vulgaris ct carvacrol

Aromatic aldehyde	Essential oil
Cinnamic aldehyde	*Cinnamomum zeylanicum* cort.

rich in monoterpenes (for example those derived from *Pinus* species and citrus fruits) is of particular relevance.

As well as essential oils given in Table 3.1, high concentrations of *Mentha piperita* (peppermint) and *Mentha arvensis* (cornmint) rich in the monoterpenol menthol, or non-aromatic aldehyde-rich oils such as *Cymbopogon flexuosus, C. citratus* (lemongrass), *Eucalyptus citriodora* (lemon scented eucalyptus), *Backhousia citriodora* (lemon myrtle) and *Litsea cubeba* (may chang) can also potentially cause irritancy particularly to mucous membranes.[22,23]

Dosages and irritation

Undiluted essential oils in baths are potentially irritating since they float on the surface of the water. It is important that they are dispersed evenly by mixing with a suitable non-polar solvent such as vegetable oil, or to some extent full cream milk before adding to bath water. Atopic and hypersensitive individuals should solubilise non-irritant oils in non-petroleum derived liquid soap to avoid filming effects which can lead to irritancy. Dispersants from natural sources, for example coconut-oil derived, are always preferable in aromatherapy to synthetic dispersants. Ethanol being both a polar and non-polar solvent can also act as a dispersant; however, since alcohol has a drying effect on the skin, dispersion in lipid emollients is favoured.

If we consider the essential oil dilution in a typical massage blend and the large area of the skin to which it is applied then the likelihood of causing irritation is low. However, the risk is increased when using topical products at much higher concentrations for small area coverage. Products containing up to 1% irritant phenols (e.g. thymol) can be considered for widespread application. This percentage can be increased for smaller localised application, to quicken the pace of healing, for example where a therapeutic antimicrobial action is indicated or counter-irritant pain relief is intended.

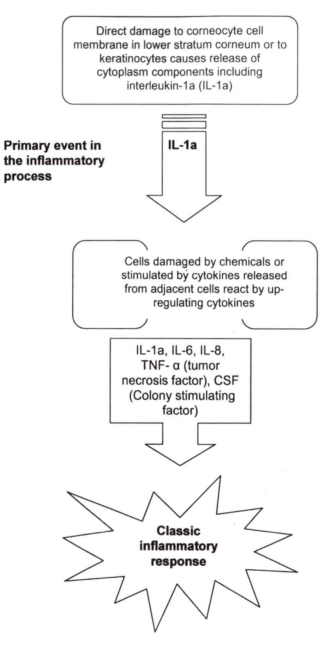

Figure 3.1 Progression of irritation response.

This intensive approach is one that is quite distinct from general aromatherapy massage applications and is reserved for limited situations. It is however recommended that the combined concentration of phenolic and aldehyde-rich oils should not exceed 20% of a formulation for use in up to 15% concentrations. Oils rich in cinnamic aldehyde such as *Cinnamomum zeylanicum* cort. (cinnamon bark) must be used with greater caution and lower doses. This intensive approach

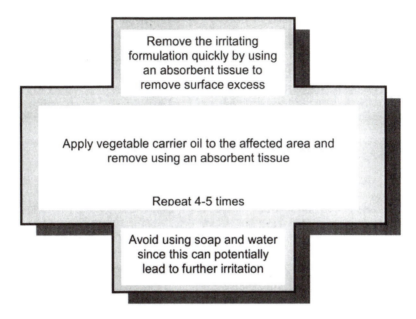

Figure 3.2 Treatment of irritation reactions.

to essential dosage is evident in the commercially available topical formulation Tiger Balm™. Indicated for arthritic and muscular pain relief by the induction of counter-irritancy, this contains potentially irritant essential oils at 60% concentration.

When formulating, in order to avoid skin irritancy always consider the following:

- potential irritancy of each oil
- potential irritancy of combined oils
- total aldehyde and phenol concentration in final product
- site and surface area to which the formulation will be applied
- skin integrity
- disorder being treated
- age, skin type and race of user
- subjective sensory skin irritancy – note that visible signs of irritancy may not be seen but burning, itching or stinging may be felt.

Irritation reactions are limited to the site of application and in the case of acute irritation the reaction will fade quickly once the irritant is removed. Figure 3.2 reviews the treatment of irritation reactions.

Skin sensitisation

A hypersensitive reaction, to be distinguished from sensitive skin as discussed earlier, is one in which the adaptive immune response is exaggerated or inappropriate. An allergy is the acquisition of an inappropriate specific immune response to a normally harmless substance. There are four main types

Table 3.2 Hypersensitivity reactions seen in aromatherapy.

Type	Reaction
Type I (immediate)	IgE is bound to the surface of mast cells. When an antigen is encountered stimulation of inflammatory mediators such as histamine, prostaglandins and leucotrienes results. The response occurs within minutes causing urticaria in the skin. Massive histamine release can lead to anaphylaxis. Common allergens are pollen grains, bee stings, house dust mites, penicillin and certain foods, e.g. nuts, eggs. Proteins contained in nut or seed carrier oils could potentially induce a response.
Type IV (cell-mediated or delayed)	Pre-sensitised T cells come into secondary contact with the antigen after it has become bound to an antigen-presenting cell. The T cells release cytokines which in turn activate other T cells and macrophages – this process takes some time and the tissue damage is most pronounced after 48–72 hours. Allergic contact dermatitis is an example of a type IV mediated response. Essential oils are potential inducers of this reaction.

of hypersensitivity response, all of which are exhibited in the skin, but it is types I and IV that may be encountered during aromatherapy practice and these are detailed in Table 3.2. Peanut and nut allergy is one of the most serious of the immediate hypersensitivity (Type I) reactions in terms of persistence and severity. In view of the preference in aromatherapy for using cold-pressed unrefined nut and seed derived carrier oils, it is appropriate to briefly review their safety.

Type I hypersensitivity

During the last decade, there has been increasing concern over the avoidable morbidity and mortality associated with allergy to nuts. There is a high incidence of sensitivity to multiple nut species and an apparent heightening of reactivity with increasing age.[24] It is therefore advisable to assume allergy to a range of nuts where there is any history of nut allergy. Clinical symptoms may develop within minutes and include oral and pharyngeal pruritus and 'tingling', a sensation of tightening of the airways, colicky abdominal pain, nausea, vomiting, cutaneous flushing, urticaria and angioedema. Progressive respiratory symptoms, hypotension and dysrhythmias develop in fatal and non-fatal cases. Biphasic reactions have been seen in up to a third of patients with fatal or near-fatal reactions. Such patients appear to have fully recovered when severe bronchospasm suddenly recurs.[25] Apart from anaphylactic reactions, for some sensitised individuals exposure to nuts may also cause exacerbation of atopic dermatitis or asthma.

Most individuals with peanut allergy avoid ingesting not only the nuts but the nut oil too. Although there is evidence to show that refined, highly processed nut and seed oils can safely be consumed by nut-allergic individuals,[26] in aromatherapy the emphasis is on using unrefined, cold-pressed oils, and it is possible these may induce allergic reactions.

Research by Lack *et al.*[27] has found the cause of increased prevalence of peanut allergy to be unrelated to maternal ingestion of peanuts and tree nuts while pregnant or breastfeeding as previously thought.[28,29] Rather, Lack suggests cutaneous exposure of ultra-low doses of nut proteins found in refined oils incorporated into creams and toiletries may induce sensitisation. His study identified children who suffered rashes over joints and skin creases had more than a two-fold increased risk of peanut allergy and in those whose rashes were oozing or crusting, the odds ratio increased to over five. In dermatitis, the skin breaks down, exposing an abundance of immune cells in the skin to allergenic substances. Interviews with parents revealed that almost all of the children with confirmed peanut allergy were exposed to creams containing peanut oil in the six months since birth. Anecdotal reports confirm that, in common with peanut allergy, the prevalence of sesame allergy is increasing, especially in infants and young children.[30] In pharmaceuticals and cosmetics, refined sesame oil is the main grade used, but hypersensitivity reactions have been reported and the oil remains an unexpected ingredient in some so-called 'allergy-tested' cosmetics.[31]

As cutaneous exposure to nut oils on inflamed skin seems to favour allergenic sensitisation and in view of the possibility that food allergy may occur via the cutaneous route rather than by ingestion, the following guidance is offered:

1   Nut and seed carrier oils are best avoided on babies and young children in the following circumstances:
    • in the case of nut or food allergic individuals
    • where there is a family history of nut or food allergy, asthma, hay fever or eczema
    • on broken or inflamed skin, for example nappy rash.
2   In the case of atopic children, care should be taken to avoid oil from the skin of other family members or carers touching the skin of the child.
3   These guidelines would also seem prudent for older children with inflamed skin or atopies.

Safe alternative fixed oils with either infrequent or no reports of allergy are *Borago officinalis* (borage), *Carthamus tinctorius* (safflower), *Cocos nucifera* (coconut), *Oenothera biennis* (evening primrose), *Simmondsia chinensis* (jojoba) and *Vitis vinifera* (grapeseed). In addition, *Calendula officinalis* (marigold) and *Hypericum perforatum* (St John's wort) infused oils are suitable if the oil used in the infusion is not obtained from nuts or seeds.

Type IV delayed hypersensitivity – skin sensitisation

Skin sensitisation describes an immunological process in which a heightened responsiveness to a chemical allergen is induced through topical exposure. The chemical allergen provokes a cutaneous immune response, which if of sufficient magnitude will result in contact sensitisation and, with enough exposure time contact dermatitis. Table 3.3 outlines the presentation of sensitisation.

To elicit an immune response the chemical must gain access to the viable epidermis. Key steps in this process can be identified:

1   The reactive sensitising agent passes across the stratum corneum barrier and persists for sufficient time and in sufficient amounts in the viable epidermis.

2 The chemical forms stable conjugates with cutaneous proteins. Skin sensitising agents (haptens) are inherently either:
   • protein reactive or
   • metabolised in the skin to a protein reactive entity.[32,33]
3 Epidermal Langerhans cells internalise and process the inducing allergen (the protein–hapten conjugate). Langerhans cells form part of a wider family of dendritic cells existing throughout the epidermis, whose function is to present antigen to the immune system.
4 A proportion of the Langerhans cell population close to the site of exposure are stimulated to migrate from the epidermis and travel via afferent lymphatics to skin draining lymph nodes where they accumulate as immunostimulatory dendritic cells which present antigen to responsive T cells.[34]
5 Allergen-responsive T cells proliferate, increasing the complement of cells (T memory cells) that are able to subsequently recognise and respond to the same inducing allergen.
6 When the now sensitised individual is once again exposed to the inducing allergen, at the same or different site, then the increased population of specific T lymphocytes will recognise and respond to the allergen in the skin at the site of contact. The activation of T lymphocytes is associated with the release of cytokines and chemokines that stimulate the influx of other leucocytes, initiating cutaneous inflammation resulting in allergic contact dermatitis.[34]

Spices and food ingredients can trigger skin reactions of a delayed type and there is a correlation between allergies to fragrances and spices due to their identical or related compounds. Clove, garlic, cinnamon, nutmeg, paprika, vanilla and ginger are the most frequent spices causing allergic contact dermatitis when ingested.[35]

The greater the exposure dose to an allergen, the more vigorous will be the induced immune response and the greater the level of sensitisation experienced.[36] Thus the induction of skin sensitisation and the elicitation of allergic contact dermatitis are a dose-dependent phenomena. In both cases, threshold concentrations can be defined below which reactions fail to develop. Under normal conditions of exposure, it is the amount of chemical allergen per unit area of skin rather than the total amount delivered that is the most important determinant in skin sensitisation induction.[36] This is also thought to be the case in elicitation of allergic contact dermatitis but has not yet been formally researched (ibid.).

Table 3.3 Presentation of sensitisation.

• When an individual is re-exposed to an essential oil to which they have become sensitised an itchy erythematous rash develops at the site of contact within 6–12 hours.
• The reaction progresses and reaches a peak between 48 and 72 hours after contact.
• Sensitivity may range from weak to strong. Even tiny amounts can elicit the same or more severe response as well as creating cross-sensitivities to other compounds.
• The induction period ranges from days to years. The establishment of immunological memory takes 8–14 days.[37]

Fragrances and essential oils in sensitisation reactions

The prevalence of sensitisation to any one chemical in allergic contact dermatitis is as much a function of exposure, nature, extent and duration of skin contact as it is the inherent potency of the chemical allergen. Illustrative of this is the fact that nickel is not a strong allergen but is the most common cause of skin sensitisation in the western world due to its widespread exposure opportunities.[38]

Fragrance allergy

Fragrances are found in a large number of consumer products with cosmetics and toiletries being the most important sources of exposure with regard to the risk of acquiring allergic contact dermatitis.[39,40] The European Union (EU) recently amended the 1976 EU law governing the manufacturing and marketing of cosmetics in Europe. The 7th Amendment to the Cosmetics Directive requires additional labelling for products containing common fragrance chemicals that can cause allergy. If a product contains any of 26 named fragrance allergens in excess of 100 ppm or 0.01% in wash-off and 10 ppm or 0.001% leave-on products then the chemical must be included in the list of ingredients.

Two diagnostic markers of perfume allergy are included in the European standard patch test series for contact allergy: balsam of Peru (BP) and the fragrance mix (FM). The ingredients of the FM are seven isolates and one extract, oak moss absolute (*see* Table 3.4).

Establishing a distinction between the uses of fragrances and aromatherapy

Frosch *et al.*[41] and Larsen[42] suggest that the single chemicals used in the FM should be supplemented with essential oils when patch testing patients with fragrance-associated problems. Frosch *et al.*,[41] following a study in six dermatological centres across Europe, lists ylang ylang I and II, lemongrass, sandalwood and patchouli essential oils, narcissus and jasmine absolutes, as potential causes of contact dermatitis 'if extensive exposure as found in aromatherapy' occurs. Larsen[42] additionally lists spearmint oil in his 'natural fragrance mix' safety net. However, products and concentrations listed as causing high reactivity by Frosch

Table 3.4 Fragrance mix ingredients.

Ingredients in FM	Concentration %	Naturally occurring
Alpha-amyl cinnamic aldehyde	1	✓
Cinnamic alcohol	1	✓
Cinnamic aldehyde	1	✓
Eugenol	1	✓
Geraniol	1	✓
Hydroxycitronellal	1	–
Isoeugenol	1	✓
Oak moss absolute	1	Extract
Sorbitan sequioleate (emulsifier)	5	–
Note: although many isolates occur naturally, synthetic isolates are used.		

bear little relevance to the vast majority of aromatherapy practices. For example, 10% occluded concentrations of ylang ylang, sandalwood and patchouli and 5% jasmine absolute are not likely to be encountered and, furthermore, narcissus absolute is not used by aromatherapists.

There is also no indication given of storage parameters for the test materials at the dermatology clinics. This is a notable omission, as the oxidation products of monoterpenes are frequently cited as sensitising agents,[43–46] leading to the possibility that this may have influenced the reactivity of the patch test materials. Other problems and limitations have been identified with the FM testing procedures, including the following:

- The components are present at insufficient concentrations for elicitation.
- The FM chemicals have not changed in 20 years, despite many new fragrance materials being introduced.
- The FM is irritant leading to false-positive interpretations.

The 26 fragrance ingredients highlighted in the 7th Amendment to the Cosmetics Directive as important causes of contact allergies arise from a report from the Scientific Committee on Cosmetics and Non-Food Products (SCCNFP). Fourteen of these ingredients, listed in Table 3.5, are naturally occurring in many essential oils used to treat skin conditions and which may contain one or often more of the chemicals at significantly higher concentrations than those stipulated.

The EU restrictions, however, are not globally anchored in scientific opinion and do not take into account whether the cosmetic uses of the restricted ingredients have any risk. Studies conducted by the Information Network of Departments of Dermatology, University of Gottingen (IVDK), demonstrate that not all single compounds identified possess the same risk. For example, iso-eugenol is a strong potent allergen whereas geraniol is less potent and should be treated less restrictively.[47] The studies that led to the current recommendations were carried out in dermatology clinics on individuals with skin barrier damage and therefore are not representative of healthy skin sensitivity.

Essential oils are not single entities, they are complex mixtures of hundreds of compounds, but no distinction between the degree of risk of 'allergens' occurring in essential oils and the same allergenic synthetic isolate is made in the EU Directive. Prediction of the sensitising potential of essential oils cannot be accurately based on the inclusion of one or more of the isolates listed in Table 3.5. The compounds and essential oils most often responsible for sensitisation reactions are listed in Table 3.6, some of which are not used in dermatological care. Other relevant oils that pose less of a risk but which may require consideration with some individuals include:

- *Pelargonium graveolens*
- *Santalum album*
- *Pogostemon cablin*
- *Cananga odorata*
- *Jasminum grandiflorum*.

Cross-sensitisation to essential oils may arise when an individual is sensitised to a particular compound in one essential oil and then reacts to another containing the same or similar compound. Additionally a cross-reaction may

Table 3.5 Fourteen ingredients found in essential oils and absolutes used in skin care, of the 26 fragrance ingredients highlighted as causes of contact allergies by the EU Scientific Committee on Cosmetics and Non-food Products (SCCNFP).

Chemical component	Examples of essential oils containing sensitisers
Benzyl alcohol	*Cananga odorata var. genuina*
	Jasminum grandiflorum
Benzyl benzoate	*Cananga odorata var. genuina*
	Cinnamomum zeylanicum fol.
Benzyl cinnamate	*Styrax benzoin* (resinoid)
Benzyl salicylate	*Cananga odorata*
	Cananga odorata var. genuina
Cinnamic alcohol	
Cinnamic aldehyde	*Cinnamomum zeylanicum* cort.
	Cinnamomum cassia
Citral	*Cymbopogon flexuosus*
	Litsea cubeba
	Melissa officinalis
Citronellol	*Cymbopogon nardus*
Eugenol	*Cinnamomum zeylanicum* fol.
	Ocimum gratissimum
	Syzygium aromaticum gem./fol.
Farnesol	*Citrus aurantium var. amara* flos.
	Rosa damascena
Geraniol	*Cymbopogon martini*
	Pelargonium graveolens
Isoeugenol	*Cananga odorata var. genuina*
d-limonene	Citrus, pine and mint oils
Linalol	*Aniba rosaeodora*
	Cinnamomum camphora var. linaloolifera
	Coriandrum sativum fol.
	Lavandula angustifolia

occur if two different compounds are metabolised in the skin to the same ultimate hapten.

Quenching

Although it is possible for a synergistic allergenic effect to occur in mixtures of essential oils, a reduction due to the influence of other compounds present in the oil or blend may also occur. Quenching is the phenomenon where allergenic compounds found in an essential oil can be nullified or 'quenched' by other components present. This concept first arose from the findings of Opdyke[48] that have since become the subject of some debate, with the literature supporting

Table 3.6 Compounds and essential oils most often responsible for sensitisation reactions, not all of which are used in aromadermatology.

Chemical component	Essential oils
Sesquiterpene lactones	Saussurea lappa*
Costuslactone	Inula helenium*
Alantolactone	
Aldehydes	
Cinnamic aldehyde	Cinnamomum cassia**
	Cinnamomum zeylanicum cort.**
Citral/citronellal	Backhousia citriodora
	Melissa officinalis*
Citral	Cymbopogon flexuosus
Oxidised hydrocarbons of	Litsea cubeba
d-limonene (hydroperoxides)	Citrus fruit oils
α- and β- pinene, δ-3-carene	Pinaceae species**
	Cupressaceae species
α-terpinene, γ-terpinene,	Melaleuca alternifolia
terpinolene (forming peroxides,	
epoxides and endoperoxides)	

IFRA recommendation: Pinus and Abies genera should only be used when the level of peroxides is kept to the lowest practical level (<10 mmol/L).
* denotes IFRA banned oils due to sensitisation potential.
** denotes IFRA restricted oils (usually concentration in final product).

varying degrees of both doubt and credibility. Sensitisation induced by citral can be quenched by the co-presence of d-limonene[49,50] while cinnamic aldehyde is quenched by an equivalent amount of eugenol.[51] Nilsson et al.[52] demonstrate a reduction in the sensitising capacity of d-carvone, a hapten, when linalol, a structurally unrelated compound, is administered in a mixture at induction. It is during induction rather than elicitation that quenching is likely to occur, but currently a full understanding of the exact mechanisms involved remains elusive.

When preparing essential oil formulations, awareness of this concept may serve to reduce sensitisation risk although the hypothesis still lacks full acceptance across the scientific community. The IFRA recognises quenching phenomena but according to Notification No. 4 of 38th Amendment to the IFRA standard, the quenching effects between eugenol and cinnamic aldehyde are unsupported.

Consequences of oxidation

Since oils that contain known sensitisers can be avoided in susceptible individuals arguably the greater risk of inducing sensitisation in aromatherapy practice is through the administration of oils that have undergone photo- or auto-oxidation. Contact allergy to oxidised d-limonene is common in cases of contact dermatitis; the hydroperoxides are considered the most important allergens,[45,53] although limonene oxide and carvone have also been identified as allergens found in oxidised limonene mixtures.[54] It is the peroxides, epoxides and endoperoxides formed from degradation of the monoterpenes alpha- and gamma–terpinene and terpinolene, which are reported to be the sensitising agents in *Melaleuca alternifolia* (tea tree) oil.[55]

Linalol readily auto-oxidises on air exposure, forming linalol hydroperoxides, which are strong sensitisers.[56] The 38th Amendment to the IFRA standard states that linalol and products rich in linalol should only be used when the level of peroxides is kept to the lowest practical level. Oils rich in linalol include *Aniba rosaeodora* (rosewood), *Cinnamomum camphora* (ho wood), *Coriandrum sativum* (coriander), *Lavandula angustifolia* (lavender), and *Thymus vulgaris* ct linalol (thyme ct linalol).

The inclusion of α-tocopherol to stabilise monoterpene and linalol-containing mediums will reduce their auto-oxidation but inevitable decomposition will occur on storage of the essential oils alone. Professional responsibility demands that oils are stored appropriately and expiry dates are monitored when working with them.

Minimisation of sensitisation risk

Sensitisation reactions in aromatherapy can develop in any healthy individual but are fortunately quite rare and may be subject to misdiagnosis. A reaction may in fact be due to irritancy and a reduction in dose would allow future use of the same essential oil. By patch testing and observing the speed of reaction and its diminution, and whether there is involvement of the skin outside the patch site, professionals working with essential oils are able to correctly assess and manage reactions.

Patch testing in aromatherapy practice

A detailed consultation is always taken and the skin problem discussed in detail with the individual or parent/guardian before starting any treatment and especially when dealing with a dermatological condition. Aside from representing normal clinical procedure, the objective is to elicit information that may indicate contact with possible allergens so that suitable protocols can be followed. Subjects discussed should include:

- the site where the rash or lesion developed and how it developed
- treatments and medications previously tried or currently using
- previous skin disease
- general health and that of family members, especially any history of asthma, hay fever or eczema
- cosmetics and toiletries used
- occupation – focusing on materials used at work and the effect of weekends and holidays on the skin condition
- hobbies.

Within aromatherapy practice, patch testing is an important and necessary safety procedure that professionals need to engage with if oils are to be used responsibly. It is not, however, necessary to routinely patch test all preparations being used. The importance for therapists is to be able to identify and thus avoid problematic agents within the context of the treatments they are providing. It is of particular use when treating individuals with increased vulnerability to irritation or sensitisation to allow a true assessment to be made of any reactions that may occur.

Testing is done on a site where no skin lesion or inflammation is apparent, ideally the upper back or outer arm. The patches must be kept dry and not exposed to sunlight or other sources of ultraviolet light for 48 hours. They are then removed and assessed for accurate testing technique such as good occlusion, good skin contact, dryness of area and so on. A final reading and interpretation occurs 96 hours to one week after patches were initially placed. Washing should be discouraged until the final reading is taken. Guidelines for the patch test procedure are as follows.

- The patch should be filter paper or an antiseptic-free pad. Ideally inert metal chambers such as Finn® chambers attached to Scanpore® tape are used. (Acrylate-based tape is best so as to avoid irritation or sensitisation to the tape itself.)
- The essential oil concentration should match that intended for treatment by dispersing in a suitable vehicle. A patch containing the vehicle alone is used as a control.
- It is recommended that a patch containing the complete formulation of oils at their appropriate concentration is also applied since synergistic irritation or sensitisation activity can then be assessed.
- Degrease the test area (upper back or outer arm) by washing.
- If applying more than one patch adjust the sequence so that those likely to cause strong reactions are not adjacent.
- Apply the patch/tape from below with mild pressure to remove air pouches and record the location of each oil tested.
- After 48 hours, remove the patches. Wait 15 minutes after removal to allow any irritation and increased blood flow to subside.
- Re-read two days later.

In conventional dermatology, for individuals with suspected contact allergy to a cosmetic or perfume it is vital to patch test with their own products and this is also true with aromatherapy formulations and essential oils they may be using at home; the importance of this is clear when the relationship between oxidation of oils and skin reactions is recalled.

Interpretation of patch test results
Any reaction can be scored according to the International Contact Dermatitis Research Group system, as follows:

- +? = doubtful reaction: mild redness only
- + = weak, positive reaction: red and slightly thickened skin
- ++ = strong positive reaction: red swollen skin with individual small water blisters
- +++ = extreme positive reaction: intense redness and swelling with coalesced large blisters or spreading reaction
- IR = irritant reaction; red skin improves once patch is removed
- NT = not tested.

Irritation reactions cause a maximum response at 48 hours, with the skin showing erythema with a fine wrinkling or 'silk paper-like' appearance which

Irritation – skin
reaction confined to
patch site

Sensitisation – skin
reaction extends beyond
patch site

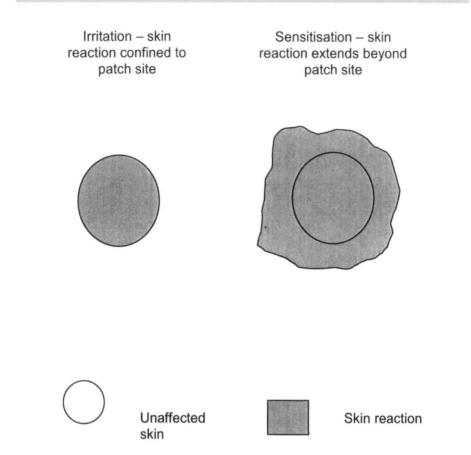

Unaffected
skin

Skin reaction

Figure 3.3 Comparison of affected skin after patch testing for irritation or sensitisation.

remains confined to the exposed patch area and fades over the next day. A sensitisation reaction may not become apparent until the second reading. Here the skin shows erythema and may be vesicular or oedematous which usually extends beyond the defined exposed area (*see* Figure 3.3). False-positive sensitisation reactions may occur where there has been current or recent dermatitis at or near the test site. The presence of a strong positive reaction at one patch site can influence reactivity of adjacent test sites producing an excited skin reaction or 'angry back' syndrome. False-negative reactions can occur in individuals who are concurrently taking oral corticosteroids or antihistamines or who may have recently applied a corticosteroid cream to the test site.

Guidelines for avoiding reactions

Aromatherapists and those regularly exposed to essential oils are most susceptible to the development of allergic contact dermatitis with cases reported in the literature.[5,57–60] Guidelines for reducing the risk of sensitisation induction both for practitioners and clients include the following:

- Minimise the use of essential oils, fragranced cosmetics and toiletries therapists use on themselves and in the home.
- Evaluate hand cleansing practices; avoid harsh detergents and excessive hand washing.
- Use a suitable barrier cream.
- When preparing blends with known sensitisers attenuate the dose used and where possible formulate with 'quenchers'.
- Minimise oxidation by storing oils appropriately and limiting air exposure. Monoterpene-rich oils are particularly vulnerable and should be replaced frequently.
- Vary the blends prepared for an individual. Discourage the use of 'favourite' or frequently used blends and oils (especially pertinent for therapists).
- Avoid all known sensitisers in those with sensitivities to cosmetics and fragrances, especially if atopic disease is also reported.
- Sensitisation reactions may take up to 96 hours after application to occur. Individuals do not always relate this to the application of essential oils, fragrances or cosmetics. Therapists should encourage skin tolerance reports following and during treatments.

Phototoxicity

Phototoxicity or photoirritation is a chemically induced non-immunologic acute skin irritation caused by a combination of a topical or oral photosensitising agent followed by the appropriate wavelength and intensity of ultraviolet (UV) light (usually within the UVA spectrum 320–400 nm). The reaction is also known as phototoxic contact dermatitis or phytophotodermatitis if caused through contact with plant-derived material. The skin response resembles exaggerated sunburn consisting of erythema (with or without blistering) and delayed hyperpigmentation. It can be evoked in all individuals providing the chemical and light wavelength doses are sufficient.

Sunlight is an abundant source of energy available to plants; absorption of a photon by a plant chemical can change its reactivity by altering its electron configuration and energy state. Many plant families produce phototoxins for resistance to pathogens, herbivores and competitors. Furanocoumarins are the major photoreactive chemicals found in essential oils. They are widely distributed in plants, but are particularly abundant in the Apiaceae, Rutaceae and Asteraceae families. Two categories are synthesised in the plant:

- linear furanocoumarins also known as psoralens, which include bergapten (5-methoxypsoralen), xanthotoxin (8-methoxypsoralen), psoralen and iso-pimpinellin
- angular furanocoumarins which include angelicin.

Clinical presentation of phytophotodermatitis

Phototoxic reactions can occur from UV radiation within 15 minutes of contact with topical furanocoumarins; UVA sensitivity peaks 30 minutes to two hours after contact.[61] Erythema, oedema and blisters appear after a latent period of 24 hours and only in sun-exposed areas; moisture and heat exacerbate the condition.[62] The inflammatory reaction peaks at 72 hours. Hyperpigmentation follows one or two weeks after UV-radiation exposure and can last for months or years. Affected areas may remain hypersensitive to UV light for years.[63]

Hyperpigmentation, also known as berloque dermatitis,* arises from several interrelated changes. After cross-linking occurs in keratinocyte and melanocyte DNA, increased mitosis of basal layer keratinocytes and melanocytes can be seen. Melanin production is heightened and packaged into an increased number of melanosomes and then transferred to the basal layer keratinocytes. In fair-skinned individuals, the distribution of melanosomes changes: instead of small clumped melanosomes in keratinocytes, large single dispersed melanosomes are seen capping the nuclei.

Phototoxic essential oils

The effect of furanocoumarins relies on their ability to absorb photons. After forming short-lived high energy states, the energy is released causing cellular damage.[61] Two distinct but concurrent reactions take place when furanocoumarin treated skin is exposed to UVA radiation.

1   In the oxygen-independent reaction, UVA alters the electron configuration and energy state of linear furanocoumarins causing covalent bonding of the furanocoumarin molecule with nuclear DNA. Cross-linking to keratinocytes DNA is the main chemical change responsible for severe damage after UVA exposure.
2   The interaction of furanocoumarins and oxygen produces reactive oxygen species which can produce clinical effects. These occur in cell nuclei, in cell membranes of epidermal, dermal and endothelial cells, and in the cytoplasm affecting enzymes, RNA (ribonucleic acid) and lysosomes.

Table 3.7 lists essential oils and absolutes that can potentially lead to phototoxic reactions. Guidelines on the IFRA website[65] for bergapten-containing (5–methoxypsoralen) fragrances that are not washed off the skin that are subsequently exposed to UV light state the total level of bergapten should not exceed 0.0015%. Some oils contain small amounts of phototoxic furanocoumarins which are not high enough to require restrictions if used alone, but in combination the total level of bergapten could exceed the recommended level. Such oils include expressed *Citrus reticulata* (mandarin and tangerine) and *Petroselinum crispum* fol. (parsley leaf).

Guidelines for using phototoxic oils

Phototoxicity potential should be reviewed when determining the concentration of oil to use. If applied to body areas exposed to sunlight the individual must be instructed to refrain from sunbathing or using UV tanning treatments for 24 hours following contact with the essential oil preparation. The use of sunscreen filtering products can be encouraged to prevent activation of phototoxic compounds. Reduced or furanocoumarin-free citrus oils are available but are

---

* This term is more correctly used to refer to perfume-related bergapten phototoxicity, with other plant-related hyperpigmentation being classified as phytophotodermatitis.[64]

Table 3.7 Phototoxic essential oils and absolutes. Many of these are not used in aromatherapy.

Common name	Plant Family
*Angelica archangelica**	Apiaceae
Apium graveolens	Apiaceae
*Citrus aurantifolia**	Rutaceae
*Citrus aurantium**	Rutaceae
*Citrus bergamia**	Rutaceae
*Citrus limon**	Rutaceae
*Citrus paradisi**	Rutaceae
Citrus reticulata var. mandarin fol.**	Rutaceae
*Cuminum cyminum**	Apiaceae
*Ficus carica***	Moraceae
*Lippia citriodora***	Verbenaceae
*Ruta graveolens**	Rutaceae
*Tagetes minuta**	Asteraceae

* IFRA provides restrictions and guidelines for these.
** IFRA prohibited oil.
Petitgrain mandarin oil is restricted due to its content of methyl N-methyl anthranilate, which is phototoxic.

aromatically inferior. Furthermore, the synergistic activity of the remaining components may be altered on distilling the expressed oil to remove the furanocoumarins. Greater reliability is achieved by selecting alternative essential oils for the case being treated.

Hypericum perforatum (St John's wort) infused oil contains the photodynamic pigment hypericin. It is known that hypericin may cause severe photodermatitis (hypericism) when large amounts of St John's wort herb are taken orally but there is no evidence that, topically, the infused oil has any notable phototoxic potential when applied to intact skin. This is probably due to poor permeation of hypericin across the epidermal barrier. However, Schempp et al.[66] warn that increased susceptibility to the photosensitising properties of hypericin may occur when applied to lesional skin and in fair-skinned individuals after extended solar irradiation.

Photocarcinogenesis

Repeated exposure of mouse skin treated with bergamot essential oil and UV light has been shown to promote skin cancer.[67] The frequency of exposure to the oil (five days per week for 75 weeks) bears little resemblance to aromatherapy practice and photocarcinogenesis is not an area of concern.

Overview of other safety issues

As stated at the start of this chapter, the intention here is not to present an all-inclusive safety review; that can be found elsewhere. However, the clinical use of essential oils in certain situations warrants further attention.

Pregnancy

The rational use of essential oils during pregnancy can help to maintain skin health and importantly may alleviate the need for prescribed drugs. It is interesting to note that a French retrospective study surveying the records of 1,000 women found 99% had received a prescription for at least one drug during their pregnancy, with an average of 13.6 medicines per woman. In addition, 59% were given drugs considered to represent a foetal risk but with a benefit that might be acceptable and 79% received drugs for which no information on safety was available from human or animal studies.[68]

So, against this background, the scarcity of evidence upon which to base professional decisions concerning the safe use of essential oils during pregnancy and breastfeeding is unsurprising. It is known that essential oil metabolites cross the blood–brain barrier and therefore accepted that they also cross the placenta. Therefore oils with any known toxicity are avoided throughout pregnancy. General guidelines for essential oil usage in pregnancy are listed in Table 3.8. When following a traditional aromatherapy approach, that is low-dose topical applications, any risk involved is considered negligible.

In dermatological care, certain conditions tend to improve during the course of pregnancy, for example psoriasis, and therefore the demand for the regular use of essential oil containing formulations may be less. Where regular topical use is indicated, for example in formulations for stretch-mark prevention, the use of only the most non-toxic essential oils is advised. Dosages throughout pregnancy are half the normal adult dose, not only for reasons of safety, but also to allow for the presence of hyperosmia, a phenomenon frequently experienced in pregnancy.

Methyl eugenol

Methyl eugenol occurs in varying amounts in several essential oils. Those of most relevance to dermatological care are *Ocimum* (basil) and *Rosa* (rose) species, plus *Laurus nobilis* (bay). Attention has recently focused on the carcinogenic potential of methyl eugenol. The IFRA 36th Amendment to the Code of Practice severely

Table 3.8 Safety guidelines for using essential oils in aromatherapy dermatological care during pregnancy.

- Essential oils should only be used under the supervision of a professional aromatherapist.
- Avoid topical exposure to essential oils at the embryonic stage or first trimester. (NB: many women using oils have been unaware of being pregnant and have used oils without ill effects.)
- Avoid all emmenagogic oils in women with poor obstetric history.
- Use half the normal adult dose.
- At every treatment, refer to the woman's medical history in case of possible further contraindications related to pregnancy.
- No authoritative list of safe and unsafe oils currently exists but oils with known toxicological concerns should be avoided.
- If a woman is breastfeeding and oils have been placed on the breast, remove using a vegetable oil before feeding.

restricts levels in finished fragrance products. It is commonly used in its natural and synthetic forms as a flavouring agent, an attractant in insecticides and a fragrance in toiletries. It has been estimated that the average human consumes 6 µg per day.[69]

Bioavailability of methyl eugenol through topical application and inhalation remains unknown. To be toxic, it needs to be activated through cytochrome p450 isoenzyme oxidation to 1'-hydroxymethyleugenol.[70] The metabolism is saturable so toxicity appears only after a certain threshold, below which methyl eugenol is eliminated before it can cause any harm. The elimination half-life in humans is 100 minutes.[71] However, Schecter et al.[71] report elevated methyl eugenol levels in a substantial number of adults in the general US population. According to other reports,[72] children are more likely to have higher concentrations, given their smaller size and the nature of some of the identified commercial sources of methyl eugenol such as ice cream, chewing gum and confectionery.

From a client's perspective any risk is minimal in view of dose and duration of treatment to which they are exposed; however, the findings of Schecter et al. and Barr et al. cannot be ignored. For therapists, until the risk associated with background levels of methyl eugenol exposure has been fully established it seems prudent to advise caution in the repeated, frequent use of methyl eugenol containing oils.

Convulsant essential oils

A survey of recorded case studies where seizures have been induced by essential oils reveals most occurred in non-epileptics and when oils had been taken orally.[22,73] However, the apparent initiation of epileptic events in a one-year-old healthy girl following five prolonged baths containing an unknown quantity of eucalyptus, pine and thyme oils over a four-day period suggests a cumulative effect is possible through repeated small-dose cutaneous applications.[73] There are very few essential oils that are indicated for dermatological care where this is likely to be a concern. Relevant oils are given in Chapter 2, Table 2.6. Their use should be avoided in undiagnosed blackouts or dizzy spells and poorly controlled epilepsy.

References

1 Wahlberg JE. Clinical overview of irritant dermatitis. In: van der Valk PGM, Maibach HI, editors. *The Irritant Contact Dermatitis Syndrome*. Florida: CRC Press; 1996. p. 1–6.
2 Draize JH, Woodward G, Calvery HO. Methods for the study of irritation and toxicity of substances applied topically to the skin and mucous membranes. *J Pharmacol Exper Ther*. 1944; **82**: 377–90.
3 Basketter DA, Reynolds FS, York M. Predictive testing in contact dermatitis: irritant dermatitis. *Clin Dermatol*. 1999; **15**: 637–44.
4 York M, Griffiths HA, Whittle E *et al.* Evaluation of a human patch test for the identification and classification of skin irritation potential. *Contact Derm*. 1996; **34**: 204–12.
5 Crawford GH, Katz KA, Ellis E *et al.* Use of aromatherapy products and increased risk of hand dermatitis in massage therapists. *Arch Dermatol*. 2004; **140**: 991–5.
6 Robinson MK. Population differences in acute skin irritation responses. *Contact Derm*. 2002; **46**: 86–93.

7 Grove GL. Age-associated changes in integumental reactivity. In: Leveque JL, Agache PG, editors. *Aging Skin. Properties and functional changes*. New York: Marcel Dekker; 1993. p. 189–92.

8 Paquet F, Pierard-Franchimont C, Fumal I *et al*. Sensitive skin at menopause; dew point and electrometric properties of the stratum corneum. *Maturitas*. 1998; **28**: 221–7.

9 Modjtahedi SP, Maibach HI. Ethnicity as a possible endogenous factor in irritant contact dermatitis: comparing the irritant response among Caucasians, Blacks and Asians. *Contact Derm*. 2002; **47**: 272–8.

10 Arakami J, Kawana S, Effendy I *et al*. Differences of skin irritation between Japanese and European women. *Br J Dermatol*. 2002; **146**: 1052–6.

11 Lamminstausta K, Maibach HI, Wilson D. Susceptibility to cumulative and acute irritant contact dermatitis. An experimental approach in human volunteers. *Contact Derm*. 1988; **19**: 84–90.

12 Frosch P, Klingman AM. A method for appraising the stinging capacity of topically applied substances. *J Soc Cosmet Chem*. 1981; **28**: 197.

13 Mcfadden JP, Wakelin SH, Basketter DA. Acute irritation thresholds in subjects with type 1 skin. *Contact Derm*. 1998; **38**: 147–9.

14 Simion P, Rau AH. Sensitive skin. *Cosmetics Toiletries*. 1994; **109**: 43–50.

15 Yokota T, Matsumoto M, Sakamaki T *et al*. Classification of sensitive skin and development of a treatment system appropriate for each group. *IFSCC Mag*. 2003; **6**: 303–7.

16 Primavera G, Berardesca E. Sensitive skin: mechanisms and diagnosis. *Int J Cosmet Sci*. 2005; **27**: 1–10.

17 Nassif A, Chan SC, Storrs FJ *et al*. Abnormal irritancy in atopic dermatitis and in atopy without dermatitis. *Arch Dermatol*. 1994; **130**: 1402–7.

18 Klas PA, Corey G, Storrs FJ *et al*. Allergic and irritant patch test reactions and atopic disease. *Contact Derm*. 1996; **34**: 121–4.

19 Uter W, Gefeller O, Schwaritz HJ. An epidemiological study of the influence of season (cold and dry air) on the occurrence of irritant skin changes of the hands. *Br J Dermatol*. 1998; **138**: 266–72.

20 Agner T, Serup J. Seasonal variation of skin resistance to irritants. *Br J Dermatol*. 1989; **121**: 323–8.

21 Basketter D, Griffiths HA, Wang XM. Individual, ethnic and seasonal variation in irritant susceptibility of skin: the implications for a predictive human patch test. *Contact Derm*. 1996; **35**: 208–13.

22 Tisserand R, Balacs T. *Essential Oil Safety. A guide for health care professionals*. Edinburgh: Churchill Livingstone; 1995.

23 Bowles EJ. *The Chemistry of Aromatherapeutic Oils*. 3rd ed. Australia: Allen & Unwin; 2003.

24 Pumphrey RS, Wilson PB, Faragher EB *et al*. Specific immunoglobulin E to peanut, hazelnut and brazil nut in 731 patients: similar patterns found at all ages. *Clin Exp Allergy*. 1999; **29**(9): 1256–9.

25 Sampson HA. Peanut allergy. *N Eng J Med*. 2002; **346**: 1294–9.

26 Hourihane JO, Kilburn SA, Nordlee JA, Hefle SL, Taylor SL, Warner JO. An evauluation of the sensitivity of subjects with peanut allergy to very low doses of peanut protein: a randomised, double-blind, placebo-controlled food challenge study. *J Allergy Clin Immunol*. 1997; **100**: 596–600.

27 Lack G, Fox D, Northstone K *et al*. Factors associated with the development of peanut allergy in childhood. *N Eng J Med*. 2003; **348**: 977–85.

28 Vadas P, Wai Y, Burks W *et al*. Detection of peanut allergens in breast milk of lactating women. *JAMA*. 2001; **285**: 1746–8.

29 Frank L, Marian A, Visser M *et al*. Exposure to peanuts in utero and in infancy and the

development of sensitisation to peanuts in young children. *Paed Allergy Immunol.* 1999; **10**: 27–32.

30 Levy Y, Danon YL. Allergy to sesame seeds in infants. *Allergy.* 2001; **56**: 193–4.

31 Spirito Perkins M. Raising awareness of sesame allergy. *Pharm J.* 2001; **267**: 757–8.

32 Basketter DA. Skin sensitisation to cinnamic alcohol. The role of skin metabolism. *Acta Derm Venereol.* 1992; **72**: 98–104.

33 Basketter DA. Skin sensitisation: risk assessment. *Int J Cosmet Sci.* 1998; **20**: 141–50.

34 Kimber I, Cumberbatch M. Dendritic cells and cutaneous immune responses to chemical allergens. *Toxicol Appl Pharmacol.* 1992; **117**: 137–46.

35 Kanerva L. Skin contact reactions to spices. A review. *Acta Dermatovenerologica* 2001; **10**(1): 1–7: www.mf.uni-lj.si/acta-apa/acta-apa-01–1/1-clanek.html (accessed 02.01.06).

36 Kimber I, Basketter DA, Berthold M *et al.* Skin sensitisation testing in potency and risk assessment. *Toxicol Sci.* 2001; **59**: 198–208.

37 Friedmann PS. Allergy and the skin. II – Contact and atopic eczema. *BMJ.* 1998; **316**(7139): 1226–34.

38 Kimber I, Basketter DA. Contact sensitisation: a new approach to risk assessment. *Human Ecol Risk Assess.* 1997; **3**: 385–95.

39 de Groot AC, Frosch PJ. Adverse reactions to fragrances. A clinical review. *Contact Derm.* 1997; **36**: 57–87.

40 Johansen JD, Andersen TE, Kjoller M *et al.* Identification of risk products for fragrance contact allergy. A case-referent study based on patients' histories. *Am J Contact Dermat.* 1998; **2**: 80–7.

41 Frosch PJ, Johansen JD, Menne T *et al.* Further important sensitisers in patients sensitive to fragrances. II Reactivity to essential oils. *Contact Derm.* 2002; **47**: 279–87.

42 Larsen WG. Fragrance testing in the 21st century. Letter to the editor. *Contact Derm.* 2002; **47**: 60–1.

43 Hausen BM, Reichling J, Harkenthal M. Degradation products of monoterpenes are the sensitising agents in tea tree oil. *Am J Contact Dermat.* 1999; **10**: 68–77.

44 Matura M, Goossens A, Bordalo O *et al.* Oxidised citrus oil (R-limonene): a frequent skin sensitizer in Europe. *J Am Acad Dermatol.* 2002; **47**: 709–14.

45 Matura M, Gossens A, Bordalo O *et al.* Patch testing with oxidised R (+) limonene and its hydroperoxide fraction. *Contact Derm.* 2003; **49**: 15–21.

46 Matura M, Skold M, Borje A *et al.* Selected oxidised fragrance allergens are common contact allergens. *Contact Derm.* 2005; **52**: 320–8.

47 Schnuch A, Lessmann H, Geier J *et al.* Contact allergy to fragrances: frequencies of sensitisation from 1996 to 2002. Results of the IVDK. *Contact Derm.* 2004; **50**(2): 65–76.

48 Opdyke DLJ. Inhibition of sensitization reactions induced by certain aldehydes. *Fd Cosmet Toxicol.* 1976; **14**: 197–8.

49 Hananu D *et al.* The influence of limonene in induced delayed hypersensitivity to citral in guinea pigs. *Acta Derm Venereol.* 1983; **63**: 1–7.

50 Basketter D. Quenching: fact or fiction? *Contact Derm.* 2000; **43**: 253–8.

51 Allenby CF, Goodwin BF, Safford RJ. Diminution of immediate reactions to cinnamic aldehyde by eugenol. *Contact Derm.* 1984; **11**: 322–3.

52 Nilsson AM, Jonsson C, Luthman K *et al.* Inhibition of the sensitizing effect of carvone by the addition of non-allergenic compounds. *Acta Derm Venereol.* 2004; **84**(2): 99–105.

53 Karlberg AT, Dooms-Goosens A. Contact allergy to oxidized d-limonene among dermatitis patients. *Contact Derm.* 1997; **36**: 201–6.

54 Karlberg AT, Magnusson K, Nilsson U. Air oxidation of d-limonene (the citrus solvent) creates potent allergens. *Contact Derm.* 1992; **26**: 332–40.

55 Hausen BM, Reichling J, Harkenthal M. Degradation products of monoterpenes are the sensitising agents in tea tree oil. *Am J Contact Dermat.* 1999; **10**(2): 68–77.

56 Skold M, Borje A, Harambasic E *et al.* Contact allergens formed on air exposure of

linalool. Identification and quantification of primary and secondary oxidation products and the effect on skin sensitization. *Chem Res Toxicol*. 2004; **17**: 1697–705.

57 Bleasel N, Tate B, Rademaker M. Case report: Allergic contact dermatitis following exposure to essential oils. *Australas J Dermatol*. 2002; **45**: 211–13.

58 Cockayne S, Gawkrodger J. Occupational contact dermatitis in an aromatherapist. *Contact Derm.* 1997; **37**: 306.

59 Schaller M, Korting HC. Allergic airborne contact dermatitis from essential oils used in aromatherapy. *Clin Experiment Dermatol*. 1995; **20**: 143–5.

60 Blisland D, Strong A. Allergic contact dermatitis from the essential oil of French marigold (Tagetes patula) in an aromatherapist. *Contact Derm*. 1990; **23**: 55–6.

61 Kavli G, Volden G. Phytophotodermatitis. *Photodermatol*. 1984; **1**: 65–75.

62 Pathak MA. Phytophotodermatitis. *Clin Dermatol*. 1986; **4**: 102–21.

63 Lovell CR. *Plants and the Skin*. 1st ed. Oxford: Blackwell Scientific Publications; 1993.

64 Chew AL, Maibach H. Berloque dermatitis. *eMedicine*: www.emedicine.com/derm/topic52.htm (accessed 01.03.06).

65. www.ifraorg.org (accessed 03.01.06).

66 Schempp CM, Ludtke R, Winghofer B *et al*. Effect of topical application of *Hypericum perforatum* extract (St John's wort) on skin sensitivity to solar simulated radiation. *Photodermatol Photoimmunol Photomed*. 2000; **16**(3): 125–8.

67 Young AR, Walker SL, Kinley JS *et al*. Phototumorigenesis studies of 5-methoxypsoralen in bergamot oil. Evaluation and modification of risk of human use in an albino mouse skin model. *J Photochem Photobiol*. 1990; **7**(2–4): 231–50.

68 Editorial: Risky drugs being given 'too frequently' to pregnant women. *Pharm J*. 2000; **265**(7125): 811.

69 Miller RC, Swanson AB, Phillips DH. Structure activity studies of the carcinogenesis in the mouse and the rat of some naturally occurring and synthetic alkenylbenzene derivatives related to safrole and estragole. *Cancer Res*. 1983; **43**: 1124–34.

70 Burkey JL, Sauer JM, McQueen CA *et al*. Cytotoxicity and genotoxicity of methyleugenol and related congeners – a mechanism of activation for methyleugenol. *Mutat Res*. 2000; **453**(1): 25–33.

71 Schecter A, Lucier GW, Cunningham ML *et al*. Human consumption of methyleugenol and its elimination from serum. *Environ Health Perspect*. 2004; **112**(6): 678–80.

72 Barr D, Barr J, Bailey SL. Levels of methyleugenol in a subset of adults in the general US population as determined by high resolution mass spectrometry. *Environ Health Perspect*. 2000; **108**(4): 323–8.

73 Burkhard PR, Burkhardt K, Haenggeli CA *et al*. Plant-induced seizures; reappearance of an old problem. *J Neurol*. 1999; **246**: 667–70.

Chapter 4

The essentials of aromatic formulations

Introduction

The dosage and vehicle used in topical aromatherapy applications largely determines their effectiveness or otherwise. In the case of skin conditions, there are multiple factors to consider, namely the nature of the condition, skin barrier integrity, the client's age and health profile, vehicle used, site of application and the aesthetics of the formulation. Client compliance is closely associated with the latter, and can be the critical factor between treatment success and failure.

Ingredients used in topical preparations

Aromatic preparations of greatest therapeutic value in skin care are usually mixtures of essential oils, vegetable oils, hydrosols, beeswax, plant waxes, butters and *Aloe vera* gel. There are additional, albeit limited, indications for using clays, oatmeal and honey with the latter being the subject of increasing interest in wound and burn care research. Ethanolic and solvent derived plant extracts (with the exception of absolutes) are outside the normal therapeutic range for aromatherapists and are not discussed here. Although the natural world offers many interesting bioactive ingredients and aromatherapy is especially rooted in the traditional use of these, there is a significant difference in the stability, purity and standardisation of these and synthetic products. Therefore, while offering exciting possibilities for future research and product development as well as in some instances demonstrating therapeutic efficacy that exceeds pharmaceuticals,[1,2] their use presents particular practical and methodological challenges that will be explored throughout this chapter.

Vegetable and infused oils

Offering an ideal therapeutic partnership for essential oils, vegetable oils are increasingly being used as key ingredients in cosmetic preparations. They interact favourably with the skin, offering excellent protective and emollient properties, which lead to a reduction in transepidermal water loss (TEWL), improved skin hydration and barrier integrity.[3] They are extracted either from the seeds, nuts, kernels, or pericarp of oil-bearing plants and for therapeutic applications cold-pressed, unrefined oils are favoured. Quality parameters, such as antioxidant content, have been shown to be adversely affected by the processes involved in refining, heat and solvent extraction.[4,5] The presence of degradation products arising as a consequence of reactions during refining are used as an indicator of contamination of unrefined oils.[6] Some oils, for example *Vitis vinifera* (grapeseed oil), are not obtainable by cold pressing.

Often referred to as 'fixed' or 'carrier' oils, vegetable oils include infused (also known as macerated) oils. Leaving plant material to infuse in suitable vegetable oil (typically sunflower seed) for a period of time, after which the mixture is filtered to remove all plant material, results in infused vegetable oils; these contain lipid-soluble constituents of the plant material, including essential oils. Infused oils of particular value in dermatology are *Calendula officinalis* (marigold flower) and *Hypericum perforatum* (St John's wort). Listed in the German Commission E Monographs of approved herbs, calendula is indicated for topical use in poorly healing wounds and inflammatory conditions, and hypericum for burns.[7] Another, readily available infused oil, useful for its anti-inflammatory activity, is produced from infusing the roots of *Daucus carota* (wild carrot).

The composition of vegetable oils

Major compounds making up 95–98% of vegetable oil composition are triglycerides (triacylglycerols) formed when long chain fatty acids esterify with hydroxyl groups of glycerol. Naturally occurring vegetable oils are complex mixtures of different triglycerides. The fatty acid content is often referred to but these do not exist in their free (unesterified) state. The remaining content is made up of minor (but often important) compounds such as wax esters, hydrocarbons, phenolic derivatives, flavonoids and vitamins.

Fatty acids

The common fatty acids of plant tissues are C16–C18 straight chain compounds with zero to three double bonds of the *cis* configuration. Fatty acids with double bonds of the *trans* configuration are occasionally found in natural lipids but are more likely to be formed during food processing (hydrogenation) – their role in nutrition remains controversial.

The most abundant saturated fatty acid in nature is hexadecanoic or palmitic acid which is designated a '16.0' fatty acid, the first numerals denoting the number of carbon atoms in the aliphatic chain, and the latter the number of double bonds. Oleic is the most common monounsaturated fatty acid designated 18:1. The C18 polyunsaturated fatty acids, linoleic (18:2) and α-linolenic (18:3) are the major components of most plant lipids and are found in many vegetable oils. They are essential fatty acids that cannot be synthesised by the body and are the biosynthetic precursors of C20–C22 polyunsaturated fatty acids with three to six double bonds; these are important constituents of membrane phospholipids and precursors of prostaglandins and eicosanoids. Polyunsaturated fatty acid rich oils such as *Carthamus tinctorius* (safflower) and *Oenothera biennis* (evening primrose) are disposed to becoming rancid since the presence of double bonds makes them open to attack by oxygen and moisture. Hence they are less stable than those high in saturated fatty acids.

Oenothera biennis (evening primrose) and *Borago officinalis* (borage) oils contain gamma-linolenic acid (GLA) and linoleic acid. GLA is not an essential dietary component but is a precursor of dihomogammalinolenic acid (DGLA) and the physiological series 1 prostaglandins (PG1) which do not possess the inflammatory effects of the PG2 series produced from arachidonic acid. The efficacy of GLA in the treatment of inflammatory skin conditions such as atopic dermatitis may in part be due to increased production of PG1 series prostaglandins at the expense of inflammatory PG2 series prostaglandins.[8] Clinical studies with GLA in inflammatory skin conditions have produced conflicting results; however, some individuals do appear to benefit.

Simmondsia chinensis (jojoba) is unique in its production of wax esters rather than triglycerides in its seeds. The liquid wax is made up of straight chain esters of monounsaturated long chain fatty acids connected directly to fatty alcohols with a total carbon chain of C42 with no side branching. It is highly resistant to rancidity due to the presence of the antioxidant α, γ, δ tocopherols.

Transdermal penetration of vegetable oils

Penetration and permeation through the skin is limited by molecular size and other physio-chemical properties.[9] The extent and rate of vegetable oil absorption into the skin remains contentious. The degree of fatty acid saturation is thought to influence the permeation extent of topically applied vegetable oils, with oils like borage (*Borago officinalis*) that are high in short chain and polyunsaturated components being favoured. However, jojoba, consisting of mainly monounsaturated fatty acids and fatty alcohols, is recognised as being readily absorbed by the skin within minutes with transdermal penetration suspected.[10]

It is currently accepted that, in the main, the permeation of many vegetable oils is restricted to the upper layers of the stratum corneum in healthy skin[9] but in areas where the skin barrier function is impaired, greater permeation will occur.[11] The topical application of oils with higher linoleic acid and lower oleic acid contents has been shown to positively influence epidermal lipids in experimentally induced irritant contact dermatitis.[3]

Fatty acids with their affinity for the lipid protein domains of the stratum corneum have been used in the transportation of some pharmaceuticals. Researchers looking for effective in vitro simultaneous transdermal delivery of the hormonal drug tamoxifen and gamma-linolenic acid (GLA) reported that complexes of tamoxifen and the polyunsaturated constituents of borage oil permeated the skin intact.[12,13] In a comparison of the penetration enhancement offered by saturated and unsaturated fatty acids, Gwak *et al.*[14] reported a very high enhancing effect on skin permeation vehicles when oleic and linoleic acids were added to the vehicles, but only a slight change with the addition of saturated fatty acids. It appears that oleic acid partitions into the lipid regions of the stratum corneum disrupting its structure and lipid fluidity, thereby enhancing penetration of drugs and other topically applied substances.[15]

Vegetable oils containing moderate to high levels of oleic and linoleic acids include *Carthamus tinctorius* (safflower), *Helianthus annuus* (sunflower), *Corylus avellana* (hazelnut), *Olea europaea* (olive), *Persea americana* (avocado) and *Prunus dulcis* (sweet almond).[16] Further research is needed if a complete, quantitative understanding of skin permeation by triglycerides and the effects on vegetable–essential oil preparations is to be reached.

Mineral oils

Mineral oils do not contain any vitamins or fatty acids and cannot be absorbed by healthy intact skin but create a thin film on the surface blocking the pores.

Mixing essential oils into mineral oils is inappropriate, as this inhibits their absorption. Although mineral oils will not go rancid they provide no nourishment to the skin and are not suitable for use in aromatherapy formulations.

Hydrosols

Also known as hydrolats (a word derived from French), these are the products of the distillation of plant material. Usually the material is being distilled to produce an essential oil, although some plants are processed only for the hydrosol and are then sometimes called plant water distillates; a well-known example is *Hamamelis virginiana* (witch hazel). Some confusion in the literature exists as to what is and is not a hydrosol and debates about the naming of these waters do not always bring clarity. Table 4.1 seeks to simplify matters for this text and we have opted to refer to these products as hydrosols in line with others; see for example Rose[17] and Catty.[18]

Unlike artificially fragranced floral waters, a true hydrosol cannot be manufactured synthetically; it has to be produced during the distillation process. During distillation, steam and essential oil compounds are in intimate contact. On condensation some essential oil compounds, namely the more water-soluble oxygenated polar compounds, dissolve in the aqueous phase and are therefore lost to the water distillate or hydrosol. As the perfumery and food industries have developed methods such as cohobation, poroplast extraction and adsorption to recover the dissolved compounds,[19,20] for use in skin care, hydrosols obtained from sources that are distilling specifically for the therapeutic value of the final products are favoured.

The composition of hydrosols

It would be incorrect to assume the same properties for hydrosols and their related essential oils, as their chemical profiles are distinctly different. For example, the primary oil of geranium (*Pelargonium ssp.*) has been found to be richer in hydrocarbons compared to the distillate, which contains greater concentrations of the oxygenated compounds linalol, citronellol and geraniol.[21] This research demonstrated that 7% of the total oil yield could be recovered from the hydrosol.

Hydrosol properties are being increasingly researched with antibacterial and anti-inflammatory effects being demonstrated.[22,23] Hydrosols are either neutral or slightly acid and according to Catty[18] the pH greatly influences the therapeutic effects; the acidic nature of *Cistus ladaniferus* (rock rose) reputedly causes the constriction of tissues (an astringent action) while *Lavandula angustifolia* (lavender), with a pH close to neutral, lacks this effect. The low levels of terpene hydrocarbons means they are very well tolerated on the skin, and throughout

Table 4.1 Defining a hydrosol.

A hydrosol is not:

- water with essential oils added
- water and essential oils with added surfactant to aid solubilisation
- water with the addition of synthetic fragrance or alcohol
- redistilled cohobated water.

this book there are examples of where they may be selected in preference to essential oils. Microbial contamination of the hydrosol is an area of concern particularly if applying topically to broken or damaged skin. It is important that steps are taken to reduce atmospheric contamination during the distillation and packaging of hydrosols and when being used in practice. They should be stored in a dark cold environment and not used beyond recommended storage times.

Cera alba (beeswax)

Glands under the abdomen of bees secrete a wax, which they use to construct the honeycomb. The wax is recovered as a by-product when the honey is harvested. It is boiled in water, filtered while warm and poured into moulds. For therapeutic use, the yellow, mildly aromatic unbleached type is preferred. Beeswax gives creams, ointments and balms their consistency and provides greater skin protection than vegetable oils because of its wax content. It is included in formulations for its soothing, softening anti-inflammatory effect; it is absorbed very slowly by the skin without blocking pores and is non-comedogenic. In 2005 the Cosmetic Ingredient Review Expert Panel concluded it was safe to be used in cosmetic products.[24]

Composition of beeswax

Beeswax is a complex lipoidal mixture, mainly composed of hydrocarbons, monoesters, diesters and free fatty acids. Adulteration of pure beeswax by the addition of petroleum waxes or fatty substances is easily detected by gas chromatography mass spectrometry[25] and waxes contaminated in this way are unsuitable for therapeutic use. The anti-inflammatory effect is due to the high molecular weight alcohol compound D-002 that has been isolated from beeswax and shown to reduce leucotriene B4 and thromboxane B2 concentrations.[26]

Plant waxes and butters

Simmondsia chinensis (jojoba)

With a unique composition, the majority of wax esters in jojoba have a chain length of C40–C42 and possess one double bond. It is exceptionally rich in *cis*-11-eicosenoic acid. Many modifications can be made at the double bond, leading to the great versatility of jojoba as an ingredient in a wide range of cosmetic and chemical products.[27]

Traditionally jojoba is used in hair care and there is abundant anecdotal evidence for its soothing properties on irritated skin conditions. Recent research offers reliable evidence for its anti-inflammatory effects.[28] It penetrates skin readily and it has been suggested that jojoba slows down sebum secretion in oily skin states, leading to it being particularly beneficial in the treatment of acne vulgaris,[29] especially in view of its non-comedogenic nature. Dweck (ibid.) suggests at least 5–10% concentration is necessary for moisturising effects; we suggest it can be used at 100% concentration if required, as it has no known contraindications. The smooth, non-greasy sensation left on the skin by jojoba makes it an especially pleasing ingredient in facial care.

Vitellaria paradoxa (*shea butter, syn. karité butter*)

Shea butter is obtained from the kernels of a sub-Saharan African tree and for centuries indigenous people have used it for cooking and medicinal purposes. The butter is rich in fatty acids – mainly oleic, stearic, linoleic and palmitic acids – plus minor amounts of sterols and esters of triterpene alcohols. In recent years, much commercial interest has been shown in shea butter and it is now a primary ingredient in many cosmetic preparations, being valued for its reputed anti-ageing, anti-inflammatory and moisturising effects. Only pure, unrefined shea butter is acceptable for use in therapeutic formulations; it can be used on its own, or as a key ingredient in creams and ointments.

Theobroma cacao (*cocoa butter*)

Like shea butter, cocoa butter is widely recognised as having skin protective benefits and has long been used in cosmetic preparations. Typically it contains oleic (37%), stearic (34%), palmitic (26%) and linoleic (2%) acids.[30] Unrefined butter remains solid at room temperature and melts at body temperature. Used with or in place of beeswax, it adds a rich consistency to creams and lotions, making them firmer. It has excellent emollient properties, softens and protects the skin and is ideal for dry skin conditions. It is widely used in baby care products.

Aloe vera (syn. Aloe barbadensis) gel

This is traditionally used topically for burns, wound healing, psoriasis, sunburn and other inflammatory conditions. There is some confusion between the leaf exudates and the gel: aloe gel is the clear gelatinous substance obtained from parenchymatous cells found in the pulp in the centre of the leaf, whereas the leaf exudates or extracts are obtained from the cells just beneath the leaf skin. This confusion may account for some of the conflicting evidence for aloe's efficacy in wound healing.[31] Others have suggested that variable results in the literature may be due to treatment of the gel following harvesting.[32]

In a review of *Aloe vera* gel research, Reynolds and Dweck (ibid.) cite evidence for its remarkable anti-inflammatory effect on burns, frostbite and wound healing; reports of antioxidant activity and restoration of cellular activity following UV radiation by aloe extracts were included and a placebo-controlled clinical trial using aloe gel had significant curative effects in psoriasis patients. The reviewers were careful to point out that the components present in the exudates and leaf gel are different and when reading the literature, it is important to keep this in mind. Although the identification of all active components in aloe is still to be completed, it seems that they include at least polysaccharides, lipids, amino acids, enzymes, sterols and glycoprotein.

Reports of adverse reactions to the cutaneous use of *Aloe vera* are rare, especially in view of the widespread use of it. A prospective multicentre trial investigating the prevalence of contact sensitisation to different *Aloe vera* preparations found no evidence of sensitising potential. The authors suggest that reports in the literature of irritation or allergy relate to the use of *Aloe* products over 15 years ago, when leaf extracts rather than gel were more commonly in use than today.[33] There is a clear role for *Aloe vera* gel in aromatherapy formulations and an essential need to ensure that, in dermatological use, only guaranteed quality assured gels are used.

Clay

The use of minerals for medicinal as well as cosmetic purposes is as old as mankind itself. There is evidence that ancient man mixed water with ochres and mud to cleanse and treat wounds and there is rich archaeological evidence for the medicinal use of clays and minerals in ancient Egypt and Mesopotamia.[34] Today, clay minerals are topically used in powders, pastes and masks and commercially are commonly found as kaolin, talc, green clay and fuller's earth. Topically, they act as drying agents, due to their high adsorbency level of skin secretions and micro-organisms, and are the active principles in face masks (ibid.). The beneficial use of clay masks is notable in conditions involving excess sebum secretion such as acne vulgaris, as well as forming part of regular skin cleansing regimens.

Honey

Like clay, honey has been used medicinally since ancient times but it is only in recent years that it has been revived as a topically therapeutic agent and subjected to research. The availability of European or CE-marked sterile honey and honey-impregnated dressings has markedly increased research interest in its wound-healing and antimicrobial activity and several studies have produced encouraging results.[26,35-39] Manuka honey has been the focus of much of this research but multifloral honeys are also effective.[26,36]

As well as some honeys possessing antibacterial constituents[40] the activity of hydrogen peroxide that is produced in honey activated on dilution by the enzyme glucose oxidase also contributes to its antibacterial efficacy.[36] Antioxidant activity has been attributed to phenolic compounds, with buckwheat honey containing large amounts and demonstrating high free radical scavenging activity.[41] In the same research, manuka honey was shown to specifically scavenge superoxide anion radicals.

As well as playing a significant role in wound care, honey has successfully treated seborrheic dermatitis and dandruff[42] and mixtures of honey, beeswax and olive oil have proven successful in the treatment of tinea infections,[26] atopic dermatitis, psoriasis[37] and nappy dermatitis.[39] Essential oils and vegetable oils mix readily with honey and the inclusion of honey in formulations for a wide range of conditions is indicated.

Avenae sativa (oatmeal)

Oats appear as an approved herb on the German Commission E Monographs for inflammatory and seborrheic skin disease, especially those accompanied by itching.[7] Vegetable oils, honey and essential oils combine well with finely ground oatmeal and can be included in face and body mask applications for a gentle exfoliating effect. Additionally adding oatmeal to baths has a soothing, antipruritic effect for dry skin or dermatitis and herpes zoster infections.

Additional ingredients

There are a number of further ingredients that do not form the mainstay of aromatic formulations, but which may be included in limited situations.

Cetyl alcohol

At room temperature cetyl alcohol takes the form of a waxy, white solid or flakes. It was traditionally obtained from the sperm whale but can now be obtained from the triglycerides of coconut oil or palm oil by a process known as hydrogenation. It is used in creams and lotions to enhance stability, improve texture and increase consistency. It has emollient properties that are due to absorption and retention of cetyl alcohol in the epidermis, where it lubricates and softens the skin, giving a characteristic velvety texture. It has been associated with sensitisation reactions in patients with eczema and cross-sensitisation with lanolin has been shown.[43]

Lanolin (wool fat)

This is a pale yellow, waxy substance with a faint characteristic odour obtained from the sebaceous secretions of sheep. It is rich in wax esters, sterol esters, triterpenes, alcohols and free acids and sterols. The fatty acid components are mainly saturated. The anhydrous or dehydrated lanolin is used in the preparation of water-in-oil (W/O) creams and ointments. When mixed with vegetable oils it produces emollient creams that penetrate the skin and facilitate absorption.[44] It has been associated with skin hypersensitivity reactions with some reports suggesting that this arises from false positives in patch testing.[45] The safety of pesticide residues in lanolin is also of concern[46] and it is now possible to obtain lanolin with minimum pesticide content.

Glycerine

This is a colourless, odourless, viscous, hygroscopic liquid which is used in skin-care formulations for its antimicrobial, emollient, humectant and plasticising properties. It occurs naturally in animal and vegetable fats and oils. At high levels (15–20%), glycerine has a preservative effect, but this benefit is offset by the increased stickiness of the product.

Lactic acid

This is a colourless, odourless, viscous, hygroscopic non-volatile liquid. It is used for its softening and conditioning effect on the skin. It is also used to regulate the pH in a formulation.

Borax (sodium borate)

This is extracted from the mineral Borin atrocalcite and is frequently used in cosmetic products since it is an effective emulsifier. However, continual use of borax-containing products is to be discouraged, as this will dry the skin.

Preservatives

When formulating with natural products, the inclusion of suitable preservatives needs to be considered, as even with good hygiene measures products will readily spoil. Any topical preparation applied to broken or diseased skin if contaminated

Table 4.2 Considerations on the need for preservatives in natural product-based formulations.

The spoilage potential of the formulation depends on a number of factors:

- the presence or absence of mediums for microbial growth, e.g. water (or hydrosol); water-based preparations have very short storage times and/or require the highest levels of preservative
- the microbial challenge present during product preparation
- the storage time and temperature of final preparation
- the pattern of normal in-use conditions to be expected and potential end-user abuse.

Preservative-free formulations may only be possible to prepare if:

- the physical and chemical properties of the final product inhibit microbial growth (e.g. water-free products; effective concentration levels of antimicrobial essential oils)
- essential oil-free products are to be used within a very short period (seven days) and limited quantities are provided.

Aromatherapy-based formulations may contain natural preservatives through:

- bactericidal, bacteriostatic, fungicidal and fungistatic essential oils at sufficient levels
- plant extracts, e.g. Biopein® or Neopein®
- honey
- alcohol.

---

could have disastrous consequences. Table 4.2 lists some points to consider when deciding upon which, if any, preservative to include. When selecting preservatives, there is a need to balance the actual levels required to work effectively with the need to avoid harm to the user. In the past, overzealous commercial producers used preservatives in dosages that prevented microbial contamination but which themselves caused skin irritation and sensitisation. Research in North America covering the period 1977–80 identified that preservatives caused the second highest incidence of skin reactions after fragrances.[47]

Bacterial spoilage of formulations is often invisible while fungal growth is indicated by blue or green discolouration on the surface. Even under refrigerated conditions, without preservatives base creams and lotions will only keep for very short periods (seven days is a conservative but safe guide). Any aqueous base product that is designed for longer-term storage without effective concentrations of antimicrobial essential oils, requires the incorporation of a preservative.

Grapefruit seed extract

Grapefruit seed extract (GSE) or Citricidal® is manufactured from the seeds and pulp of grapefruit and has gained a popular reputation for being an effective broad-spectrum bactericide, fungicide, antiviral and antiparasitic compound with low toxicity and irritancy. It is frequently advocated as a natural alternative to synthetic preservatives due to its broad-spectrum bactericidal effects[48,49] and for its apparently beneficial effects in wound healing.[50] However, research has revealed that some of these products are not as natural as claimed. A 1996 study into a commercially available GSE found methyl-p-hydroxybenzoate and triclosan (synthetic preservatives) to be present and similar findings were reported in 2001.[51,52]

The 2001 paper also rebuts the suggestion which is sometimes made that the active substance in GSE is simply chemically related to benzethonium chloride (a preservative which has been found in some extracts). In other work, researchers found that out of six commercially available GSEs five contained the preservatives triclosan, methyl paraben or benzethonium chloride. The preservative-free sample, along with a self-made extract included in the study, showed no antimicrobial activity.[53] On such evidence the validity of using GSE in the belief that this is providing a natural option to preservation is highly dubious.

Parabens

Preservatives commonly used in pharmaceutical and commercial cosmetic preparations are parabens, chlorocresol, sorbic acid and propylene glycol. All of these can cause sensitisation and subsequent allergic contact dermatitis. Parabens are esters of para-hydroxybenzoic acid. They have a broad spectrum of antibacterial activity and are the most commonly used preservatives found in skin-care products. They are found in nature, but for commercial purposes are synthetically produced. Common parabens include methyl parabens, ethyl parabens (E214), propyl parabens (E126) and butyl parabens. They are generally better tolerated than potassium sorbate and sodium benzoate, but do have the potential in some individuals to cause irritation. Sodium benzoate is a natural product but like parabens is normally produced synthetically and its availability is subject to restrictions.

There has been concern expressed about the possible link between parabens in underarm products and breast cancer. The European Scientific Committee on Consumer Products (SCCP) adopted an opinion in 2005 saying there was insufficient evidence to make any link between the use of parabens-containing products and breast cancer. Parabens are regulated by Cosmetic Directive 76/768/EEC, Annex VI, part 1, reference 12. According to this, they can be used as a preservative up to a maximum concentration of 0.4% for one ester and 0.8% for mixtures of esters.[54]

Plant extracts and essential oils as preservatives

In the search for natural preservatives, specially formulated commercially available plant extracts may offer interesting potential. Two examples are the products *Biopein*® and *Neopein*®, which contain antimicrobial compounds from the extracts of plants such as *Thymus vulgaris* (thyme), *Cinnamomum zeylanicum* (cinnamon), *Rosmarinus officinalis* (rosemary) and *Hydrastis canadensi* (golden seal) plus others. A similar product on the market is Melaleucol®, an extract created from *Melaleuca alternifolia* (tea tree). Essential oils themselves possess broad-spectrum antimicrobial activity (*see* Chapter 7) and their preservative role in pharmaceutical and cosmetic preparations has been investigated. In a microbial challenge test carried out according to European Pharmacopoeia (EP) Commission preservation standards, *Thymus vulgaris* (thyme) at 3% in oil-in-water (O/W) and water-in-oil (W/O) vehicles demonstrated effective preservative activity against *Staphylococcus aureus*, *Pseudomonas aeruginosa* and *Escherichia coli*. Against *Candida albicans*, the thyme and W/O combination showed immediate inhibitory activity while the O/W combination kept microbial growth low, but not sufficiently low to meet the EP criteria.[55]

A combination of *Laurus nobilis* (bay), *Salvia officinalis* (common sage) and *Eucalyptus globulus* (blue gum eucalyptus) showed effective inhibition of microbial growth in oil-in-water skin cream and hydrogel formulations at varying degrees of concentration and against different pathogens. Synergistic activity was noted in the study both within combinations of the essential oils and with a standard preservative, methyl-p-hydroxybenzoate (MBP). Interestingly, the essential oils were found to be capable of reducing the amount of MBP normally required as a preservative by up to 200-fold in some cases.[56] This leads to the valid possibility of reducing the use of synthetic preservatives by the synergistic activity offered by essential oils if used in effective concentrations.

Antioxidants

These are frequently added during the preparation of lipid-rich formulations to prevent oxidation reactions; polyunsaturated fatty acids being particularly vulnerable when exposed to air and light. However, while adding an antioxidant will help to prolong the shelf-life of preparations through slowing oxidation, it will do nothing to inhibit microbial spoilage. Vitamin E and vitamin C are commonly used for antioxidant activity.

Essential measures in product preparation

As outlined above, the issue of preservatives is far from straightforward if the aim is to minimise the use of synthetic chemicals and there is plenty of debate as to why this may be desirable which lies outside the scope of this text.[57–60] When choosing to use formulations based entirely on natural materials, it is vital that good practice measures are observed during their preparation. To reduce or eliminate spoilage organisms in products the following observations can be made.

- Ensure aseptic conditions are maintained during preparation.
- Both in preparation and during use do not contaminate the product by direct contact with fingers.
- Avoid exposing the product to UV radiation, air, heat and moisture.
- Lessen the total water content.
- Refrigerate the finished product.
- If the nature of the skin condition for which the preparation is to be used allows it, include essential oils with antimicrobial activity at greater than 3% of the total product.
- Consider the inclusion of natural preservatives, the claims for which are backed up by independent research.
- If formulating with hydrosols or water, preservatives are essential, not optional, if the product is to be used beyond seven days.
- Observe strict shelf-life periods for individual ingredients as well as finished products.

The packaging of the final preparation also affects how well microbial contamination is controlled. Clearly, the sterility of the container is essential, but beyond this, the type of packaging has a heavy influence. Wide-necked jars with shives (cardboard or plastic inserts) present a large surface area for air to attack, plus the plastic covers may accumulate condensation, the cardboard harbours organisms and both provide a potentially rich microbial environment. Modern airless pump dispensers are available that allow efficient dispensing of even viscous material and are a good option especially as they prevent the user scooping out the product and causing contamination. Tubes are an alternative, especially for smaller quantities, and are available with non-return valves that stop air from entering thus maximising their efficiency in respect of minimising the microbial challenge to the product.

Choice of vehicles

As the relative solubility of essential oils in the base vehicle influences skin penetration, the selection of these is extremely important for successful therapy. However, in addition to maximising delivery of active components, the base vehicle itself often plays an important therapeutic role having valuable properties of its own (*see* Table 4.3). The incorrect choice of vehicle may also cause harm. Choice of vehicle depends upon:

- action required which is determined by the nature of the condition
- site of application
- speed of onset of condition
- skin type
- availability
- messiness
- ease of application and client preference
- cost.

Creams

Creams are used for their cooling, moisturising and emollient effect. They are either oil-in-water emulsions (O/W) or water-in-oil emulsions (W/O). In O/W emulsions the oil is surrounded by water which results in a preparation that feels less greasy. These rub into the skin easily and readily wash off, but they may have a drying effect. W/O emulsions have the water surrounded by oil and are greasier, although the extent of this depends on the relative proportions of oil, wax and water. These prevent surface loss of moisture from the skin, making them suitable for conditions characterised by dryness and flaking.

Lotions

Watery lotions evaporate and cool inflamed sites. As the oil content increases, evaporation slows and skin moisture is maintained. Shake lotions are watery lotions to which powder has been added so that the area for evaporation is increased. These lotions dry wet weeping skin but clumping and abrasion can occur.

Table 4.3 Vehicles and their properties.

Vehicle	Application	Effects and benefits	Problems
Dusting powders	Flexures	Lessens friction	If too wet: can clump and irritate.
Lotions and shake lotions	Acutely inflamed exudative skin	Drying, soothing, cooling	Prone to fungal and bacterial contamination. Tedious to apply. Powder in shake lotions may clump.
Creams	Both moist and dry skin	Cooling, emollient, moisturising	Prone to fungal and bacterial contamination.
Ointments	Dry, scaly skin	Occlusive and emollient	Messy to apply.
Pastes	Dry, lichenified and scaly skin	Protective and emollient. Most protective if applied correctly.	Messy and tedious to apply.
Hydrosol sprays	Weeping, acutely inflamed skin.	Drying, non-occlusive. No need to touch skin to treat it.	Vehicle evaporates quickly. Prone to microbial spoilage.
Compresses	Hypersensitive skin. Scalp.	Cool: cooling, soothing, drying. Warm: loosens crusts, debrides.	Messy and time consuming to apply.
Gels	Exudative, acutely inflamed skin. Wounds. Face and scalp.	Cooling, soothing, drying. Can cover with make up.	May sting inflamed skin.

Gels

These are semi-colloids, which liquefy on contact with the skin. They are commonly used in anti-acne and scalp preparations. They have soothing, cooling effects and are used on open wounds, burns and irritated lesions. In a poorly healing wound site, they help to maintain the locally moist environment that is essential for healing to progress. In widespread applications though they tend to be drying and need to be used in moderation if excessive drying of the skin or scalp is to be avoided.

Ointments

Ointments are used for their occlusive and emollient properties. They allow skin to remain pliable, by preventing evaporation of water from the stratum corneum. Their greasiness and difficulty in application makes them less user-friendly than creams and lotions, and poor patient compliance may result. The lipid-rich environment of an ointment slows the rate of movement of essential oils through the vehicle to the stratum corneum interface hence reducing their availability for absorption through the skin. They are best used for small areas and are a perfect medium for nail-care treatments.

Pastes

These are formed from powder and oil. The powder lessens the occlusive effect of oil and such preparations are used for their protective and emollient properties. They are messy to use and like ointments may result in poor compliance.

Dusting powders

These are used in folds to lessen friction between opposing surfaces. They may repel water (e.g. talc) or absorb it (e.g. cornstarch). Powders should not be overused in moist areas where they tend to cake or abrade; however, moderate use may be indicated in certain conditions such as tinea pedis but careful guidance is required.

Selecting the vehicle

Vehicle selection by skin type follows the general principles:

- normal to oily skin types – gels and lotions are preferred
- normal to dry skin types – lotions or creams are preferred
- dry skin – ointments and creams are preferred.

In addition the skin site to be treated affects the choice:

- hairy areas – use lotions, gels or sprays
- intertriginous areas – creams, lotions and powders are indicated.

It is mainly the therapeutic rationale for the type of lesion that guides the choice of vehicle for clinical treatment, rather than for cosmetic purposes.

Wet, exudative lesions: These require initial treatment with tepid to cool compresses to suppress inflammation and debride crusts. The repeated wetting and drying cycles will eventually dry the lesions and the application of compresses is then stopped. Excessive use must be avoided as severe drying and chapping may occur. Once the exudative phase of the condition is controlled, the lost lipids are restored with the liberal use of emollient creams and lotions. *See* Table 4.4 for guidelines to using compresses.

Dry, thickened scaly lesions: Loss of water and epidermal lipids requires treatment with rich, emollient fatty ointment, paste and oil formulations. Applying emollients to moist skin, for example after bathing, is most effective. Emollients need to be applied as frequently as required to keep the skin moist.

Bathing

Daily bathing helps to remove crusts, scales and medicaments. For full-body application of preparations bathing provides an ideal opportunity for maximum

Table 4.4 Preparation and application of compresses.

To make and apply a compress:

- fold sterile gauze to make several layers and cut to fit an area slightly larger than the affected site
- temperature of solution is determined by therapeutic aim: tepid to debride crusts and cool to suppress inflammation
- immerse in the solution and wring out until still wet, but not dripping
- place wet compress on affected area, leaving in place for 30 minutes to one hour
- do not pour solution over the compress once in place, as this will affect the concentration of the solution; if it dries out, replace with a fresh compress
- stop using the compresses once the lesion has dried; excessive drying will lead to cracking and possibly fissures developing.

Effects of compresses:

- antibacterial activity from essential oils and hydrosols
- gentle removal of crusts when the compress is lifted
- a cooling, soothing, anti-inflammatory effect arises from the evaporation of water and via the action of selected oils and hydrosols which constricts the superficial blood vessels
- excellent for antipruritic effects.

coverage and absorption. Oily, emollient preparations are added to warm (not hot) baths in the treatment of dry, flaking conditions such as dermatitis and psoriasis, leaving the skin with a light oily covering and allowing gentle removal of scales. Cooling, soothing antipruritic benefits are achieved by cool water bathing and the cleansing effects are obvious and indicated in infections, acne vulgaris and general skin hygiene practices. Foot-baths are especially important in conditions like pitted keratolysis and tinea pedis. Essential oils can be added to a full-fat milk base for dispersion in the water when an emollient effect is not the primary goal of the bath; otherwise mixing them with carrier oils, honey or oatmeal all contribute healing effects. (Chapter 5 gives sample formulations for bathing.)

Variables associated with topical application

As previously elaborated, the decision on which vehicle to use for a particular condition depends on a number of factors. In addition to these considerations, there are specific factors that are outlined here, which affect the treatment following application of the preparation. Chapter 3 discusses the safety aspects of topical applications.

The effects of occlusion

Occlusion can significantly affect skin permeation of essential oils and if it causes extended hydration of the skin this may be problematic. Occlusion can be inadvertent, such as following the application of a nappy-rash preparation by wearing tightly fitting pants. The possibilities of irritancy or toxicological concerns need to be taken into account when formulating. The effects of occlusion on the skin are usually reversible but in addition to the risk of irritation, microbial growth may also be encouraged. On the other hand, occlusion can be valuable when increased essential oil flux into the skin is required to achieve a therapeutic effect.

The effects of a repairing barrier on dosage requirements

When treating conditions where the skin barrier is compromised, the repair of the barrier on treatment may require dosage and formulation changes to be made, since essential oil permeation through the tissue will change. In conditions ranging from psoriasis and eczema to ulcers and infections, the stratum corneum may be compromised and hence essential oil permeation through the tissue may be considerably greater than when the condition is resolved. By contrast, it is also possible that essential oil delivery to abnormal skin is reduced compared to that in normal tissue, for example where the skin is thickened but intact, as in lichenified skin.

As the barrier repairs itself, it may either be that the therapeutic essential oil dosage can be reduced as the condition improves, or it might be necessary to adjust the dosage upwards to continue the same rate of essential oil delivery throughout the whole treatment process. Constant delivery through a repairing barrier requires a range of formulations (usually increasing the percentage of essential oil) to be used over the treatment period.

Release of essential oil at the stratum corneum interface

Absorption of essential oils through the skin is dependent on their release from the vehicle. This occurs at the interface of the stratum corneum and the applied layer of preparation. The physical–chemical relationship between the essential oil and the vehicle determines the rate and amount of oil released to the stratum corneum. Oils with a strong affinity for the vehicle have a lower rate and extent of absorption than oils with a weaker affinity.

Dosage approaches

The subject of essential oil dosage is perhaps one of the most difficult areas in modern aromatherapy on which to obtain unanimous opinion from experts. Contemporary aromatherapists base their clinical decisions concerning dose against a background of different philosophies underlying the therapy's evolution. Over the past 40 years in Britain, the aesthetic nature of aromatherapy has influenced an inherently low-dose cosmetic style of application, popularised by numerous publications largely written for a lay readership. This has characterised the British approach to the therapy over the years, which has since been exported to Asia, North America and Australia.

Mainly because of the dominance of this aesthetically biased approach, training for therapists in the past lacked scientific rigour. As a result, information on dosages, both for essential oils and hydrosols (which are by their nature an already dilute therapeutic form), remains doggedly attached to the esoteric, energetic, homoeopathic-inspired model. Even as recently as 2002, a small-scale survey of UK aromatherapists[61] found that reasons given for either increasing or decreasing dosages in practice were general and non-specific and lacked credible scientific rationale. Furthermore, confusion existed over the actual dosages being used, with many therapists surveyed not being trained to work with percentage dilutions and not able to recognise the distinction between high and low dilutions.

On the other hand, influences from the French high-dose style of practice are beginning to appear more frequently in English-language aromatherapy literature.[62–64] In French aromatic medicine, the concentration of oils for topical application can range from 0.1 to 100%. In addition, dosages usually far exceed recommendations appearing in mainstream English texts for essential oils that are often regarded as being only suitable to use in minute proportions (for example phenol, ketone, ether and aldehyde-rich oils). Table 4.5 gives examples of French topical dermatology formulas. Guba[62] describes the French approach as a 'realistic view of the safe uses and potential toxicity of essential oils for all practitioners'. This view is qualified by the absolute necessity for practitioners to be thoroughly knowledgeable about chemistry, toxicology and pharmacology of the essential oils they use in their practice.

Dosage guidelines

It would be inappropriate, in this book, to dogmatically promote the benefits of one system over the other, as there are undoubtedly experienced and knowledgeable practitioners all along the high to low dose spectrum adhering to their preferred approach and able to demonstrate clinical effectiveness.

In this text, the approach to dosages is consistent with:

- traditional models where appropriate
- findings from pharmacological and clinical research
- clinical experience
- full knowledge of chemical profiles of essential oils.

Table 4.5 French approaches to dosages and formulations.[65]

---

1. Insect/mosquito bite[65]

Essential oils:

- *Pelargonium asperum* 5 ml
- *Eucalyptus citriodora* 4.5 ml
- *Tanacetum annuum* 0.5 ml.

Apply two or three drops to the affected area three times a day.

2. Acne treatment[65]

Essential oils:

- *Hyssopus officinalis ssp. officinalis* 2 ml
- *Mentha piperita* 0.5 ml
- *Melaleuca alternifolia* 6 ml
- *Lavandula latifolia spica* 1 ml
- *Matricaria recutita* 0.5 ml.

Apply neat to individual spots morning and evening until healed.

With regard to the latter point, in practice this cannot be assumed and should be confirmed with batch-specific analyses to avoid the risk of using adulterated or poor quality oils. Every case that is being treated requires consideration of all factors that are detailed throughout this text and dosages are decided upon following a full evaluation. Guidelines follow that can be adapted to suit each individual clinical situation.

The recommended dosages in Table 4.7 for children are based on body surface area (*see* Table 4.6) and are applicable for widespread applications, since many physiological phenomena correlate better to this measurement compared to body weight. The adaptation and maturation of skin enzymes and epidermal barrier function in the developing child has been taken into account. Note that, for localised applications, body surface area is not relevant. It is necessary when viewing the recommendations to contextualise them rather than to regard them in abstract terms. Specifically, the intention is that, for each clinical case, the guidelines are interpreted after full consideration of all relevant factors.

Body surface area calculations for widespread applications

To calculate the dosage for children the following approach is used in Table 4.7, columns A and B:

$$\text{Children's dosage} = \frac{\text{surface area of patient}(m^2) \times \text{adult concentration}}{1.8}$$

It must be emphasised that the above recommendations are guidelines and the following also require thorough consideration before utilising the recommended dosages, both in adults and children.

1 Skin condition: acute or chronic, extent of skin barrier disruption.
2 Application to atopic dermatitis.
3 Total surface area of skin lesion(s).
4 Frequency of applications and vehicle medium.
5 Chemical profile of individual oils: irritant and/or sensitisation potential.
6 Other medical conditions and general health of the individual.

Table 4.6 Body surface area based on 'average' body weight and height.

Age	Ideal body weight kg	Height cm	Body surface m²
Newborn*	3.5	50	0.23
1 month*	4.2	55	0.26
3 months*	5.6	59	0.32
6 months	7.7	67	0.40
1 year	10	76	0.47
3 years	15	94	0.62
5 years	18	108	0.73
7 years	23	120	0.88
12 years	39	148	1.25
Adult (male)	68	173	1.80

* Figures provided assume the infant was full term. Reduced barrier function and use of essential oils in premature babies is discussed in Chapter 8.

Table 4.7 Recommended maximum essential oil % concentration for non-occluded widespread dermal application in children based on body surface area estimates and suggested maximum % concentrations for non-occluded localised application.

	A Full-body application	B Widespread application to skin lesions covering 3/5 of body surface	C Localised lesions* (body surface calculations are not applicable here)
Newborn	N/A	N/A	N/A
1 month	0.1	0.1	0.1
3 months	0.35	0.8	0.8
6 months	0.45	1.0	1.0
1 year	0.5	1.3	2.0
3 years	0.7	1.7	3.0
5 years	0.8	2.0	5.0
7 years	1.0	2.5	7.5
12 years	1.5	3.5	10
Adult	2%	5%	25%

* Relevant for lesions where skin barrier function is disrupted. As lichenified skin (and warts) increases resistance to absorption, dosages that are required are likely to be greater. In infections affecting children under 1 year medical care is required and essential oils may act as adjunctive therapy.

Table 4.8 is a quick reference guide to concentrations and quantities.

How much to supply

It is extremely important that the client knows which preparation to apply to each body site and how much to use. Generally formulations should be applied sparingly, with the exception of those intended as emollients. It is important that enough is provided so that there will be no break in treatment before the agreed follow-up date but excessive quantities should be avoided. It is believed by many that efficacy will be increased by applying increasing amounts of a topical formulation. While this approach is unlikely to be harmful with emollient preparations containing low concentrations of essential oils, the risk of adverse reactions from aqueous-based formulations containing higher concentrations of

Table 4.8 Amount of essential oil (ml) in total product or applied to skin.

Concentration in total product or applied	5 ml	10 ml	15 ml	25 ml
0.1%	0.005	0.01	0.015	0.025
0.5%	0.025	0.05	0.75	0.125
1%	0.05	0.1	0.15	0.25
2%	0.1	0.2	0.3	0.5
5%	0.25	0.5	0.75	1.25
10%	0.5	1.0	1.5	2.5
25%	1.25	2.5	3.75	6.25

Table 4.9 Minimum amount of cream (g) required for twice-daily application for one week.

Age	Whole body	Trunk	Both arms and legs
6 months	35	15	20
4 years	60	20	35
8 years	90	35	50
12 years	120	45	65
Adult (70 kg male)	170	60	90

oils will be increased. It is not always an advantage to supply excessive quantities as this can lead to substantial waste. It also encourages the individual to apply more frequently than suggested, keep products well beyond the shelf life or share with friends and family. The amount required for treatment is often under-estimated. Lotions go further than creams, which go further than ointments. Table 4.9 gives guidelines to the quantity of a cream formulation to supply.

In order to assess compliance with a formulation, it may be helpful to provide trial sizes of different mediums for a period in order to allow the client to experiment with those they prefer, while taking into account the best medium for the condition.

The frequency of application naturally depends on several factors, principally:

- nature and severity of the condition
- duration of the condition
- sites involved
- convenience
- common sense!

When supplying preparations following one-to-one consultations, labels and information leaflets need to be fully completed and it is strongly recommended that the following information always be given:

- name and contact details of practitioner supplying the preparation
- name of person for whom it is intended
- quantity supplied
- method of application, along with frequency
- limitations on usage and cautions, e.g. for external application only, keep out of the eyes
- active ingredients such as essential oils, preservatives, etc. listed in order of concentration with the highest given first
- storage conditions
- use-before date/discard-by date.

The need for correct labelling is clear but, to summarise, good practice in this area ensures:

- the user is fully informed as to method of usage and restrictions on this
- the storage conditions and use-before dates are clearly given, thus avoiding risk of microbial contamination and pathological sequelae and limiting the occurrence of degradation products which may act as sensitisers

- demands of regulatory bodies are met
- misunderstandings do not arise as to the purpose for which the preparation has been supplied.

Base product recipes

Simple cream base (without preservative)

8 g beeswax.
10 g cocoa butter or shea butter.
40 ml vegetable oils.
42 ml purified water BP or hydrosol.

Simple ointment base (without preservative)

20 g beeswax.
80 ml vegetable oil.

Simple lip balm (without preservative)

15 g beeswax.
10 g cocoa butter.
25 ml vegetable oils.

Gels

A gel is usually semi-opaque or clear and made from water and a thickening agent. The addition of 1–5% vegetable oil can prevent the skin becoming too dry if the gel is applied frequently. The thicker the gel is, the more vegetable oil and essential oil it will be able to carry. Natural polysaccharides act as thickening agents and are extracted from plants or algae. Examples include:

- cellulose gum (extracted from wood fibre)
- pectin (extracted from citrus peel)
- alginates (extracted from different algae)
- carrageen (extracted from the seaweed carrageen)
- Xanthan gum (fermentation of glucose by bacteria, *Xanthomonas compestris*).

Basic gel

98 ml purified water BP.
1 g (2 ml) Xanthan gum.
1–5% vegetable oil may be added to a gel to provide a less drying formulation. Gels are able to carry an essential oil content up to 5% depending on the viscosity of the gel.

Powders

Ingredients that can be incorporated into powder formulations include corn-starch, zinc oxide and magnesium stearate. Essential oil concentration is kept to a maximum of 2% to avoid clumping.

Sample powder

Zinc oxide 15%.

Magnesium stearate 85%.

Mix all ingredients together and shake thoroughly. Shake well before each use.

References

1 Dryden MS, Dailly S, Crouch M. A randomised, controlled trial of tea tree topical preparations versus a standard topical regimen for the clearance of MRSA colonization. *J Hosp Infect.* 2004; **56**: 283–6.

2 Caelli M, Porteous J, Carson CF *et al.* Tea tree oil as an alternative topical decolonisation agent for methicillin-resistant *Staphylococcus aureus. J Hosp Infect.* 2000; **46**: 236–7.

3 Schliemann-Willers S, Wigger-Alberti W, Kleesz P *et al.* Natural vegetable fats in the prevention of irritant contact dermatitis. *Contact Derm.* 2002; **46**: 6–12.

4 Tobares L, Guzman C, Maestri D. Effect of the extraction and bleaching processes on jojoba (*Simmondsia chinensis*) wax quality. *Eur J Lipid Sci Technol.* 2003; **105**: 749–53.

5 Alpaslan M, Tepe S, Simsek O. Effect of refining processes on the total and individual tocopherol content in sunflower oil. *Int J Food Sc Technol.* 2001; **36**: 737–9.

6 Moreda W, Pérez-Camino MC, Cert A. Gas and liquid chromatography of hydrocarbons in edible vegetable oils. *J Chromatogr A.* 2001; **936**: 159–71.

7 Blumenthal M, editor. *The Complete German Commission E Monographs.* Austin, Texas: American Botanical Council; 1998.

8 Mason P. *Evening Primrose Oil in Dietary Supplements.* 2nd ed. London: Pharmaceutical Press; 2001.

9 Zatz JL. Scratching the surface; skin permeation. *Cosmet Toil.* 1990; **105**(8): 39–50.

10 Wilson RJ. Jojoba oil seen ready to prosper with green. *Jojoba Happening.* 1992; Jul 5–6.

11 Lack G, Fox D, Northstone K. Factors associated with the development of peanut allergy in childhood. *N Eng J Med.* 2003; **438**: 977–85.

12 Karia C, Harwood JL, Heard CM *et al.* Simultaneous permeation of tamoxifen and γ linolenic acid across excised human skin. Further evidence of the permeation of solvated complexes. *Int J Pharm.* 2004; **271**: 305–9.

13 Heard CM, Gallagher SJ, Congiatu C *et al.* Preferential π-π complexation between tamoxifen and borage oil / γ linolenic acid: transcutaneous delivery and NMR spectral modulation. *Int J Pharm.* 2005; **302**: 47–55.

14 Gwak HS, Chun IK. Effect of vehicles and penetration enhancers on the in vitro percutaneous absorption of tenoxicam through hairless mouse skin. *Int J Pharm.* 2002; **236**: 57–64.

15 Oh HJ, Oh YK, Kim CK. Effects of vehicle and enhancers on transdermal delivery of melatonin. *Int J Pharm.* 2001; **212**: 63–71.

16 Sakurai H, Pokorny J. The development and application of novel vegetable oils tailor-made for specific dietary needs. *Eur J Lipid Sci Technol.* 2003; **105**: 769–78.

17 Rose J. 375 *Essential Oils and Hydrosols.* California: Frog Ltd; 1999.

18 Catty S. *Hydrosols: The next aromatherapy.* Vermont: Healing Arts Press; 2001.

19 Bohra P, Vaze AS, Pangarker VG *et al.* Adsorptive recovery of water soluble essential oil components. *J Chem Technol Biotechnol.* 1994; **66**: 97–102.

20 Machale KW, Niranjan K, Pangarkar VG. Recovery of dissolved essential oils from condensate waters of Basil and *Mentha arvensis* distillation. *J Chem Technol Biotechnol.* 1977; **69**: 362–6.

21 Rao BR, Kaul PN, Syamasunder KV *et al.* Water soluble fractions of rose-scented geranium (Pelargonium species) essential oil. *Bioresour Technol.* 84(3): 243–6.

22 Sagdic, O, Ozcan, M. Antibacterial activity of spice hydrosols. *Food Control.* 2003; **14**: 141–3.

23 Sagdic, O. Sensitivity of four pathogenic bacteria to Turkish thyme and oregano hydrosols. *Lebensmittel-Wissenschaft und-Technologie.* 2003; **36**(5): 467–73.

24 Anon. Annual review of cosmetic ingredient safety assessments – 2002/2003. *Int J Toxicol.* 2005; **24**(Suppl. 1): 1–102.

25 Jiménez JJ, Bernal JL, Aumente S *et al.* Quality assurance of commercial beeswax Part 1. Gas chromatography – electron impact ionisation mass spectrometry of hydrocarbons and monoesters. *J Chromatogr A.* 2004; **1024**: 147–54.

26 Al-Walili NS. An alternative treatment for pityriasis versicolor, tinea cruris, tinea corporis and tinea faciei with topical application of honey, olive oil and beeswax mixture: an open pilot study. *Complement Ther Med.* 2004; **12**: 45–7.

27 Palzkill DA. Jojoba. In: www.accessscience.com (accessed 16.01.06).

28 Habashy RR, Abdel-Naim AB, Khalifa AE *et al.* Anti-inflammatory effects of jojoba liquid wax in experimental models. *Pharmaco. Res.* 2004; **51**(2): 95–105.

29 www.dweckdata.com/Lectures/In_Shape_97.pdf (accessed 16.01.06).

30 Robbers JE, Speedie MK, Tyler VE. *Pharmacognosy and Pharmacobiotechnology.* Baltimore: Williams & Wilkins; 1996.

31 Orafidiya LO, Agbani EO, Oyedele AO *et al.* The effect of aloe vera gel on the anti-acne properties of the essential oil of *Ocimum gratissimum* Linn leaf – a preliminary clinical investigation. *Int J Aromatherapy.* 2004; **14**: 15–21.

32 Reynolds T, Dweck AC. Aloe vera leaf gel: a review update. *J Ethnopharmacol.* 1999; **68**: 3–37.

33 Reider N, Issa A, Hawranek T *et al.* Absence of contact sensitisation to *Aloe vera* (L.) Burm. F. *Contact Derm.* 2005; **53**: 332–4.

34 Carretero MI. Clay minerals and their beneficial effects upon human health. A review. *Appl Clay Sci.* 2002; **21**: 155–63.

35 O'Connell N. It's all the buzz. *Nursing Standard.* 2005; **20**(8): 22–4.

36 Bang LM, Bunting C, Molan P. The effect of dilution on the rate of hydrogen peroxide production in honey and its implications for wound healing. *J Altern Complement Med.* 2003; **9**(2): 267–73.

37 Al-Waili NS. Topical application of natural honey, beeswax and olive oil mixture for atopic dermatitis or psoriasis: partially controlled, single-blinded study. *Complement Ther Med.* 2003; **11**: 226–34.

38 Al-Walili NS. Mixture of honey, beeswax and olive oil inhibits growth of *Staphylococcus aureus* and *Candida albicans. Arch Med Res.* 2005; **36**: 10–13.

39 Al-Waili NS. Clinical and mycological benefits of topical application of honey, olive oil and beeswax in diaper dermatitis. *Clin Microbiol Infect.* 2005; **11**: 160–3.

40 Russel KM, Molan PC, Wilkins AL *et al.* Identification of some antibacterial constituents of New Zealand manuka honey. *J Agric Food Chem.* 1990; **38**: 10–13.

41 Inoue K, Murayama S, Seshimo F *et al.* Identification of phenolic compound in manuka honey as specific superoxide anion radical scavenger using electron spin resonance (ESR) and liquid chromatography with colometric array detection. *J Sci Food Agric.* 2005; **85**: 872–8.

42 Al-Waili NS. Therapeutic and prophylactic effects of crude honey on chronic Seborrheic dermatitis and dandruff. *Eur J Med Res.* 2001; **6**(7): 306–8.

43 van Ketel WG, Wemer J. Allergy to lanolin and lanolin free creams. *Contact Derm.* 1983; **9**(5): 420.

44 Rowe RC, Sheskey PJ, Wellar P. *Handbook of Pharmaceutical Excipients.* 4th ed. London: Pharm Press; 2003

45 Klingman AM. The myth of lanolin allergy. *Contact Derm.* 1998; **39**: 103–7.

46 Clark EW. Estimation of the general incidence of specific lanolin allergy. *J Soc Cosmet Chem.* 1975; **26**: 323.

47 Rodford R. Safety evaluation of preservatives. *Int J Cosm Sci.* 1997; **19**: 281–90.

48 Sachs A. *The Authoritative Guide to Grapefruit Seed Extract*. Mendochine: LifeRhythm; 1997.

49 Sharamon S, Baginski BJ. *The Healing Power of Grapefruit Seed*. Twin Lakes, WI: Lotus Light Publications; 1995.

50 Guba R. Wound healing. *Int J Aromatherapy*. 1999; **9**(2): 67–74.

51 Sakamoto S, Sato K, Maitani T *et al*. Analysis of components in natural food additive 'grapefruit seed extract' by HPLC and LC/MS. *Eisei Shikenjo Hokoku*. 1996; **114**: 38–42.

52 Takeoka G, Dao L, Wong RY *et al*. Identification of benzethonium chloride in commercial grapefruit seed extracts. *J Agric Food Chem*. 2001; **49**(7): 3316–20.

53 Von Woedtke T, Schluter B, Pflegel P *et al*. Aspects of the antimicrobial efficacy of grapefruit seed extract and its relation to preservative substances contained. *Pharmazie*. 1999; **54**(6): 452–6.

54. http://europa.eu.int/comm/health/ph_risk/committees/04_sccp/docs/sccp_q_019.pdf (accessed 03.03.06).

55 Manou I, Bouillard L, Devleeschouwer MJ *et al*. Evaluation of the preservative properties of *Thymus vulgaris* essential oil in topically applied formulations under a challenge test. *J Appl Microbiol*. 1998; **84**: 368–76.

56 Maccioni AM, Anchisi A, Sanna A *et al*. Preservative systems containing essential oils in cosmetic products. *Int J Cosm Sci*. 2002; **24**: 53–9.

57. www.ewg.org/reports/skindeep/ (accessed 22.01.06).

58 www.toxicsinfo.org/personal/BeautyAndTheBeast.htm (accessed 22.01.06).

59. www.chooseorganics.com/organicarticles/cosmetic_safety.htm (accessed 22.10.06).

60. www.cosmeticsaresafe.org/ (accessed 22.01.06).

61 Mann, S. Current practice on essential oil dilutions. *In Essence*. 2002; **1**(3): 26–9.

62 Guba, R. Toxicity myths – the actual risks of essential oil use. *Int J Aromatherapy*. 2000; **10**(1/2): 37–49.

63 Chanus H. Essential oils and their practical applications in childhood pathologies. *Int J Clinical Aromatherapy*. 2005; **2**(2): 20–5.

64 Hadji-Minaglou F, Bolcato O. The potential role of specific essential oils in the replacement of dermacorticoid drugs (strong, medium and weak) in the treatment of acute, dry or weeping dermatitis. *Int J Aromatherapy*. 2005; **15**(2): 66–73.

65 Baudoux D, Zhiri A. *Les Cahiers Pratiques d'Aromathérapie Selon l'école Française*. Vol. 2. Luxembourg: Edition Inspir; 2003.

Chapter 5

Skin-care essentials

Introduction

Looking after our skin by following an appropriate regular skin-care regime pays dividends beyond the cosmetic benefits this confers. By nurturing skin using natural products, we provide optimal support for it to perform its vital functions such as protection, sensory perception and thermoregulation, as well as improving its aesthetic qualities. It is helpful to remember that as skin reflects our general health, externally applied products are only a part of the story; good nutrition is essential for good skin health and the reader is advised to consult nutritional texts for further detailed information in this area. This chapter concentrates on routine skin care with an emphasis on facial skin and will discuss the possibilities for using natural approaches to delay the visible signs of ageing.

Cleanse, moisturise, protect – the mantra

Fundamental to good skin health is protecting the barrier by achieving cleanliness without sterility, coupled with balanced hydration. Forming a remarkable protective barrier throughout the human life cycle in the face of numerous endogenous and exogenous challenges, the skin undergoes a host of complex processes at any given moment in time. Essential to achieving homeostatic balance and a healthy skin, the stratum corneum is constantly striving to maintain correct moisture levels in the presence of highly variable environmental conditions; when it loses the battle, dry, flaking skin conditions result. It is therefore essential that anything that is applied to the skin positively affects, or at least minimally interferes with, the structure and function of the stratum corneum, while performing the task for which it is applied.

Cleansing

Effective cleansing removes dirt and debris that continually accumulates on the skin from the combination of sebum, sweat, environmental pollutants, microbes and unshed corneocytes. Since cleansing interacts with the proteins and lipids of the stratum corneum the barrier can be weakened to a greater or lesser extent. Therefore the type of cleanser used, alongside the frequency of use, largely determines whether skin is dry or normal.

Skin types

There are two common skin classification systems: first, one based upon the amount of sebum secretion experienced which we will briefly review here and, second, one developed to assess an individual's response to sunlight which we will look at later in this chapter.

In the sebum secretion classification model, skins are cosmetically classified into three main types according to an individual's subjective evaluation of sebum secretion, leading to dry, normal and oily categories. Variations on these exist, which have been developed to meet the needs of the cosmetic industry, including combination, severely dry, mildly dry, mildly oily and severely oily.[1] However, individual assessments are by their nature subjective and it has been shown that people generally consider their skin type to be drier than accurate sebum measurements indicate (ibid.); this limits the analytical value of this system, but for basic skin type assessment, it offers a straightforward, easily understood tool.

Types of cleansers

Ideal cleansers are lipid based, emollient and able to minimise barrier disruption while performing their cleansing function. Much commercial soap is formulated from surfactants, which, while providing effective cleansing, have harshly drying effects on the skin. Consumers may accept the resultant dryness as their 'skin type', little realising the extent of the contribution that their cleansing routine makes.[2]

Body washes and liquid cleansers tend to contain less damaging surfactants than soaps and there are commercially available moisturising cleansers that contain more emollients than surfactants, designed to leave an emollient deposit on the skin. Cleansers for the face should be specially formulated to contain milder surfactants and ideally be non-soap based. However, not all soap needs to be abandoned, as there is a huge difference between poor quality soaps rich in animal fats, synthetic fragrances and aggressive surfactants and those that are specially prepared from plant oils and extracts.

Ideal mediums for facial cleansing are those that interact favourably with the lipids of the skin: lotions, gels and creams containing essential oils are good options for regular use, followed by removal with cotton wool soaked in hydrosol. Table 5.1 gives suggestions for natural cleansers, which can be used as alternatives to commercial products, and Table 5.2 provides a basic cleansing cream recipe which can be individually adapted. If skin feels tight or irritated following cleansing, it is an indicator that the lipid balance has been negatively affected and switching to a richer, more emollient cleanser is advisable. *Simmondsia chinensis* (jojoba), *Prunus dulcis* (sweet almond) and *Persea gratissima* (avocado) oils will remove make-up naturally, but care needs taking around the eye area to avoid irritation.

The use of fruit acids or alpha-hydroxy acids (AHAs) in cosmetics has developed in recent years, with desquamatory efficacy being shown.[3] When applied to the epidermis, they weaken intercorneocyte cohesion and contribute to desmosome dissolution, aiding the removal of cells from the skin surface and promoting cell renewal. Easily available sources are pineapple, papaya and citrus fruits, all of which can be used once a day for gentle exfoliation on non-inflamed skin. Oatmeal has a long history in cosmetics, being used in baths and facial masks for its soothing, hypoallergenic properties and is recommended by the German Commission E for cases of skin irritation.[4]

Table 5.1 Simple cleansers and exfoliators.

Plain live organic yoghurt
Persea gratissima oil
Prunus dulcis oil
Simmondsia chinensis liquid wax
Corylus avellana oil
Finely ground oatmeal
Pineapple juice*
Papaya juice*
Inside skin of lemon*

* Not suitable for use on inflamed, irritated skin.

Table 5.2 Cleansing cream recipe.

10 g beeswax
20 ml *Helianthus annuus* oil
20 ml *Corylus avellana* oil
45 ml hydrosol

Exfoliators and masks

Exfoliation – the sloughing of dead skin cells – is a valuable part of effective cleansing when done regularly and non-aggressively, with the routine use of natural exfoliators (*see* Tables 5.1 and 5.3). Irritation should not result from correct exfoliation but for highly sensitive or inflamed skin, even the gentlest exfoliation may provoke an inflammatory response and extra care needs to be taken, desisting from use if necessary, until the skin condition improves.

The simplest exfoliation is washing the skin using a cotton flannel or muslin gauze, and this may be all that sensitive skin needs, but for more targeted effect different mediums are used. Gently massaging with fixed plant oils provides superb exfoliation as they seep into the sebaceous glands, permeating the layers of the epidermis and mix with skin lipids, exerting their dual cleansing and emollient effects where needed. They are easily removed with hydrosol-soaked cotton wool, taking away grime and dead cells while leaving behind a fine lipid layer. For extra benefit, a small quantity of finely ground oatmeal can be added to the oil before applying. Table 5.3 provides a sample formulation which is suitable for body and facial skin. It can readily be adapted to include any of the ingredients in Table 5.1.

Clay has been used for centuries to draw impurities from the skin and is traditionally used in face masks and body packs, each clay having its own particular balance of minerals and cleansing effects. The most commonly used clays are kaolin, green clay and fuller's earth. Green clay is traditionally used for oily skin types and acneic skin, but is equally beneficial for rejuvenating dry, dull skin. Essential oils and hydrosols mix well with clays and basic clay mask recipes can easily be tailored for individual needs. *See* Tables 5.4 and 5.5.

Table 5.3 Exfoliating base suitable for use on the face and body. Quantity is sufficient for one full body application. Unsuitable for inflamed skin conditions.

1 tablespoon finely ground oatmeal
1 teaspoon green clay
5 ml freshly squeezed lemon juice
5 ml organic clear honey
20 ml unrefined *Persea gratissima* oil
3 drops *Lavandula angustifolia* essential oil
10 ml *Lavandula angustifolia* hydrosol

Mix together the oatmeal and clay. In a separate bowl, mix the remaining ingredients and when well combined add to the dry ingredients, mixing until a smooth paste forms. Apply thoroughly to damp skin with small circular massage movements. Rinse thoroughly, pat dry and follow with liberal application of moisturiser. If a more liquid mix is preferred, increase the hydrosol and avocado oil proportionally or omit the clay.

Table 5.4 Clay masks.

Mask for weekly application to oily skin
1 tablespoon green clay or fuller's earth
15 ml *Mentha piperita* hydrosol
15 ml *Lavandula angustifolia* hydrosol
2 drops *Melaleuca alternifolia* essential oil

Mix the essential oil with the green clay or fuller's earth. Combine together the hydrosols and add to the powder, until a thick paste forms. Apply a layer to the skin and leave in place for 10 minutes then rinse off and finish with a final spray of lavender hydrosol.

Mask for weekly application to normal or dry skin
1 tablespoon green clay or fuller's earth
1 tablespoon organic clear honey
15 ml *Lavandula angustifolia* hydrosol
10 ml *Rosa damascena* hydrosol
2 drops *Cymbopogon martini* essential oil

Mix the essential oil with the honey and then mix with the green clay or fuller's earth. Combine together the hydrosols and add to the clay mixture, until a thick paste forms. Apply a layer to the skin and leave in place for 10 minutes then rinse off and finish with a final spray of rose hydrosol.

Moisturising

Moisturising is the process of restoring the ability of the stratum corneum to hold and retain moisture, so alleviating dryness. However, dry skin is more than a mere lack of water in the cells; it arises from disturbances in key processes of the stratum corneum, namely the barrier lipids and natural moisturising factors (NMF). The symptoms of dry skin – scaling, roughness, flaking – occur because skin cells accumulate at the skin surface rather then being shed; corneocyte shedding is regulated by enzymes which are inactive in dry conditions.[2] Lack of moisture reduces the suppleness and plasticity of the skin, with contracted

Table 5.5 Hydrosols and essential oils for use in cleansing routines.

Skin type	Essential oils	Hydrosol
Dry	*Anthemis nobilis* *Boswellia carterii* *Citrus aurantium* flos. *Cymbopogon martinii* *Pelargonium graveolens* *Pogostemon cablin* *Rosa centifolia* *Santalum album*	*Anthemis nobilis* *Lavandula angustifolia* *Matricaria recutita* *Rosa centifolia*
Oily	*Citrus aurantium* fol. *Citrus limonum* *Cupressus sempervirens* *Melaleuca alternifolia* *Rosmarinus officinalis*	*Cupressus sempervirens* *Juniperus communis* *Melaleuca alternifolia* *Mentha piperita* *Salvia officinalis* *Salvia sclarea*
Normal	*Daucus carota* *Cymbopogon martinii* *Lavandula angustifolia* *Pelargonium graveolens* *Rosa centifolia*	*Hamamelis virginiana* *Lavandula angustifolia* *Pelargonium graveolens*

corneocytes producing the characteristic tight feeling of dry skin progressing to cracking and fissuring.

The regulation of water loss by the stratum corneum is determined by several factors with the following known to result in increased water loss and dry skin:

- ageing
- low environmental humidity
- low environmental temperature
- increased pH.

Optimal skin hydration occurs when in addition to balancing water loss, the stratum corneum also maintains levels of NMF. Unique to the stratum corneum, NMF represents between 10 and 30% of the dry weight of the stratum corneum and there is a significant age-related decline in levels,[5] accounting in part for the dryness associated with ageing skin. Dry environmental conditions include centrally heated or air-conditioned buildings as well as climatic dryness, leading to the requirement for more emollient, lipid-rich moisturisers in these conditions.

Ingredients in moisturisers

Although the term 'moisturiser' suggests we are adding water to the skin, this is slightly misleading, as a good moisturiser contains both humectants and lipids, and perhaps the term 'emollient' is closer to what is being applied. Effective emollients partly act by forming an oily layer over the skin by using occlusive ingredients that are hydrophobic, thus preventing water loss from the stratum corneum. The occlusive effect happens quickly and soon fades if the formulation penetrates the lipid layers of the stratum corneum. Examples of natural occlusive agents include beeswax, lanolin and vegetable oils. With improved knowledge of stratum corneum physiology, moisturisers are now designed to be more than occlusive. Physiologic lipid mixtures as used for example in aromatherapy practice can supplement the barrier lipids by direct application and benefit the skin in a natural way. This traditional aromatherapy approach is mirrored by the current direction of cosmetic research, which is increasingly focused on identifying and formulating with active functional ingredients.[3]

Humectants attract water to the epidermis, usually being drawn from the dermis, rarely from the environment. They mimic natural hydrophilic humectants found in the stratum corneum and include amino acids, alpha-hydroxy acids (which include lactic, glycolic and tartaric acids), propylene glycol, glycerol, panthenol and urea (some of these are components of NMF). Other ingredients found in commercial moisturisers include those that emulsify, stabilise, suspend or disperse ingredients to create a more aesthetically pleasing product. Many body moisturisers contain between 65 and 85% water: the high water content of these lotions promotes good dispersion of the ingredients, absorption of some components and easy application over a larger area. For facial use, cream forms are favoured which contain less water and greater lipid content.

Table 5.6 gives a sample formula for a natural basic cream recipe; increasing or decreasing the hydrosol/water content determines the final texture and can be adapted according to personal preference and body-site application. Table 5.7 gives a basic bath exfoliating blend that can be adapted according to skin type and desired effect. The combination of oatmeal and vegetable oils is often more acceptable to those who dislike the oily effect left by the use of vegetable oils alone.

Protection

Along with ensuring suitable cleansing and moisturising routines are followed, protecting against sun and ultraviolet (UV) exposure is essential if integrity of the stratum corneum is to be maintained and skin health achieved. Modern skin-care products reflect the growing awareness of the damage caused by sun exposure and sunscreen filters are routinely added to products.

Table 5.6 Basic cream formula.

8g beeswax
10 g cocoa butter or shea butter
40 ml vegetable oils
42 ml hydrosol or purified water BP
To extend the short life of this base cream, the addition of a preservative is required and guidance in their selection is given in Chapter 4.

Table 5.7 Exfoliating and moisturising bath blend.

1 tablespoon finely ground oatmeal
10 ml suitable vegetable carrier oil (e.g. jojoba, avocado, olive, sunflower)
0.5 ml non-irritant essential oils
Mix together the essential and vegetable oils and then blend thoroughly with the oatmeal before adding the mixture to running bath water. The oatmeal absorbs the oils, facilitating even dispersion in the water, and has a gentle exfoliating effect.

Table 5.8 Skin type classification according to sunburn and tanning history.[7]

Skin type reaction to sun exposure
Type 1: Always burns, never tans
Type 2: Always burns, sometimes tans
Type 3: Sometimes burns, always tans
Type 4: Never burns, always tans
Type 5: Brown skin (e.g. Asian)
Type 6: Black skin (e.g. Black African)

Skin phototypes

Developed by Fitzpatrick, in the 1970s a classification system for assessing an individual's response to sunlight proposed sun-reactive types I–IV for white-skinned individuals based upon their susceptibility to sunburn and capacity to tan[6]. The lower the skin type number, the greater the sun sensitivity. This system was further developed as a six-group classification and included a category each for brown and black skin (*see* Table 5.8) and it has since undergone further revisions. Although not wholly reliable and the subject of continuing revisions (ibid.), a system based upon phototype is a simple tool, which can be used to reduce harmful sun exposure by using appropriate sunscreens for the skin type involved. However, the effectiveness of sunscreen products for preventing long-term damage is debatable and sun avoidance is increasingly advocated as the best approach.[2]

Preventing skin ageing

Several factors determine the way skin ages: principally genetics, chronological age, amount of exposure to sun and environmental pollutants, smoking, psychological stress, bouts of significant weight gain and loss and the nature of exercise taken. Cutaneous changes arising from these factors can be understood as two independent but overlapping processes (*see* Figure 5.1):

- extrinsic ageing
- intrinsic ageing.

Although many of the histological changes seen in the skin are similar in both cases, significant differences exist between them, an understanding of which helps in the development of skin-care products for delaying ageing.

Extrinsic ageing and the effects of sun

Mainly referring to changes associated with exposure to UV radiation, extrinsic ageing also encompasses exposure to air pollution, tobacco smoke, and extreme temperatures as well as poor or imbalanced nutrition. Focusing on UV exposure, UVB rays are more biologically active, but less penetrating than UVA rays, with 90% of received UVB being confined to the epidermis.[8] Skin is far more reactive to UVB rays and the main risk for burning and skin cancer development arises

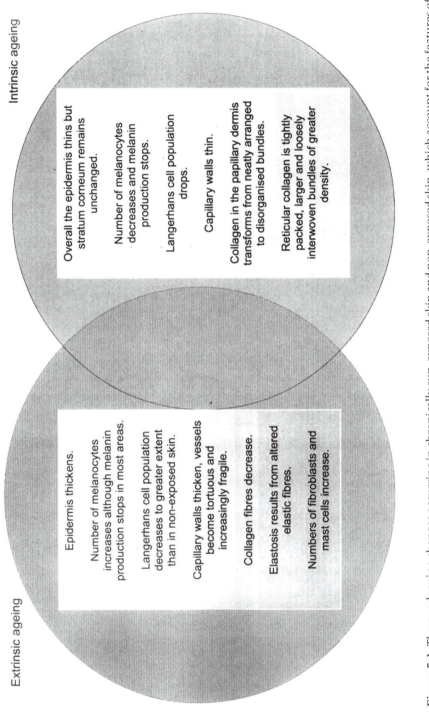

Intrinsic ageing

Overall the epidermis thins but stratum corneum remains unchanged.

Number of melanocytes decreases and melanin production stops.

Langerhans cell population drops.

Capillary walls thin.

Collagen in the papillary dermis transforms from neatly arranged to disorganised bundles.

Reticular collagen is tightly packed, larger and loosely interwoven bundles of greater density.

Extrinsic ageing

Epidermis thickens.

Number of melanocytes increases although melanin production stops in most areas.

Langerhans cell population decreases to greater extent than in non-exposed skin.

Capillary walls thicken, vessels become tortuous and increasingly fragile.

Collagen fibres decrease.

Elastosis results from altered elastic fibres.

Numbers of fibroblasts and mast cells increase.

Figure 5.1 The overlapping changes occurring in chronically sun-exposed skin and non-exposed skin, which account for the features of aged skin.

from this exposure. On the other hand, skin ageing is more closely associated with the damage caused by UVA. Although researchers have clearly identified the role of UVB in skin cancer development, UVA is also widely believed to be carcinogenic albeit to a lesser extent (ibid.).

Following acute sun exposure, changes in the epidermis are well known and most apparent: inflammation and thickening, followed by tanning. Severe oxidative stress occurs, resulting in both transient and permanent damage. Even mild doses of UV radiation damage the stratum corneum, by blocking the processes involved in NMF production, causing a layer in the mid stratum corneum to be devoid of NMF. As this layer moves to the surface, it prematurely breaks, causing corneocytes above to shed in fine sheets – the characteristic skin peeling associated with sunburn.[2]

Extrinsically aged skin is characterised by a leathery and coarse texture, sagging and wrinkling, discolouration and irregular pigmentation, telangiectasia, benign, pre-malignant and malignant neoplasms. These signs take years to become clinically apparent, but several histological changes have been identified which precede the obvious signs of photoageing.

- UVA damages collagen and elastin fibres in the dermis, leading to the characteristic dermal elastosis consisting of thickened, tangled, non-functional elastic fibres arising from abnormal elastin.[9]
- At the same time, there is a decrease in collagen fibres and bundles, with degraded and deformed fibres being found in the papillary dermis.[10]
- Stiffness associated with photoaged skin is in part due to an increase in collagen cross-links.
- There is an increase in the number and activity of fibroblasts, inflammatory cell infiltrates and lower numbers of blood vessels.[10]
- UVB damages epidermal cells, their DNA and their cell membranes and hyperplasia and thickening of the stratum corneum develops.
- Langerhans cell population drops.
- Levels of vitamins A and E and other antioxidants fall.
- Melanocytes increase in number, but do not continue to produce melanin in sufficiently protective quantities.

Intrinsic ageing

Normally aged skin is characterised by generalised wrinkling and an increasingly dry appearance. The normal degenerative processes of tissue ageing, which are governed largely by hereditary factors, when affecting the skin, overlap with the extrinsic changes previously outlined. Cell turnover slows from around the age of 40 and there is an overall loss of extracellular matrix. The epidermal–dermal junction flattens and elastic fibres in the reticular dermis become irregularly thickened and lose their organised distribution. Changes in the connective tissue arise with an increase in enzymes – elastase and collagenases – that are responsible for breaking down elastin and collagen.[11]

Can aromatherapy delay skin ageing?

Skin ageing cannot be entirely prevented but it can certainly be delayed if the causes are avoided. A great deal of effort by cosmetic companies is channelled into the search for the ultimate anti-ageing, anti-wrinkle products. Although for commercial reasons many of the findings of this research are closely protected, some evidence is available that points to the efficacy of topical products. Namely, the topical use of enzyme inhibitors and antioxidants has been shown to slow some aspects of skin ageing[12–17] and yields an interesting picture for the potential benefit of essential oils.

Essential oils potentially prevent wrinkles and stretchmarks

Elastase activity increases with age, fragmenting collagen and elastin, leading to a reduction in the elasticity of the skin and in the appearance of wrinkles and stretchmarks.[15] Essential oils may be useful anti-ageing agents by acting as elastase inhibitors, with *Citrus limon* (lemon), *Juniperus communis* (juniper), *Citrus paradisi* (grapefruit) and *Piper nigrum* (black pepper) all showing strong in vitro inhibition (ibid.). In this particular work, it was shown that for the citrus oils, the complete oils had more effect than their main isolated component limonene, a finding that confirms how it is often the synergy of all the constituents within essential oils that provides therapeutic efficacy. In other work,[17] marjoram and chamomile oils demonstrated anti-elastase activity in vitro. Although this work failed to specify the botanical origin of all the oils, the level of esters present in the chamomile suggests the findings relate to *Anthemis nobilis* (Roman chamomile) rather than *Matricaria recutita* (German chamomile).

Antioxidant aromatherapy

In a quest to find effective topical photoprotective agents, plant-derived products have been researched for their antioxidant activity and the use of natural antioxidants in skin-care products is increasing.[14] This has implications beyond the cosmetic treatment of wrinkles as effective agents could be used to prevent ultraviolet radiation (UVR)-induced skin cancer. Effective botanical antioxidant compounds are widely used in traditional medicine and include tocopherols, flavonoids, phenolic acids, nitrogen-containing compounds (indoles, alkaloids, amines and amino acids) and monoterpenes.[14,18] As the topical supplementation of antioxidants has been shown to substantially modulate the antioxidant network in the skin,[12] applying aromatherapy formulations that are rich in antioxidant materials offers interesting avenues for future research.

Some essential oils have demonstrated antioxidant activity (*see* Table 5.9) and have potential in this area. It is worth noting that significant differences in antioxidant activity have been identified between various plant extracts including essential oils. For example, antioxidant activity in a hexane-extracted product does not necessarily correlate with similar efficacy in the steam-distilled essential oil of the same plant origin. This has notably been identified in extracts of ginger and rosemary, with hexane extracts of the latter being a more potent antioxidant than the steam-distilled essential oil.[19]

The generic term 'vitamin E' consists of a group of eight isomers naturally present in vegetable oils named tocopherols, all of which possess antioxidant properties.[3] In both animal and human studies, topical application of vitamin E has been shown to decrease the severity of UV-induced skin ageing, with reductions being shown in depth and length of wrinkles as well as inflammation, oedema and skin roughness.[3,12–14]

Table 5.9 Essential oils in common use in aromadermatology possessing antioxidant activity.

Achillea millefolium ssp. millefolium[20]
Boswellia thurifera (frankincense)[21]
Boswellia serrata (frankincense)[22]
Cananga odorata (ylang ylang)[21,23]
Citrus limonum (lemon)[21]
Commiphora myrrh (myrrh)[22]
Cymbopogon citratus (lemongrass)[23]
Majorana hortensis (marjoram)[21]
Ocimum basilicum (basil)[21]
Pistacia lentiscus var. Chia (mastic gum)[22]
Rosmarinus officinalis (rosemary)[19,21,23]
Thymus vulgaris (thyme)[23,24]

Triticum vulgare (wheatgerm) oil is particularly rich in vitamin E and for many years the aromatherapy literature has advocated mixing it with other carrier oils to extend their storage times.[25–28] Modern aromadermatological practice builds upon this limited recommendation by utilising the antioxidant promise of this vitamin E-rich oil in topical anti-ageing formulations. The value that aromatherapists place upon using cold-pressed, unrefined carrier oils is given contextual support from evidence that antioxidant components are damaged by heat extraction and refining processes. For example, the total amounts of antioxidant phenolic compounds and tocopherols are highest in cold-pressed, unbleached *Simmondsia chinensis* (jojoba) wax.[29] Extra virgin *Corylus avellana* (hazelnut) oil has good levels of tocopherols with α-tocopherol being the main component of the total tocopherols.[30–32] *Helianthus annus* (sunflower)[32,33] and *Sesamum indicum* (sesame) oils[34] are also useful sources of α-tocopherol and well established in aromatherapy practice.

Although not yet commonly used in aromatherapy, *Cucurbita pepo* (pumpkin) seed oil deserves greater recognition. With a lipid profile containing high levels of linoleic acid (43–53%),[35] it contains two classes of antioxidant compounds: tocopherols and phenolics, which account for 59% of the antioxidant effects.[36] It is especially valued in the healing folklore of Eastern and Central Europe and the Middle East for its nutritious benefits and is used both topically and systemically for a range of medical conditions. Due to the strong, rich aroma, it is only used in small proportions in topical formulations.

Oil extracted from the fruits and pulp of *Hippophae rhamnoides* (sea buckthorn) has long been used in dermatology practices in Turkey, China and Russia[37,38] and represents interesting possibilities for future research in developing aromatic anti-ageing formulations. There are over 300 sea buckthorn derived medicinal preparations in the literature and over the past 50 years in China and Russia these have been used to treat, among other things, radiation damage, burns, oral inflammation and gastric ulcers.[39] The antioxidant, anti-inflammatory, anti-microbial, photoprotective and regenerative properties of the plant extracts are well documented.[18,37] The fruit oil is a good source of hydrophilic and lipophilic antioxidants such as carotenoids, ascorbic acid and tocopherols. In addition, it contains high levels of linoleic (30–40%) and α-linolenic (23–36%) acids.[36]

Beta-carotene and other carotenoids have been intensively studied as potential natural sunscreens and protectors against extrinsic damage. Although oral beta-carotene supplementation has been shown to have little effect as a sunscreen, topical application either alone or with α-tocopherol over a period of three months has demonstrated a reduction in solar light-induced erythema.[14] *Sesamum indicum* (sesame) oil is used in modern sunscreens and in traditional Ayurvedic medicine for skin protection. Edwards Smith *et al*.[40] found that sesame oil selectively inhibited malignant melanoma growth over normal melanocytes and suggested it may have potential usefulness as a chemoprotective agent. *Persea americana* (avocado) oil is rich in vitamin E and beta-carotene[41] and offers considerable benefits when added to preparations.

While aromatic skin care certainly has much to offer in the quest to prevent skin ageing and photochemoprotection, without doubt the single most important factor involved in extrinsic ageing is photodamage and daily UV protection is vital. Although natural oils offer some degree of sun protection, they cannot be regarded as an alternative to regular sunscreen, or sun avoidance. Table 5.10

Table 5.10 Steps to reduce UV-radiation exposure.

- Limit time spent in the sun between 10 am and 4 pm.
- Seek shade whenever possible.
- Use a broad-spectrum sunscreen with sun protection factor (SPF) of 15+.
- Cover all exposed skin liberally and remember ears, backs of knees, feet and hands.
- Reapply sunscreen every two hours, after being in the water, or after exercising and sweating.
- Use sunscreen even on cloudy days as even in cloudy conditions 30–60% of UV rays can penetrate the earth's surface.
- Do not use sunscreen as method of extending sun exposure such as prolonged sunbathing.
- Wear a wide-brimmed hat.
- Wear tightly-woven, preferably unbleached cotton clothing as loose weaves ineffectively block UV. (Clothes made from polyester crepe, bleached cotton or viscose offer little protection because they are transparent to UV rays.)
- Wear UV-protective sunglasses.
- Avoid sun lamps and sun beds.
- Remember that *limited* exposure to sunlight is healthy; it is necessary in the manufacture of vitamin D.
- Use the UV index as a guide. The index goes from 0 to 20, although in Europe it's unlikely to hit levels over 10, and indicates the following:
  - **1–2**: the sun is unlikely to cause harm, so everyone is at low risk (e.g. typically during British winters)
  - **3–4**: low risk for most people, except those with very sensitive skin, who should use protection
  - **5–6**: everyone with white or brown skin needs protection if in the sun; low risk for those with black skin
  - **7+**: everyone, regardless of skin colour, is at risk and should cover up.
  Those with white skin have a high or very high risk; people with brown skin have a medium risk and at level 10 this rises to a high risk and people with black skin are at medium risk up to 10.

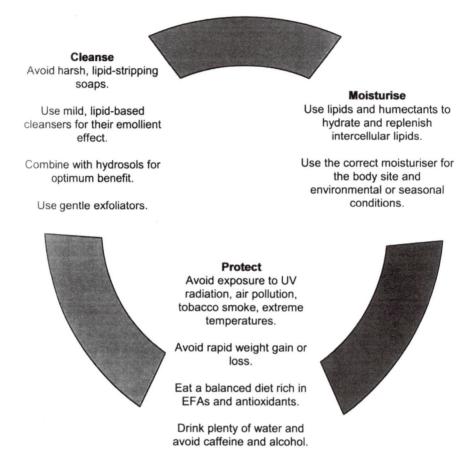

Cleanse
Avoid harsh, lipid-stripping soaps.

Use mild, lipid-based cleansers for their emollient effect.

Combine with hydrosols for optimum benefit.

Use gentle exfoliators.

Moisturise
Use lipids and humectants to hydrate and replenish intercellular lipids.

Use the correct moisturiser for the body site and environmental or seasonal conditions.

Protect
Avoid exposure to UV radiation, air pollution, tobacco smoke, extreme temperatures.

Avoid rapid weight gain or loss.

Eat a balanced diet rich in EFAs and antioxidants.

Drink plenty of water and avoid caffeine and alcohol.

Figure 5.2 Following these fundamental approaches to routine skin care may delay cutaneous ageing.

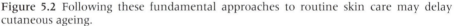

provides simple advice for reducing exposure which, used in combination with an holistic approach to maintaining good health such as adopting balanced nutritional habits, a healthy lifestyle and a good skin-care regime, may delay cutaneous ageing (*see* Figure 5.2).

References

1 Youn SW, Kim SJ, Hwang IA *et al*. Evaluation of facial skin type by sebum secretion: discrepancies between subjective descriptions and sebum secretion. *Skin Res Technol*. 2002; **8**(3): 168–72.
2 Johnson AW. Overview: fundamental skin care – protecting the barrier. *Dermatol Ther*. 2004; **17**: 1–5.
3 Rona C, Vailati F, Berardesca E. The cosmetic treatment of wrinkles. *J Cosmet Dermatol*. 2004; **3**: 26–34.
4 Blumenthal M, editor. *The Complete German Commission E Monographs*. Austin, Texas: American Botanical Council; 1998.

5 Rawlings AV, Harding CR. Moisturization and skin barrier function. *Dermatol Ther.* 2004; **17**: 43–8.

6 Guinot C, Latreille J, Morizot F *et al*. Assessment of sun reactive skin type with multiple correspondence analysis, hierarchical and tree-structured classification methods. *Int J Cosm Sci.* 2002; **24**(4): 207–16.

7 Gawkrodger DJ. *Dermatology, An Illustrated Colour Text.* 3rd ed. Edinburgh: Churchill Livingstone; 2002.

8 Nole G, Johnson AW. An analysis of cumulative lifetime solar ultraviolet radiation exposure and the benefits of daily sun protection. *Dermatol Ther.* 2004; **17**: 57–62.

9 El-Domyati M, Attia S, Saleh F *et al*. Intrinsic aging vs photoaging: a comparative histopathological, immunohistochemical, and ultrastructural study of skin. *Exp Dermatol.* 2002; **11**: 398–405.

10 Wulf HC, Sanby-Moller J, Kobayashi T *et al*. Skin aging and natural photoprotection. *Micron.* 2004; **35**: 185–91.

11 Benaiges A, Marcet P, Armengol R *et al*. Study of the refirming effect of a plant complex. *Int J Cosm Sc.* 1998; **20**: 223–33.

12 Biesalski HK, Berneburg M, Grune T *et al*. Oxidative and premature skin ageing. *Exp Dermatol.* 2003; **12**(Suppl. 3): 3–15.

13 Chiu A, Kimball AB. Topical vitamins, minerals and botanical ingredients as modulators of environmental and chronological skin damage. *Br J Dermatol.* 2003; **149**: 681–91.

14 F'guyer S, Afaq F, Mukhtar H. Photochemoprevention of skin cancer by botanical agents. *Photodermatol Photoimmunol Photomed.* 2003; **19**: 56–72.

15 Mori M, Ikeda N, Kato Y *et al*. Inhibition of elastase activity by essential oils in vitro. *J Cosm Dermatol.* 2003; **1**: 183–7.

16 Lee KK, Kim JH. Inhibitory effects of 150 plant extracts on elastase activity and their anti-inflammatory effects. *Int J Cosm Sci.* 1999; **21**: 71–82.

17 Étienne JJ, Pham Duc TL. New and unexpected cosmetic properties of perfumes. Effects upon free radicals and enzymes induced by essential oils, absolutes and fragrant compounds. *Int J Cosm Sci.* 2000; **22**: 317–28.

18 Arora R, Gupta D, Chawla R *et al*. Radioprotection by plant products: present status and future prospects. *Phytother Res.* 2005; **19**: 1–22.

19 Dang MN, Takacsova M, Nguyen DV *et al*. Antioxidant activity of essential oils from various spices. *Nahrung/Food.* 2001; **45**(1): 64–6.

20 Candan F, Unlu M, Tepe B *et al*. Antioxidant and antimicrobial activity of the essential oil and methanol extracts of *Achillea millefolium subspecies millefolium* Afan (Asteraceae). *J Ethnopharmacol.* 2003; **87**: 215–20.

21 Baratta M, Damien Dorman HJ, Deans SG *et al*. Antimicrobial and antioxidant properties of some commercial essential oils. *Flav Fragr J.* 1998; **13**: 235–44.

22 Assimopoulou AN, Zlatanos SN, Papageorgiou VP. Antioxidant activity of natural resins and bioactive triterpenes in oil substrates. *Food Chemistry.* 2005; **92**: 721–7.

23 Sacchetti G, Maietti S, Muzzoli M *et al*. Comparative evaluation of 11 essential oils of different origin as functional antioxidants, antiradicals and antimicrobials in food. *Food Chemistry.* 2005; **91**: 621–32.

24 Dapkevicius A, Venskutonis R, van Beek TA *et al*. Antioxidant activity of extracts obtained by different isolation procedures from some aromatic herbs grown in Lithuania. *J Sc Food Agric.* 1998; **77**: 140–6.

25 Price L, Price S, Smith I. *Carrier Oils for Aromatherapy and Massage.* Stratford-upon-Avon: Riverhead Publishing; 1999.

26 Price S. *Aromatherapy Workbook.* London: Thorsons; 1993.

27 Earle L. *Vital Oils.* London: Vermilion; 1992.

28 Worwood VA. *Aromatherapy for the Beauty Therapist.* Australia: Thomson Learning; 2001.

29 Tobares L, Guzman C, Maestri D. Effect of the extraction and bleaching processes on jojoba *(Simmondsia chinensis)* wax quality. *Eur J Lipid Sci Technol*. 2003; **105**: 749–53.

30 Bada JC, Léon-Camacho M, Prieto M *et al*. Characterization of oils of hazelnuts from Asturias, Spain. *Eur J Lipid Aci Technol*. 2004; **106**: 294–300.

31 Parcerisa J, Richardson GD, Rafecas M *et al*. Fatty acid, tocopherol and sterol content of some hazelnut varieties *(Corylus avellana* L.) harvest in Oregon (USA). *J Chromatogr*. 1998; **5**: 259–68.

32 Aturki Z, D'Orazio G, Fanali S. Rapid assay of vitamin E in vegetable oils by reversed-phase capillary electrochromatography. *Electrophoresis*. 2005; **26**: 798–803.

33 De Greyt WF, Kellens MJ, Huyghebaert AD. Effect of physical refining on selected minor components in vegetable oils. *Fett/Lipid*. 1999; **11**: 428–32.

34 Yoshida H, Takagi S. Antioxidative effects of sesamol and tocopherols at various concentrations in oils during microwave heating. *J Sci Food Agric*. 1999; **79**: 220–6.

35 Younis YMH, Ghirmay S, Al-Shihry SS. African *Cucurbita pepo* L.: properties of seed and variability in fatty acid composition of seed oil. *Phytochem*. 2000; **54**: 71–5.

36 Fruhwirth GO, Wenzl T, El-Toukhy R *et al*. Fluorescence screening of antioxidant capacity in pumpkin seed oils and other natural oils. *Eur J Lipid Sci Technol*. 2003; **105**: 266–74.

37 Cakir A. Essential oil and fatty acid composition of the fruits of *Hippophae rhamnoides* L. (sea buckthorn) and *Myrtus communis* L. from Turkey. *Biochem Syst and Ecol*. 2004; **32**: 809–16.

38 Yang B, Kalimo KO, Tahvonen RL *et al*. Effect of dietary supplementation with sea buckthorn *(Hippophae rhamnoides)* seed and pulp oils on the fatty acid composition of skin glycerophospholipids of patients with atopic dermatitis. *J Nutr Biochem*. 2000; **11**: 338–40.

39 Negi PS, Chauhan AS, Sadia GA *et al*. Antioxidant and antibacterial activities of various sea buckthorn *(Hippophae rhamnoides* L.) seed extracts. *Food Chem*. 2005; **92**: 119–24

40 Edwards Smith D, Salerno JW. Selective growth inhibition of a human malignant melanoma cell line by sesame oil in vitro. *Prostaglandins Leukot Essent Fatty Acids*. 1992; **46**(2): 145–50.

41 Ozdemir F, Topuz A. Changes in dry matter, oil content and fatty acids composition of avocado during harvesting time and post-harvesting ripening period. *Food Chem*. 2004; **86**: 79–83.

Chapter 6

Skin and the psyche

Introduction

Due to close connections with the nervous system, human skin is acutely sensitive to emotional states. Although most organs can react to emotional disturbances, the skin is unique in its exposure to the outside world. According to Field, the skin has been described as the 'shock organ' for emotional stress, manifesting in the form of several skin diseases.[1] Clinical observations have identified psychological stress as either precipitating, aggravating or prolonging many skin diseases and the psychosomatic aspects of many disorders have been the subject of research in recent years. Stress has been shown to delay skin barrier recovery, a delay which is blocked by sedative drugs, which is an outcome that has been reproduced with the inhalation of sedative aromas.[2] The potential of aromatherapy is great as it offers a unique intervention by aromatically targeting the physical symptoms while addressing the psychological realm.

Mind and skin associations

Although an awareness of the associations between the mind and body has been the foundation of traditional medicine and alternative practice for centuries, the developing interdisciplinary field of psychoneuroimmunology (PNI) is beginning to provide complex physiological explanations for these interactions. It is now beginning to be understood how through brain pathways, which control thoughts, emotions and behaviour, extensive control is exerted on the immune and endocrine systems. Sharing a language of neuropeptides, cytokines, glucocorticoids and other effector molecules, these intimately linked systems determine daily health and subjective well-being (*see* Figure 6.1). PNI examines, in scientific terms of some complexity, the commonly held precept that good emotional health is essential for good physiological health. It also presents insights into how the pleasurable nature of aromatherapy is translated into measurable physical and psychological effects, which support those achieved through essential oil pharmacology.

PNI connections

If we consider how this discipline advances our understanding of the skin, it is known that through complex multidirectional communication pathways involving the endocrine, immune and central nervous systems the skin maintains internal homeostasis. Brazzini *et al.*[3] propose that the skin should be viewed as 'an active neuro-immuno-endocrine interface' or neuroendocrine organ, exhibiting

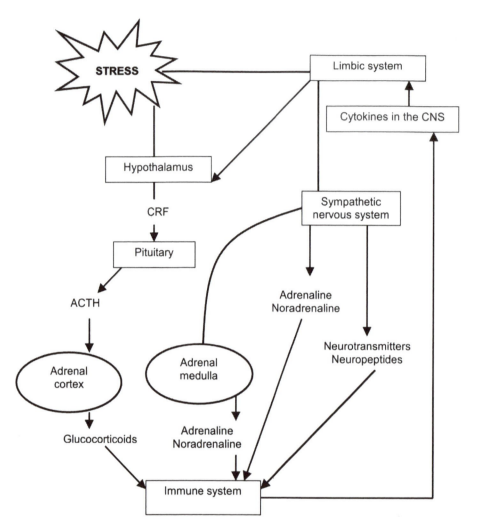

Figure 6.1 A simplified overview of the channels of communication between the immune, endocrine and central nervous (CNS) systems in the stress response.

multidirectional and local communication, which is made possible by the production in the skin of cytokines, hormones and neurotransmitters, and anatomical links between the central nervous system (CNS) and skin. In addition, circulating immune cells, recruited in the skin, express receptors for a variety of neuropeptides, cytokines, neurotransmitters and hormones, identical to those expressed centrally, allowing the CNS to communicate with the skin (ibid.). This means that systemic signals affecting the skin initiate a flow of information between this and other organs, leading to modulation of local immune activity, vascular functions, sensory reception, thermoregulation, exocrine secretion and maintenance of skin barrier integrity.

It is known for example that the CNS seems to be actively involved in reducing inflammatory reactions produced in the skin by locally applied irritants, an effect which can be modulated by psychological intervention (ibid.). This leads to the suggestion that cutaneous inflammation could be controlled via anti-inflammatory agents targeting not only the skin, but the CNS as well.

With the growing accumulation of data detailing the presence and function of epidermal nerves, immune cells, cutaneous neuropeptides and other intercellular messengers, the complex picture of how the skin neuro-immuno-endocrine interface communicates with itself and within other systems is becoming better understood. As pathways of neuroimmunomodulation are explained, this increasingly accounts for the widely held belief that psychological stress lowers immune function, which has implications for a host of immune-related skin conditions.

Aromatherapy and the mind

Aromatherapy practice has long been valued as a stress-reduction therapy. This is particularly the case in countries where aromatherapists traditionally favour massage as the primary application method for essential oils, as in Britain. Essential oils are increasingly being recognised for their capacity to alter emotional states, as well as being able to affect physiology, as a growing body of evidence supports traditional claims.[4-6]

The psychophysiological effects of essential oils occur both via the inhalation of volatile chemical constituents and through cutaneous absorption of constituents when applied to the skin. Research has identified changes in both autonomic nervous system parameters and mental-emotional conditions following massage using sandalwood oil.[7] When essential oils are applied with massage, the therapeutic effects of massage are potentially enhanced. It is important to remember, however, that aromatherapeutic approaches to skin conditions go beyond massage; in fact, in some conditions massage may be contraindicated.

The olfactory system and limbic brain

Aside from the specific activity of essential oils, of additional interest are the potential links between the olfactory side of aromatherapy and managing cutaneous pathology. Unlike other senses, which have processing structures, uniquely the sense of smell has a direct pathway to the brain, with the olfactory bulb being part of the limbic system, described by many as the emotional brain. There are numerous neural connections between the olfactory system, hypothalamus, hippocampus, temporal cortex, amygdala, and other limbic structures, which all affect mood, emotion, memory storage, behaviour and immunity. Effects of essential oil odours are mediated by the complex chemical activity of their aromatic molecules interacting with a host of neurochemical mechanisms along these pathways. The diversity of reactions and memories arising from olfactory input can be explained by these close links, with abundant evidence now available showing mood and behaviour to be directly affected by odour.[4,5,8-11]

Aromas and the skin

As the mind affects the skin, and aromas affect the mind, could it be possible that aromas can induce changes in the skin? It has been shown that sedative drugs can block the delay in skin barrier repair caused by psychological stress.[2] This finding prompted research into whether inhaled sedative fragrances would have similar effects on skin barrier homeostasis (ibid.). In both mice and humans, recovery to barrier disruption and transepidermal water loss (TEWL) measurements following tape stripping improved when sedative odours were inhaled.

Skin barrier disruption is associated with various common skin diseases such as dermatitis and psoriasis and involves exogenous and endogenous factors, for example environmental humidity and ageing. Research has demonstrated that inhalation of a component of Bulgarian rose oil, dimethoxymethylbenzene (DMMB), which had previously been found to have a sedative effect, accelerated skin barrier repair in human subjects, unlike the inhalation of non-sedative odour and no inhalation which both produced no change in barrier recovery rates.[12]

This research holds great potential for using essential oils to mitigate the added effects of psychological stress on the deterioration of skin barrier homeostasis. Many essential oils have traditionally been used as natural sedatives and relaxants. The use of fragrance for instilling a sense of calm is reflected in the incense traditions of many religious and cultural practices, with *Boswellia carterii* (frankincense) and *Commiphora myrrha var. molmol* (myrrh) having a long history in the Christian church, and *Santalum album* (sandalwood) and *Vetiveria zizanioides* (vetiver) being valued in eastern traditions.

There is now some evidence to support the traditional use of herbal aromatics as sedatives and it has been shown that a wide variety of essential oils have the capacity to depress the function of the CNS such that sedation is produced.[2,13] Classifications for oils in this area include anxiolytics, relaxants, sedatives and soporifics. Although each action is distinct in terms of strict pharmacological definitions, in the context of aromatherapy practice, and with the dosages that are used, it is likely that the effects of each are broadly similar. Table 6.1 lists essential oils which are traditionally valued in this area.

It should be noted that as well as specific pharmacological actions, whether an odour has a stimulating or sedating effect might depend on a number of other factors: odour associations and conditioning, cultural perceptions, placebo effects and expectations. A detailed account of each of these is outside the scope of this

Table 6.1 Essential oils with sedative properties.

Anthemis nobilis[16,17]
Citrus aurantium ssp. aurantium flos.[21]
Citrus bergamia[18]
Citrus sinensis[5]
Commiphora myrrha var. molmol
Lavandula angustifolia[15,19,20,22]
Matricaria recutita
Origanum majorana
Pelargonium graveolens
Santalum album[7]
Valeriana officinalis[14]
Vetiveria zizanioides

Table 6.2 Examples of psychodermatologic disorders.[24]

Primary psychiatric	Secondary psychiatric	Psychophysiologic
Delusions of parasitosis	Alopecia areata	Acne
Dermatitis artefacta	Cystic acne	Alopecia areata
Dysmorphophobia	Hemangiomas	Atopic dermatitis
Neurotic excoriations	Ichthyosis	Psoriasis
Trichotillomania	Psoriasis	Psychogenic purpura
	Vitiligo	Rosacea
		Seborrheic dermatitis
		Urticaria

book; however, the following research findings illustrate the complexity involved. In Japanese experiments, floral fragrances often result in stimulation, while citrus and herbaceous aromas elicit relaxation, but in European studies this is reversed.[23] This does not negate research findings into pharmacological effects of essential oils, which occur irrespective of these factors,[7] but it does illustrate that when considering psychological responses to aroma, there are several factors to take into account.

Psychodermatologic disorders

Located at the boundary between psychiatry and dermatology, a psychodermatologic disorder is one involving a close interaction between the mind and the skin. These disorders can be classified into three broad categories, outlined with examples in Table 6.2.

Primary psychiatric disorders

These skin conditions are self-induced, because of psychiatric disorder. One of the most common forms of disorder in this category is *delusions of parasitosis*. These patients believe that an organism infests their bodies, describing symptoms such as crawling, biting and stinging sensations. Obsessive-compulsive disorders (OCDs) are one important group of primary psychiatric disorders. Some OCDs express themselves as skin disorders, as listed in Table 6.3.

The incidence of OCD is much higher than originally thought: studies have shown the prevalence in the general population as ranging from 2 to 3% although how many involve the skin has not been identified.[25] Clearly, OCD presents complex clinical challenges, not least because the majority of sufferers tend to minimise their symptoms and are not always ready to acknowledge and address their condition. In a review of OCD in dermatology, Monti *et al.*[25] highlight the drawbacks when patients are directly referred by their dermatologist to a psychiatrist when addressing OCD-related conditions as this can easily be perceived as a refusal of care and set up a position of conflict. The benefits of frequent examinations and changes of topical preparations that involve the patient are highlighted as being useful in establishing good relationships between clinicians and patients.

Table 6.3 Examples of cutaneous expressions of obsessive-compulsive disorder.[25]

Representative obsessional worries	Representative compulsive behaviours
Losing hair	Hair pulling (trichotillomania)
Looking ugly	Lip licking
Early skin ageing	Neurotic excoriations
Facial hirsutism	Irritant dermatitis due to hand washing
Greasy skin	Dermatitis caused by repeated mechanical
Skin cancer	gestures
Infestations	Localised neurodermatitis
Scarring from acne	
Germs, dust, dirt being contaminated/	
contaminating	

Therefore, within the context of aromatherapy practice, the trusting therapeutic relationship which typically characterises the client–therapist dynamic may provide substantial benefit. Although aromatherapy alone may not resolve the psychiatric condition, the inherently caring nature of the approach, which concurrently addresses psychological and physical aspects, is profoundly valuable. It is reasonable to suggest that aromatherapists can use the unique nature of the therapy to help individuals to recognise the need for and to accept appropriate treatment that addresses the psychological as well as physical manifestations of their condition.

Secondary psychiatric disorders and quality of life

In this category are disorders that tend to be disfiguring and which have a significant psychological impact. For humans, body image is an important part of self-perception, maintaining or destroying feelings of self-esteem and closely affecting quality of life.[26,27] Patients with skin conditions suffer significant psychological distress and although most skin conditions are not life threatening, the impact on an individual's quality of life can be profound. Taking one of the most prevalent skin disorders, acne vulgaris, in surveys approximately 30 to 50% of those with acne between the ages of 12 and 20 show psychological responses such as low self-esteem, lack of self-confidence, perceived social rejection, anxiety and depression.[28] In a survey of 2,144 psoriasis patients, more than 40% associated the development of plaques with concurrent emotional stress.[29]

In recent years, researchers have developed valid and reliable quality of life tools. As well as generic tools such as the Sickness Impact Profile, there are disease-specific measures such as the Psoriasis Disability Index and the Infant's Dermatitis Quality of Life Index that facilitate greater understanding of the impact of skin disease.[30,31] One result of this is that a patient-centred approach is adopted, as they are encouraged to express the impact the skin disease has on their lives, and furthermore such measures can be useful tools in evaluating the effectiveness of interventions.

Undoubtedly the psychological impact of a disfiguring skin disease is profound and few would argue that the emotional state of an individual suffering from such a condition should be carefully monitored. However, the impact on those with relatively common and apparently 'normal' skin conditions such as acne vulgaris may be overlooked. In a study that looked at the accuracy of dermatologists' opinions about the impact of various skin conditions on patients' lives and the frequency of psychiatric morbidity, an underestimation of the frequency of depression and anxiety by dermatologists was observed in many diagnostic categories.[32]

The following psychosocial effects associated with common skin disorders have been reported:

- low self-esteem
- social isolation and anxiety
- altered self-image and lack of self-confidence
- depression, anxiety, embarrassment
- relationship and work problems
- self-consciousness.

Unsurprisingly, those whose skin condition is most visually obvious or severe are affected more seriously. It has been found for example that facial disfigurement leads to patients experiencing lower career aspirations and having negative expectations about forming long-term relationships. It is also recognised that sufferers are more likely to play down the positive aspects of their appearance and personality, complying with restricted social standards when referring to attractiveness. For many, a heightened sense of body awareness and self-image can have a profound impact on their willingness to participate in activities such as swimming and sports.

Psychophysiologic disorders and the 'itch–scratch cycle'

These are conditions which, although not directly related to the mind, are frequently caused or worsened by emotional stress. A number of studies have looked not only at the role of stress on cutaneous pathology but personality as well, revealing possible relationships in a range of conditions.[33] In chronic conditions, emotional stress is implicated in the initiation of the notoriously distressing 'itch–scratch cycle'. Although itching (pruritus) can be a sign of several systemic and infective conditions (*see* Table 6.4), and therefore may be said to be an innate defensive mechanism, all too often in skin diseases, it seems to have no positive role. It does however significantly contribute to the patients' psychological distress, not least because it seriously disrupts sleeping patterns.

If we return to consider the skin as a neuro-immuno-endocrine interface we can explain the itch–scratch cycle as a manifestation of quite complex interactions. Although the mechanisms involved in itch are not yet fully understood, endogenous agents that have been implicated include histamine, serotonin, prostaglandins, proteases, cytokines, leucotrienes, neuropeptides, opioids and endorphins. Of these, the strongest evidence for a causal role exists for histamine.

At a simple level, scratching or rubbing the skin causes local irritation which, as a result, causes the release of inflammatory mediators such as histamine and substance P, which provoke the skin's itch receptors, believed to be located in the lower epidermis and dermoepidermal junction. Itch sensation is transmitted by peripheral sensory non-myelinated C-fibres to the spinal cord, thalamus and

Table 6.4 Examples of systemic disease associated with itching.

Diabetes mellitus
Hypo- and hyper-thyroidism
Liver disease
Primary biliary cirrhosis
Chronic renal failure
Polycythaemia
Lymphoma
Hodgkin's disease
Parasitosis

---

cerebral cortex. In addition, immunocompetent cells may cross the blood–brain barrier, consequently affecting the CNS, which may respond by releasing neurotransmitters further initiating motor behaviours such as picking or scratching, so continuing the cycle.

Aromatherapy to control itching

Targeting therapy towards controlling pruritus can have a profound effect on the quality of life of those for whom this is a clinical feature. Itching should always be viewed as symptomatic of another problem and responsible treatments seek to eliminate the cause. However, too often precise triggers remain elusive and symptom control is the best that can be achieved. A number of approaches are needed to address both the symptoms and causes.

- Where possible identify and eliminate triggers.
- Take cool showers or tepid baths (maximum 30 minutes).
- Limit the use of soaps and cleansers.
- Moisturise frequently and always after bathing.
- Avoid contact with irritants and allergens.
- Wear cotton and silk; avoid wool and synthetic fibres close to the skin.

A small study investigated the effects of aromatherapy on pruritus in 29 patients with chronic renal failure undergoing haemodialysis.[34] A seven-minute aromatherapy massage was given three times a week for four weeks to those in the experimental group, while those in the control group received standard care. Lavender and tea tree essential oils (5%) were mixed with sweet almond and jojoba oils (no specific dosages, or botanical sources given). There was a statistically significant reduction in pruritus scores for the experimental group. Despite the small study size and failure to separate the effects of the essential oils from the effects of massage, this study presents some interesting possibilities for using aromatherapy massage to reduce pruritus.

Aromatherapeutic approaches include formulating with anti-inflammatory oils and hydrosols using cooling application methods such as gels, lotions, cool compresses and hydrosol sprays. This approach is concordant with medical advice, which includes keeping the skin cool by taking short, cool showers or baths together with using prescription anti-inflammatories and corticosteroids as well as non-prescription traditional products such as calamine lotion.[35,36]

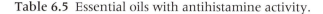

Table 6.5 Essential oils with antihistamine activity.

Curcuma longa[41]
Lavandula angustifolia[39]
Matricaria recutita, Chamomilla recutita (German chamomile)[40,42]
Melaleuca alternifolia[37,38]

Table 6.6 Essential oils traditionally used for topical cooling and anti-inflammatory effects.

Achillea millefolium
Anthemis nobilis[16,17]
Boswellia carteri
Cedrus deodara[43]
Commiphora myrrha var. molmol[42]
Cymbopogon martinii[44]
Helichrysum italicum[42]
Melaleuca quinquenervia
Mentha piperita
Pelargonium graveolens
Pogostemon cablin[42]
Rosa centifolia; R. damascena
Santalum album[42]

For histamine-mediated disorders (these are usually accompanied by a wheal and flare response as in urticaria), *Melaleuca alternifolia* (tea tree) essential oil is indicated. It has been shown to reduce histamine-induced wheal and flare in human skin; specifically, terpinen-4-ol is identified as the most active component.[37] In this particular study, terpinen-4-ol and tea tree oil at 100% concentration were used, with no adverse effects reported with undiluted use. Table 6.5 shows other oils with proven antihistamine activity.

Pruritus is a complex, poorly understood condition and, although histamine is thought to be the primary mediator of itch, there are many other possible mediators involved in both allergic and non-allergic conditions. Therefore, it cannot be assumed that the demonstrated antihistamine activity of certain essential oils will automatically be able to control itching. Oils which are traditionally used in skin care for their anti-inflammatory effect are also deemed suitable for the potential control of pruritus and are listed in Table 6.6. Itching and the recommended use of carrier oils and hydrosols are further discussed in Chapter 8.

Body image and self-esteem

Whether we like it or not, modern western culture is a culture of youth, with social advantages for those considered physically attractive, which generally excludes the elderly. As society increasingly places importance on concepts of beauty, equating this with desirability and success, a disparity exists with an increasingly aged population where such qualities are changing. In an article exploring the psychosocial aspects of ageing and the skin, Caroline Koblenzer[45] discusses how experiences very early in life shape the developing self-esteem, integrity of the body image, personal identity and determine an individual's capacity to adapt positively to changing circumstances which inevitably includes ageing.

Pertinent to aromatherapy practice, she stresses that early tactile stimulation is associated with meeting the emotional needs of infants and, if provided in an accepting environment, children learn to view their bodies and personalities as admirable and worthy of respect, establishing foundations for positive self-esteem later in life. The greater the area of skin touched, the more favourably children view themselves and the more accurate and stable the body image develops. Furthermore, Koblenzer asserts that the capacity to maintain stable emotional and physical boundaries of the self requires early positive tactile experience; difficulties in accepting the changes of ageing are associated with poor body image and less stable boundaries. Inadequate touching and holding has also been linked with obsessional concerns about body image and aspects of OCD.[25] This essential need for tactile stimulation is as important in maintaining self-esteem later in life as it is in childhood, particularly in light of the physical changes which occur in the skin, which in some individuals may contribute to anxiety about ageing.

The importance of control

The perception of control – or loss of control – that an individual has while experiencing symptoms of a disease appears to have a central role in determining the emotional impact the condition produces.[46] Control relates to many aspects of our social and personal lives, and includes the general society we live in, work and social interactions, family relationships, religious and spiritual beliefs, ideas and feelings about ourselves as well as our general health. A sense of loss of control in any of these leads to feelings of stress and anxiety. A locus of control refers to a personality trait which helps to determine how an individual copes with stressors. Those with an internal locus of control feel largely in control of themselves and the environment in which they live, have fewer psychosomatic symptoms and are able to deal with stressful events better than those who feel they are controlled by unpredictable external forces. Although a strong internal locus of control helps an individual cope with a broad range of stressors, it may also lead to an exaggerated sense of responsibility, producing tension or pain syndromes (ibid.).

Wherever an individual's locus of control is, when developing therapeutic strategies, we should remember that they are attempting to maintain or regain their own sense of control. The objective must be to support this attempt by encouraging and strengthening a feeling of self-confidence in being able to cope with the symptoms or disease; this is especially important in chronic or recurring conditions. A strong therapeutic relationship between therapist and client goes a long way to achieving this goal. The incorporation of quality of life tools discussed earlier in this chapter is a part of developing this client-focused approach. Furthermore, involving the client in the planning of treatment, ensuring essential oil formulations are aesthetically pleasing and in a medium that they find acceptable are all vital features of re-establishing their perception of control.

Focus on aromatherapeutic approaches

Discussions regarding the most appropriate methods of using oils for specific conditions lie elsewhere in this book. Here, we summarise the value of incorporating psychological considerations into the treatment strategy. Consider the following suggestion:

> Since many dermatologic treatments are topical, the addition of specific olfactory cues may maximize the therapeutic value of these agents, particularly when the agents are used for conditions with strong presumptive mind-body connections (e.g. allergic dermatitis, psoriasis, eczema, pruritus, urticaria, atopic dermatitis, and inflammatory dermatoses).[47]

In essential oils, we find olfactory cues co-existent with the therapeutic properties of a topical agent. When used within an aromatherapeutic regimen, which embraces a broad range of application methods, they have the potential to bring maximum relief to sufferers of skin disease.

To summarise, the key benefits of using holistically focused aromatherapy approaches are as follows.

- If used with massage, aromatherapy is able to reduce any sense of embarrassment about being touched which may be present. It also helps to foster an improved sense of self-esteem and emotional well-being.[45]
- Wherever possible, essential oils are selected which will address both physical symptoms of the skin disorder as well as the individual's psychological state, which should be explored within the therapeutic encounter.
- If skin barrier disruption or inflammation are clinical features of the condition, consider using oils with sedative effects.
- The application method needs to include self-administration of inhalation of essential oil aromas for optimal benefit: supplying pocket diffusers or inhalation sticks makes this practicable.
- Encouraging self-administration of formulations which clients find acceptable helps to foster and encourage a sense of self-confidence and perception of control. Avoid using mediums that are greasy and difficult to apply wherever possible, as this has been shown to limit compliance with treatment regimes and can exacerbate feelings of anxiety and depression.
- Using essential oils as mood-enhancers leads to a general improvement in the overall health profile of an individual and immune modulation, which is relevant in many immune-related skin disorders. There are strong associations between pleasing aromas and mood-enhancement.
- As an adjunct to pharmacological approaches, aromatherapy leading to stress reduction will, in turn, control stress-related cutaneous symptoms, which subsequently may lead to a reduction in medication.

References

1 Field T. *Touch Therapy*. Edinburgh: Churchill Livingstone; 2000.
2 Denda M, Tsuchiya T, Shoji K *et al*. Odorant inhalation affects skin barrier homeostasis in mice and humans. *Br J Dermatol*. 2000; 142: 1007–10.

3 Brazzini B, Ghersetich I, Hercogova J *et al*. The neuro-immuno-cutaneous-endocrine network: relationship between mind and skin. *Dermatol Ther*. 2003; **16**: 123–31.

4 Holmes C, Hopkins V, Hensford C *et al*. Lavender oil as a treatment for agitated behaviour in severe dementia: a placebo controlled study. *Int J Geriatr Psychiatry*. 2002; **17**: 305–8.

5 Lehrner J, Eckersberger C, Walla P *et al*. Ambient odor of orange in a dental office reduces anxiety and improves mood in female patients. *Physiol Behav*. 2000; **71**: 83–6.

6 Saeki Y, Shiohara M. Physiological effects of inhaling fragrances. *Int J Aromatherapy*. 2001; **11**(3): 118–25.

7 Hongratanaworakit T, Heuberger E, Buchbauer G. Evaluation of the effects of east Indian sandalwood oil and α-santalol on humans after trans dermal absorption. *Planta Med*. 2004; **70**: 3–7.

8 Knasko S. Ambient odour effects on human behaviour. *Int J Aromatherapy*. 1997; **8**(3): 28–33.

9 Itai T, Amayasu H, Kuribayashi M *et al*. Psychological effects of aromatherapy on chronic hemodialysis patients. *Psychiatry Clin Neurosci*. 2000; **54**(4): 393–7.

10 Louis M, Kowalski SD. Use of aromatherapy with hospice patients to decrease pain, anxiety, and depression and to promote an increased sense of well-being. *Am J Hosp Palliat Care*. 2002; **19**(6): 381–6.

11 Diego MA, Jones NA, Field T *et al*. Aromatherapy positively affects mood, EEG patterns of alertness and math computations. *Int J Neurosci*. 1998; **96**(3–4): 217–24.

12 Joichi A, Yomogida K, Nakamura S *et al*. The scent of roses: tea-scented modern roses and ancient Chinese roses. In: Proceedings of the 20th International Federation of the Societies of Cosmetic Chemists (Cannes) 1998; cited in Denda M, Tsuchiya T, Shoji K *et al*. Odorant inhalation affects skin barrier homeostasis in mice and humans. *Br J Dermatol*. 2000; **142**: 1007–10.

13 Buchbauer G, Jirovetz L, Jager W *et al*. Fragrance compounds and essential oils with sedative effects upon inhalation. *J Pharm Sci*. 1993; **82**(6): 660–4.

14 Buchbauer G, Jager W, Jirovetz L *et al*. Effects of valerian root oil, borneol, isoborneol, bornyl acetate and isobornyl acetate on the motility of laboratory animals (mice) after inhalation. *Pharmazie*. 1992; **47**(8): 620–2.

15 Buchbauer G, Jirovetz L, Jager W *et al*. Aromatherapy: evidence for sedative effects of the essential oil of lavender after inhalation. *Z Naturforsch C*. 1991; **46**(11–12): 1067–72.

16 Rossi T, Melegari M, Bianchi A *et al*. Sedative, anti-inflammatory and anti-diuretic effects induced in rats by essential oils of varieties of *Anthemis nobilis*: a comparative study. *Pharmacol Res Commun*. 1988; **20**(Suppl. 5): 71–4.

17 Melegari M, Albasini A, Pecorari G *et al*. Chemical characteristics and pharmacological properties of the essential oils of *Anthemis nobilis*. *Fitoterapia*. 1989; **59**(6): 449–55.

18 Occhiuto F, Limardi F, Circosta C. Effects of the non-volatile residue from the essential oil of *Citrus bergamia* on the central nervous system. *Int J Pharmacognosy*. 1995; **33**(3): 198–203.

19 Karamat E, Ilmberger J, Buchbauer G *et al*. Excitatory and sedative effects of essential oil on human reaction time performance. *Chem Senses*. 1992; **17**: 847.

20 Sugano H. Effects of odours on mental function. *Chem Senses*. 1989; **14**(2): 303.

21 Jager W, Buchbauer G, Jirovetz L *et al*. Evidence of the sedative effects of neroli oil, citronellal and phenylethyl acetate on mice. *JEOR*. 1992; **4**: 387–94.

22 Elizabetsky E, Brum LF, Souza DO. Anticonvulsant properties of linalool in glutamate-related seizure models. *Phytomedicine*. 1999; **6**(2): 107–13.

23 Jellinek S. Odours and mental states. *Int J Aromatherapy*. 1998/9; **9**(3): 115–20.

24 Koo J, Lebwohl A. Psychodermatology: the mind and skin connection. *Am Fam Physician*. 2001; **64**(11): 1873–8.

25 Monti M, Sambvani N, Sacrini F. Obsessive-compulsive disorders in dermatology. *J Eur Acad Dermatol Venereol*. 1998; **11**:103–8.

26 Wittkowski A, Richards H, Griffiths C *et al*. The impact of psychological and clinical factors on quality of life in individuals with atopic dermatitis. *J Psychosom Res*. 2004; **57**(2): 195–200.

27 Hutchings C, Shum K, Gawkrodger D. Occupational contact dermatitis has an appreciable impact on quality of life. *Contact Dermatitis*. 2001; **45**(1): 17.

28 Henkel V, Moehrenschlager M, Hegerl U *et al*. Screening for depression in adult acne vulgaris patients: tools for the dermatologist. *J Cosmetic Dermatol*. 2002; **1**: 202–7.

29 Farber EM, Bright RD, Nall ML. Psoriasis: a questionnaire of 2144 patients. *Arch Dermatol*. 1968; **98**: 248–59; cited in: Sullivan RL, Lipper G, Lerner EA. The neuro-immuno-cutaneous-endocrine network: relationship of mind and skin. *Arch Dermatol*. 1998; **134**: 1431–5.

30 Halioua B, Beumont M, Lunel F. Quality of life in dermatology. *Int J Dermatol*. 2000; **38**(11): 801.

31. www.ukdermatology.co.uk/ (accessed 17.03.05).

32 Sampogna F, Picardi A, Melchi CF *et al*. The impact of skin diseases on patients: comparing dermatologists opinions with research data collected on their patients. *Br J Dermatol*. 2003; **148**: 989–95.

33 Saez-Rodriguez M, Noda-Cabrera A, Alvarez-Tejera S *et al*. The role of psychological factors in palmoplantar pustulosis. *J Eur Acad Dermatol Venereol*. 2002; **16**: 325–7.

34 Ro YJ, Ha HC, Kim CG. The effects of aromatherapy on pruritus in patients undergoing hemodialysis. *Dermatol Nurs*. 2002; **14**(4): 231–9.

35 Millikan LE. Alternative therapy in pruritus. *Dermatol Ther*. 2003; **16**: 175–80.

36 Charlesworth EN, Beltrani VS. Pruritic dermatoses: overview of etiology and therapy. *Am J Med*. 2002; **113**(9A): 25S–33S.

37 Khalil Z, Pearce AL, Satkunanathan N. Regulation of wheal and flare by tea tree oil: complementary human and rodent studies. *J Invest Dermatol*. 2004; **23**: 683–90.

38 Koh KJ, Pearce AL, Marshman G *et al*. Tea tree oil reduces histamine-induced skin inflammation. *Br J Dermatol*. 2002; **147**: 1212–17.

39 Kim H-M, Cho S-H. Lavender oil inhibits immediate-type allergic reaction in mice and rats. *J Pharm Pharmacol*. 1999; **51**(2): 221–6.

40 Miller TM, Wittstock U, Lindequist U *et al*. Effects of some components of the essential oil of chamomile, *Chamomilla recutita*, on histamine release from rat mast cells. *Planta Med*. 1996; **62**(1): 60–1.

41 Chandra D, Gupta SS. Anti-inflammatory and antiarthritic activity of volatile oil of *Curcuma longa* (Haldi). *Indian J Med Res*. 1972; **60**(1): 138–42.

42 Baylac S, Racine P. Inhibition of 5-lipoxygenase by essential oils and other natural fragrant extracts. *Int J Aromatherapy*. 2003; **13**(2/3): 138–42.

43 Shinde UA, Kulkarni KR, Phadke AS *et al*. Mast cell stabilising and lipoxygenase inhibitory activity of *Cedrus deodara* (Roxb.) Loud. Wood oil. *Ind J Exp Biol*. 1999; **37**: 258–61.

44 Krishnamoorthy G, Kavimani S, Loganathan C. Anti-inflammatory activity of the essential oil of *Cymbopogon martini*. *Ind J Pharm Sci*. 1998; **60**(2): 114–16.

45 Koblenzer C. Psychologic aspects of aging and the skin. *Clin Dermatol*. 1996; **14**: 171–7.

46 Melmed RN. *Mind, Body and Medicine: an integrative text*. Oxford: Oxford University Press; 2001.

47 O'Sullivan RL, Lipper G, Lerner EA. The neuro-immuno-cutaneous-endocrine network: relationship of mind and skin. *Arch Dermatol*. 1998; **134**: 1431–5.

Chapter 7

Skin infections

Introduction

As a barrier to infection, the skin is crucial; however, if its defences are disrupted, a variety of micro-organisms can cause disease. It has been suggested that, globally, skin infection is responsible for more discomfort and illness than any other disease process.[1] The aim of this chapter is not to provide information on every skin infection; rather we will examine both the independent and adjunctive roles which aromatherapy can play in the management and treatment of some of the most common as well as identifying its limitations. It is not the intention to suggest that effective conventional treatments be replaced; rather we will suggest how and when aromatherapy can support these.

Normal skin microflora

Normal skin has a resident flora of micro-organisms, including bacteria, yeasts and mites, collectively termed commensals (viruses are not thought to inhabit the skin surface as commensals). These are found on the surface and deep in the pores and ducts of sweat and sebaceous glands. The numbers of bacteria vary from a few hundred per square centimetre on the forearm and back, to tens of thousands in the moist areas of the axillae, feet, perineum and groin. Different skin areas play host to different flora, being largely determined by local humidity: exposed dry areas have fewer flora compared with moister areas. The presence of these micro-organisms plays an important role in preventing foreign organisms from colonisation, although a balance does need to be maintained (*see* Table 7.1). The disadvantages of the normal flora lie mainly in the potential for spreading into otherwise sterile sites, for example when skin integrity is breached.

Bacterial infections

Bacteria are classified by the nature of their cell walls as either gram-positive or gram-negative, according to their reaction to a stain in microbiological identi-

Table 7.1 Factors maintaining skin's microbial balance.

Low humidity of area.
Acid pH of normal skin.
Surface temperature which remains too low for microbial growth.
Excretion of sebum, fatty acids, urea and sweat.
Competition between species.

fication procedures. The main structural component of the cell wall is peptido-glycan, a compound unique to bacteria, which in gram-positive bacteria forms a thick layer, external to the cell membrane; in gram-negative species, the layer is thin and covered by an outer membrane, attached to lipoprotein molecules in the peptidoglycan. The peptidoglycan layer is highly polar, giving gram-positive bacterium a thick hydrophilic surface. Lysozyme, an enzyme found in body secretions, digests the layer, thus having a bactericidal effect. In gram-negative bacteria, the lipopolysaccharide content of the outer membrane gives it hydro-phobic properties. Interactions with the cell wall structures of bacterium play a key role in determining the activity of antibiotics, including essential oils.

As commensals of healthy intact skin, staphylococci and streptococci are common causes of skin infections such as boils, pustules, carbuncles and post-operative wound infections. It is possible for the same organism to cause different infections in different layers of the skin and soft tissue. For example, *Streptococcus pyogenes* causes both impetigo and cellulitis. A common feature of a staphylo-coccal infection is acute inflammation and the presence of pus as these organisms are pyogenic. The most important pathogenic staphylococcal organism is *Staphylococcus aureus*, which is carried by around 30% of healthy people.[2] This has gained major resistance to antibiotic therapy – the resistant form being known as MRSA (methicillin resistant *Staphylococcus aureus*). Staphylococcal and strepto-coccal infections of the skin can be primary or secondary, for example super-infection of eczema, psoriasis or leg ulcers. *Proprionibacterium acnes* is a normal commensal found on healthy intact skin, but its proliferation is one of the causative factors in the development of the inflammatory lesions of acne vulgaris.

Immuno-compromised individuals, the non-active elderly and hospitalised patients are all highly susceptible to bacterial skin infections, some of which have serious or fatal outcomes, and correct medical treatment must be sought. In an age of growing antibiotic resistance, prevention of infection is one of the great challenges of modern healthcare. The following section provides an overview of some of the most common bacterial infections and their causative organisms. It is not intended that this be used as a reference for differential diagnosis and it must always be remembered that some common bacterial skin infections can have serious complications, which require prompt medical attention.

Impetigo

Impetigo is the most common, highly contagious skin infection affecting chil-dren.[3] Infection is superficial, remaining in the outer layers of the epidermis. Symptoms of impetigo are honey-coloured crusted sores often on the face between the mouth and upper lip that develop from discharging red spots or blisters. It is caused by one of two bacteria, *S. aureus* and less frequently *Strep. pyogenes*. Streptococcal infection forms tiny blisters which erupt exposing wet patches of red skin that gradually become covered by a yellowish crusting. Staphylococcal infection produces larger blisters that remain intact for longer (bullous type impetigo). Infection spreads from site to site and between persons either by direct contact or indirectly through clothing, toys, towels, or bed linen that has been in contact with the infected person. However, the value of disinfecting measures to control infection has recently been questioned.[4] For people with limited disease antibiotic creams have been found to be equally or more effective than oral antibiotic treatment (ibid.). Impetigo is a complication of atopic dermatitis due to the constant scratching of the skin and resulting excoriation.

Since children are found to comply better with topical rather than oral treatment and where the infected areas are small, initial topical aromatic treatment can safely be considered. The crusts of impetigo act as a barrier to essential oil formulations and therefore need to be removed. Soaking with a disinfecting warm hydrosol–essential oil compress can do this. Following debridement, a cream or lotion formulation is applied several times a day. Essential oils with activity against *S. aureus* and *Strep. pyogenes* are given later in Table 7.5 and precise selection and dosage is made after full consideration of all factors.

Since the nose is commonly the source of the infecting bacteria, the area between the upper lip and the nose needs to be kept clean with hydrosol-soaked wipes. A thin layer of essential oil formulation can be placed under the nose to prevent spreading. If impetigo is not improved after four days, or any new infected areas appear, medical treatment should be sought.

Pitted keratolysis

Pitted keratolyis is a superficial bacterial skin infection that produces crateriform pitting and depressed discoloured areas, particularly on the pressure-bearing aspects of the feet. Sweaty feet and occlusive footwear encourage overproliferation of skin organisms, namely *Micrococcus sedentarius*, *Dermatophilus congolensis*, *Corynebacterium* and *Actinomyces* species. These bacteria produce proteases that destroy keratin in the stratum corneum, creating pits. The characteristic malodour associated with the condition is thought to be due to the production of sulfur-containing by-products. Since these keratolytic bacteria are limited to the stratum corneum, topical aromatic treatment using gel or lotion formulations can be considered; gels and watery lotions are the preferred medium since their drying and cooling action will discourage bacterial proliferation.

There has been little research to date investigating essential oils with activity against the causative pathogens of pitted keratolysis. However, by using essential oils and hydrosols that possess broad-spectrum antibacterial activity this provides a sound therapeutic approach. To prevent recurrence and to achieve successful cure, excessive perspiration (hyperhidrosis) needs to be controlled (*see* Table 7.2). *Cupressus sempervirens* (cypress), *Citrus aurantium ssp. amara* fol. (petitgrain), *Pinus*

Table 7.2: Aromatic management of pitted keratolysis.

- Limit the use of occlusive footwear.
- Prevent foot friction by wearing correctly fitting footwear.
- Change socks frequently to prevent excessive moisture. Wool socks remove moisture more efficiently than cotton.
- Use antibacterial washes, either hydrosols or essential oils dispersed in warm water, as part of an improved hygiene regimen.
- Apply aromatic gel formulation containing antibacterial oils three times a day.
- Odour and lesions should clear in three to four weeks.

sylvestris (pine) and *Cymbopogon citratus* (lemongrass) essential oils are tradition-ally used as antisudorifics and deodorants; using them in foot-baths offers useful adjunctive therapy.

Cellulitis and erysipelas

Cellulitis is an acute spreading bacterial infection causing inflammation of the dermis and subcutaneous tissue. Many different bacteria may cause it, with the most common being streptococci. Small breaks in the epidermis allow entry of the causative organism. Hypostatic oedmatous areas, such as the legs, are particularly vulnerable to the development of cellulitis. Initial symptoms are redness, pain and tenderness. The infected skin becomes hot and swollen and may look slightly pitted. Erysipelas is a more superficial subcutaneous strepto-coccal infection causing intense erythema with a sharp demarcated border. Fluid-filled blisters sometimes appear on the infected skin. The first warning of an attack is often flu-like symptoms: fever, malaise and shivering. As the infection spreads, nearby lymph nodes are affected, becoming enlarged and tender.

Both erysipelas and cellulitis require prompt antibiotic treatment to prevent spread and the development of complications such as lymphaginitis, bacteremia, sepis and skin abscesses. The infected part of the body should be kept immobile and elevated to control swelling. Since the infection affects the subcutaneous tissue and progresses rapidly, using topical essential oil based treatment alone would have little impact on its course. However, as adjunctive therapy, the application of cool hydrosol compresses to the infected area will ease discomfort and may quicken the pace of healing.

Hair follicle infection

Folliculitis is inflammation of the hair follicles that arises following damage to them, either from a blockage or from friction caused by shaving or clothing. The injured hair follicle becomes susceptible to infection by bacteria, fungi or yeasts. *S. aureus* and *Pseudomonas aeruginosa* cause superficial bacterial folliculitis which presents as pus-filled itchy lumps. Antibacterial gel washes containing essential oils with known activity against the suspected infecting bacteria (*see* Table 7.5 later) can be used to prevent spread and recurrence. The application of cool compresses, prepared using essential oils and/or hydrosols, applied three to six times a day, may help to heal the pustules and relieve itching.

Furuncles or boils affect the hair follicle at a deeper level than folliculitis. The causative organism is usually *S. aureus* which produces a red, tender nodule that enlarges over five to seven days forming a yellow–white tip that ruptures and drains leaving a scar. Many furuncles are self-limited and like folliculitis respond well to frequent warm hydrosol–essential oil based compresses that encourage pointing of the infection. Carbuncles are the result of a deeper and more severe infection. A group of hair follicles infected deeply by *S. aureus* produces a large swollen suppurating lesion that discharges pus from several sites. They heal more slowly than boils, often causing considerable pain and possibly systemic symp-toms. Carbuncles require topical and oral antibiotic treatment, but adjunctive

Table 7.3: Common bacterial diseases of the skin.

Disease	Depth of infection	Causative organism
Impetigo	Superficial epidermis	*S. aureus* *Strep. pyogenes*
Pitted keratolysis	Superficial epidermis (stratum corneum only)	*Micrococcus sedentarius* *Dermatophilus congolensis* *Corynebacterium ssp.* *Actinomyces ssp.*
Erysipelas	Dermis Superficial subcutaneous	*Strep. pyogenes*
Cellulitis	Subcutaneous tissue involvement	Streptococci, staphylococci or other organisms
Folliculitis (bacterial)	Superficial follicle involvement	*S. aureus* *Ps. aeruginosa*
Furunculosis (boils)	Deep follicle involvement	*S. aureus*
Carbuncle	Deep follicle involvement of a group of adjacent hair follicles	*S. aureus*

aromatic care using essential oils with analgesic, anti-inflammatory and anti-bacterial activity against *S. aureus* can relieve some discomfort.

Table 7.3 summarises the depth of infection and likely causative organisms of some common bacterial diseases of the skin.

Antibacterial aromatherapy

For years, the antimicrobial activity of a wide variety of plant extracts and essential oils has been studied, and the rise of multiresistant organisms has added impetus to research efforts to find alternatives to conventional agents. Coupled with the fact that many people increasingly prefer natural alternatives,[5] the need for in vitro, in vivo and safety information has driven many researchers to undertake work in this field; a convincing amount of data now exists to confirm the potential for using essential oils as effective therapeutic agents. Although evidence from controlled clinical trials is still relatively scarce, there is some which shows essential oil based topical treatments to be equally or more effective than conventional treatments, for example in the control of acne[6] and MRSA.[5,7]

Essential oils and MRSA

The potential for using *Melaleuca alternifolia* (tea tree) essential oil as an agent against MRSA has been recognised for some years, with it being mentioned in revised guidelines issued by the Combined Working Party of the Hospital Infections Society, the British Society for Antimicrobial Chemotherapy and the Infection Control Nurses Association.[8] Dryden *et al.*[9] compared two topical MRSA eradication regimes in a randomised controlled trial of 224 hospital patients colonised with MRSA. The standard treatment regimen comprised

Table 7.4: Essential oils with
inhibitory effects against MRSA.

Melaleuca alternifolia[5–7,9–13]
Mentha piperita[5]
Lavandula angustifolia[5]
Ocimum basilicum[15]
Origanum vulgare[14]
Satureja montana[16]
Thymus vulgaris[5]

mupirocin 2% nasal ointment, chlorhexidine gluconate 4% soap and silver sulfadiazine 1% cream all applied for five days. This was compared with a five-day tea tree oil regimen, which comprised 10% tea tree cream applied to the anterior nostrils, 5% tea tree body wash and 1% tea tree cream. Results showed mupirocin to be significantly more effective than tea tree cream in the nostrils, but with mupirocin resistance increasing, the researchers suggested that tea tree offered a useful alternative in areas of high resistance. At other superficial body sites including open skin lesions the tea tree preparations were more effective than chlorhexidine soap or silver sulfadiazine. Both treatment regimes achieved clearance rates of 40–50%. There were no adverse effects reported and it is possible that higher concentrations of tea tree could achieve greater clearance rates.

Table 7.4 lists essential oils which have inhibitory effects against MRSA and Table 7.5 lists those active against a range of bacteria involved in common skin infections.

Table 7.6 lists individually active components of essential oils but it is important to note that it has been shown that minor components in oils contribute to their overall actions[14,29] and it is not necessarily desirable to focus on the individual components for maximum therapeutic effectiveness.

The aromatogram

This is a laboratory procedure, based upon the antibiogram, which is used to test the effectiveness of antibiotics against pathogens. Used in French medical aromatherapy, aromatograms are used to determine which essential oils are most effective in specific clinical situations. The test involves taking a germ sample from the patient and putting this in contact with a culture medium such as agar-agar in a Petri dish. Figure 7.1 illustrates the procedure. Several paper discs, each impregnated with a different essential oil, are placed on the medium. Following this, the Petri dish is incubated. Given optimal growth conditions, the microbes grow, except in the circles around the impregnated discs where essential oils are active.

When the results are read the halo surrounding the discs is measured. Each inhibitory halo demonstrates the effectiveness of a particular oil against a particular pathogen, allowing an assessment to be made of the in vitro anti-microbial activity of each essential oil being tested. It is possible for results to show an oil to be inactive on its own, but which becomes active when in close

Table 7.5: Essential oils with antibacterial activity relevant to dermatology.

Organism	Essential oil
Pseudomonas aeruginosa	Backhousia citriodora[23]
	Cymbopogon citratus[25]
	Lavandula officinalis[18]
	Melaleuca cajuputi[17]
	Melissa officinalis[18]
	Ocimum basilicum[15]
	Ocimum gratissimum[26]
	Origanum vulgare ssp. hirtum[27]
	Pelargonium graveolens[27]
	Rosmarinus officinalis[18]
	Syzygium aromaticum[27]
	Thymus vulgaris[27]
Staphylococcus aureus	Backhousia citriodora[23]
	Cymbopogon citratus[25]
	Cymbopogon martinii[25]
	Lavandula angustifolia[24]
	Lavandula latifolia[24]
	Melaleuca alternifolia[21]
	Melaleuca cajuputi[17]
	Ocimum basilicum[15]
	Ocimum gratissimum[26]
	Origanum vulgare ssp. hirtum[27]
	Origanum vulgare[14]
	Pelargonium graveolens[25,27]
	Piper nigrum[27]
	Pogostemon patchouli[25]
	Santalum album[25]
	Syzygium aromaticum[27]
	Thymus vulgaris[25,27]
	Vetiveria zizanioides[25,28]
Staphylococcus epidermidis	Melaleuca alternifolia[21]
	Ocimum basilicum[15]
	Origanum vulgare[14]
Streptococcus pyogenes	Lavandula angustifolia[24]
	Lavandula latifolia[24]
	Melaleuca alternifolia[19]
	Melaleuca cajuputi[17]
	Thymus capitatus[20]
Propionibacterium acnes	Backhousia citriodora[23]
	Melaleuca alternifolia[21,22]

proximity to another oil. Similarly, two oils combined may give a large inhibitory area, but singly have no activity – examples of essential oil synergy. It can be seen how useful aromatograms can be in practice, enabling the most effective selection of essential oils in terms of antimicrobial activity for individual infections.

Table 7.6 Essential oil components with antibacterial activity relevant to dermatology.

carvacrol[14,27,28]
geraniol[27]
linalol[17,27]
terpinen-4-ol[17,21,27,29]
α-terpineol[17,21,27]
α-pinene[21,27]
1,8 cineole[17]
citral[23,27]
citronellal[27]
thymol[14,30]
eugenol[30]

Modes of action of essential oils

Although evidence exists to confirm the broad-spectrum antibacterial effects of many essential oils, the exact mechanisms of action are not yet fully understood. It is known that much of the activity results from their ability to disrupt the permeability barrier of membrane structures and interfere with the enzymes embedded in it.[31,32] In tests with the sesquiterpenoid compounds nerolidol, farnesol and bisabolol, their ability to disrupt the barrier function of bacterial cell membranes was most marked in gram-positive bacteria, explained by the presence of the outer membrane in gram-negative bacteria.[33] The ineffectiveness of one of the most antimicrobially active oils, *Melaleuca alternifolia* (tea tree), against some strains of *Pseudomonas aeruginosa* has been attributed to the nature of its gram-negative outer membrane, which is composed mainly of lipopoly-saccharide. It has been shown that when permeabilising agents (with no anti-microbial activity) are used in conjunction with tea tree, the minimum inhibitory and minimum bactericidal concentration (MIC/MBC) values of tea tree against normally tolerant *Ps. aeruginosa* strains are similar to those for more tea tree-sensitive species.[30] In this particular study, it was also shown that normally inactive components in the oil showed increased activity against permeabilised cells, suggesting that increased diffusion through the outer membrane allowed toxic levels to accumulate in cytoplasmic membranes.

The lipophilic nature of cyclic monoterpenes results in their preferential partitioning from an aqueous phase into membrane structures, leading to membrane expansion, increased membrane fluidity and inhibition of a membrane-embedded enzyme.[34] The more lipophilic a compound is, the more preferentially it partitions into the cell membranes, thus damaging its structure and function. Tea tree oil has been shown to stimulate leakage of cellular potassium ions and to inhibit respiration in bacterial cells at MIC/MBC levels, leading to the conclusion that the disruption in cell membrane structures and permeability with attendant loss of chemiosmotic control indicate the most likely source of the oil's lethal action.[32] Tests on essential oil compounds have shown that their chemical structures, functional groups and configurations all influence their antibacterial activity. Components with phenolic structures, such as

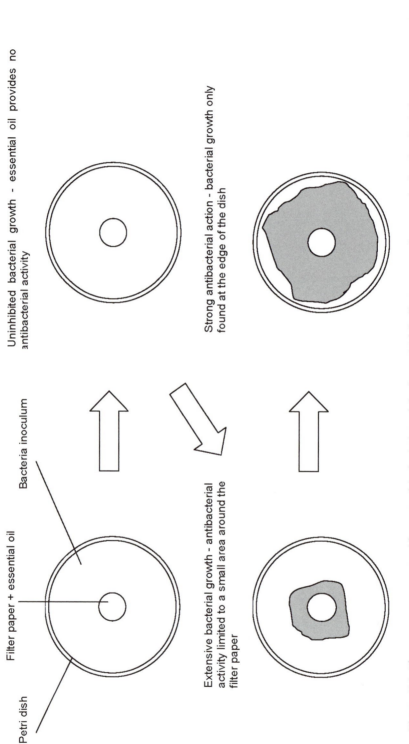

Petri dish

Filter paper + essential oil

Bacteria inoculum

Uninhibited bacterial growth - essential oil provides no antibacterial activity

Extensive bacterial growth - antibacterial activity limited to a small area around the filter paper

Strong antibacterial action - bacterial growth only found at the edge of the dish

Figure 7.1 The aromatogram provides a graphic depiction of the bactericidal effectiveness of essential oils. The shaded area indicates the area of inhibition.

carvacrol, eugenol and thymol, show the greatest activity, with the concentration used determining the bacteriostatic or bactericidal activity. Both the presence and position of the hydroxyl group in the phenolic structure are known to be influential in the effectiveness of components.[27]

Using essential oils effectively

Before using essential oils to treat infections, the clinical significance of any condition must be assessed and conditions requiring medical treatment identified. If essential oil therapy is appropriate, first the infection must be treated with sufficiently powerful high-dose formulas: if we use sub-therapeutic concentrations, we run the risk that the infection will not be eradicated and resistance may develop. This targeted, high-dose approach should only be used for short periods, and be based upon a sound understanding of essential oil chemistry and safety (*see* Chapters 2 and 3). This is followed by lower-dose, supportive formulas over the long term, following traditional aromatherapy practices. By combining high- and low-dose formulas we address the need not only to attack the micro-organism, but, importantly, to support the general health of the individual leading to an overall improvement in long-term therapeutic effectiveness. Where appropriate this aromatic approach is a useful adjunct to conventional medical treatment.

As a guide, for widespread application in adults a maximum 25% essential oil concentration in the final product is indicated, of which the proportion of dermo-reactive oils (e.g. phenol and aldehyde rich oils) should not exceed 20% (*see* formula 1 in Table 7.7). In localised applications, for example the short-term treatment of a carbuncle, depending on the safety profile of the oils chosen, age, health and skin reactivity of the individual, the essential oil concentration may be much higher.

To optimise the antibacterial activity of formulas, combinations of, rather than single, essential oils are used. As essential oils work in different ways with different bacteria, this allows the maximum range of organisms to be targeted,

Table 7.7 Sample formulations.

1. Broad-spectrum antibacterial formula	2. Folliculitis formula
Essential oils:	Essential oils:
Thymus vulgaris ct thymol 10%	*Ocimum gratissimum* 5%
Syzygium aromaticum gem. 5%	*Melaleuca alternifolia* 40%
Lavandula angustifolia 40%	*Pogostemon patchouli* 20%
Melaleuca alternifolia 45%	*Lavandula angustifolia* 35%
Add 15% of this formula to a suitable medium and apply to the local area three times daily for seven days.	Add 5% to gel base and apply to lesions twice daily after cleansing wash and compress application.
3. Hydrosol spray or facial wash	4. Clearance of MRSA colonisation[7]
Hydrosols:	*Melaleuca alternifolia* essential oil:
Mentha piperita 50%	10% cream applied to anterior nostrils
Origanum majorana 50%	5% body wash, all over body
Use as topical spray, foot-bath or facial wash twice daily.	10% cream applied to all skin lesions and as an alternative to body wash for groin and axillae. Treatment consists of once-daily application for five days.

thus providing a broad-spectrum approach, whilst minimising the chance of resistance developing. It is worth noting that although the chemical complexity of essential oils has led to the assumption that resistance is unlikely, incidents of MRSA resistance to tea tree have been reported[35] and it might be assumed that this will happen with other essential oils in future if they are commonly used. It is, however, prudent to limit the number of essential oils in a formula to between three and five, with each chosen to enhance the others, as it is possible to dilute the overall activity of the final formula. When combining essential oils the goal is to create effective synergies and to avoid antagonism, both within the essential oils and between the medium and essential oils.

Mediums

Mediums need careful selection, as certain bases will inhibit the antibacterial activity of essential oils. For example, ointments have been shown to inactivate *Ocimum gratissumum* (clove basil), an oil with excellent antibacterial effects.[26] Hydrophilic bases such as lotions, creams and gels are recommended. However, the greater the essential oil concentration that is required in the final preparation, the less likely a gel base will be used. Each case should be examined carefully and all factors considered, especially user compliance with the treatment regime. If formulas are unpleasant to use, there is less likelihood of them being used correctly and an increased chance of ineffective treatment resulting. Depending on the infection, different approaches will be indicated (*see* Figure 7.2). For example, it may be that crusts require softening with compresses (e.g. impetigo infection), followed with application of a lotion. Daily foot-baths are indicated for pitted keratolysis together with gel or lotion applications. In cases of dryness, the use of emollient creams is essential.

Antibacterial hydrosols

The antibacterial activity of hydrosols has been demonstrated, including against micro-organisms involved in skin infections. *Satureja hortensis* (summer savory) is active against *S. aureus* in vitro[36] as are thyme and oregano species (*Thymus vulgaris, Thymus serpyllum, Origanum onites, Oregano majorana*) with the oregano being more antibacterial than the thyme.[37] As with essential oils, the concentrations determine bacteriostatic or bactericidal effects. There is evidence that some phenol-containing essential oils and hydrosols have the same active substances, with a lower concentration in the hydrosol. For example, in the case of *Origanum compactum* hydrosol, the compounds thymol and carvacrol form more than 95% of the total aromatic fraction, which is relatively high with approximately 500 mg/l.[38]

In some circumstances, hydrosols may be indicated for antibacterial therapy either as alternatives to essential oils or in combination. For example:

- in the preparation of antibacterial washes, e.g. facial washes, foot-baths
- as active ingredients in water–oil bases or gels
- in the preparation of compresses
- in wound irrigation
- paediatric treatments
- topical sprays – this is especially useful if itching is present and hydrosols with both anti-inflammatory and antibacterial properties are combined.

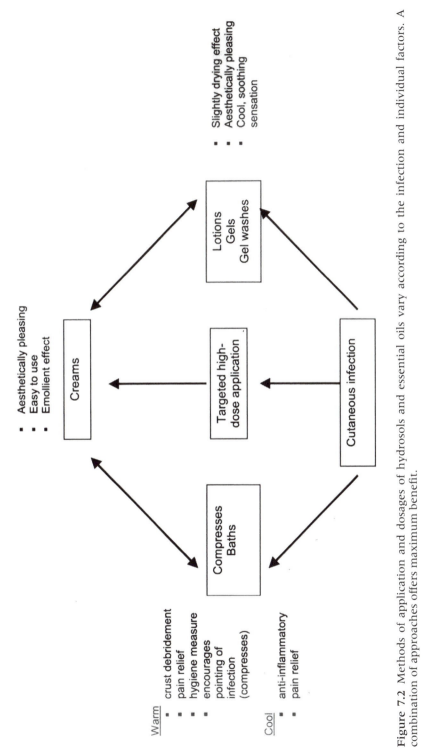

Figure 7.2 Methods of application and dosages of hydrosols and essential oils vary according to the infection and individual factors. A combination of approaches offers maximum benefit.

The long-term use of phenol-containing hydrosols presents fewer safety concerns, compared with essential oils of the same plant origin.

Safety

When using high-dose formulations, judgements must be made between achieving therapeutic efficacy and skin toleration. It is always necessary to use essential oils in the full knowledge of their individual and collective chemical, toxicological and pharmacological profiles. Treatment of children requires particular care and this is discussed fully in Chapter 8.

The validity of using essential oils on a regular basis may be questioned when we consider the importance of maintaining the resident flora. Work from Hammer et al.[39] has demonstrated that tea tree can effectively remove transient flora while maintaining commensal populations. As there is currently no definitive answer as to whether the benefits of using oils outweigh the potential for interfering with the commensal population, it is advisable to reserve essential oils with strong antimicrobial properties for when they are needed and to avoid their indiscriminate or excessive use.

Fungal infections

Fungal infections of the skin are very common and are increasingly affecting individuals, especially the immuno-compromised. Most frequently, they are restricted to the stratum corneum, nails and hair and are termed superficial mycoses, but they can penetrate other tissues, thus becoming deep mycoses. Infections tend to be chronic and difficult to eradicate, sometimes requiring long-term systemic medication. Two main groups of fungi are involved in cutaneous infections:

- dermatophytes
- yeasts.

Dermatophyte infections (ringworm)

Three genera cause infections, which are then named according to the anatomical location of the infection with the Latin prefix, *tinea* (*see* Figure 7.3).

- Dermatophytes:
  - *Microsporum*: infect skin and hair
  - *Trichophyton:* infect skin, hair and nails
  - *Epidermophyton*: infect skin and nails.
- Infections:
  - tinea capitis (scalp)
  - tinea corporis (trunk, limbs)
  - tinea cruris (groin)
  - tinea facei and barbae (face and beard area)
  - tinea manuum (hand)
  - tinea pedis (feet)
  - tinea unguium (nails).

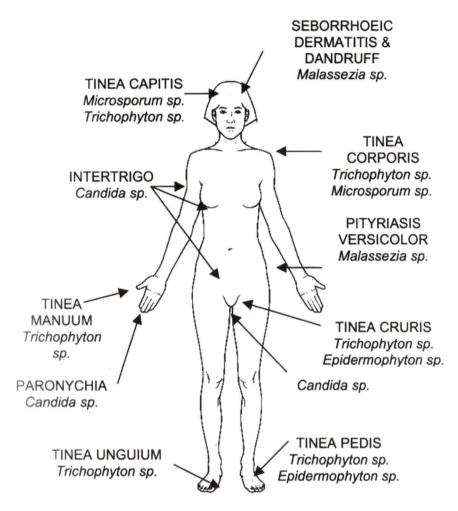

TINEA CAPITIS
Microsporum sp.
Trichophyton sp.

SEBORRHOEIC DERMATITIS & DANDRUFF
Malassezia sp.

TINEA CORPORIS
Trichophyton sp.
Microsporum sp.

INTERTRIGO
Candida sp.

PITYRIASIS VERSICOLOR
Malassezia sp.

TINEA MANUUM
Trichophyton sp.

PARONYCHIA
Candida sp.

TINEA CRURIS
Trichophyton sp.
Epidermophyton sp.

Candida sp.

TINEA UNGUIUM
Trichophyton sp.

TINEA PEDIS
Trichophyton sp.
Epidermophyton sp.

Figure 7.3 Superficial mycoses.

Within each genus, dermatophytes are categorised according to their origin: zoophilic, anthropophilic or geophilic (animal, human, soil) (*see* Table 7.8). It is possible for zoophilic dermatophytes to infect human hosts, for example we can catch ringworm from domestic pets; generally zoophilic species produce more inflammation than human-only species. Geophilic dermatophytes (*Microsporum gypseum*) are uncommon causes of human infection, but are sometimes seen in those exposed to soil, for example gardeners or agricultural workers.

Dermatophytes reproduce by spore formation and are keratin-loving organisms; hence, they readily invade the keratinised structures of the body. Arthrospores are the reproductive cells produced by dermatophyte hyphae, which adhere to keratinocytes, germinate and invade, eventually being shed from the body surface in skin scales and hair, thus spreading infection. The arthrospores can survive for long periods, even through low-temperature washing machine cycles.

Table 7.8 Dermatophytes and their natural hosts.

Anthropophilic dermatophytes	Zoophilic dermatophytes
Trichophyton rubrum	Microsporum canis (dogs and cats)
Trichophyton mentagrophytes var. interdigitale	Trichophyton equinum (horses)
Trichophyton mentagrophytes var. mentagrophytes	Trichophyton verrucosum (cattle)
Trichophyton schoenleinii	
Trichophyton tonsurans	
Microsporum audouinii	
Epidermophyton floccosum	

The typical dermatophyte lesion is an annular scaling patch with a raised margin. The exact features will depend on the site affected but itching is a main symptom, although this does vary in severity. The degree of inflammation also depends on the infecting species, but can be severe, especially in chronic infections. If the hair is involved, permanent hair loss may occur in serious cases. Table 7.9 gives an overview of the presenting features of dermatophyte infections; microscopy and culture of skin scrapings is required for clinical diagnoses.

Yeast infections

Candida albicans is a yeast which is found in low numbers on healthy intact skin, but which rapidly proliferates on damaged skin, causing candidiasis infections when conditions are favourable (*see* Tables 7.10 and 7.11). Cutaneous lesions due to *Candida albicans* are generally a glazed brick-red colour and are characterised by 'satellite lesions' and sometimes pustules around the main site of infection. Painful fissures commonly form in the affected body folds and can be resistant to treatment. *Malassezia furfur* is also found in commensal populations. Members of the genus *Malassezia* were formerly classified as *Pityrosporum* yeast species, but it is now generally accepted that *Malassezia* is the correct name.*[40–42] It produces the infection Pityriasis versicolor and is involved in seborrhoeic dermatitis and dandruff (*see* Chapter 11). Pityriasis versicolor is a chronic infection, characterised by changes in pigment. Most typically, the presentation is of slightly scaly patches on the upper trunk, upper arms and neck. In pale skin, the patches appear a slightly dirty brown colour, while in darker skins the areas are hypopigmented due to the inhibition of melanogenesis.

Antifungal aromatherapy

Essential oils

Many essential oils have been successfully tested both in vitro and in vivo for their antifungal activity. Although currently there are relatively few controlled

---

* The taxonomy of the genus has recently been revised into ten species: *M. globosa, M. restricta, M. furfur, M. sympodialis, M. slooffiae, M. obtusa, M. nana, M. dermatis, M. japonica,* and the sole non-lipid-dependent species, *M. pachydermatis.*

Table 7.9 Common presenting features of dermatophyte infections.

Disease	Organism	Comments
Tinea barbae, facei (beard)	Zoophilic *Trichophyton* species	Patches of inflammation, sometimes with follicular pustules develop in beard area (outside beard area = facei). Easily misdiagnosed as eczema or bacterial folliculitis; should be suspected in those in contact with cattle or other animals. Can also affect those in long-stay communal living arrangements.
Tinea capitis (scalp)	*M. canis* *M. audounii* *T. tonsurans* *T. verrucosum*	Usually affects children. Main feature is hair loss with variable degrees of inflammation and scaling. Anthropophilic species cause defined scaly areas with slight inflammation and alopecia. Zoophilic infections cause an acutely inflamed, boggy, pustular swelling (kerion) which requires correct medical intervention, but which is often misdiagnosed.
Tinea corporis (trunk, limbs)	*T. rubrum* *T. verrucosum* *M. canis*	Single or multiple plaques with scaling and erythema. Lesions are often annular, enlarge slowly with a central clearing, leaving a classic 'ring-like' pattern. Often starts in the body folds.
Tinea cruris (groin)	*T. rubrum* *T. interdigitale* *E. floccosum*	Most common in men. Infection of groin, upper and inner thigh. Typical lesion is red, marginated eruption which spreads outwards from groin crease with edges which may be scaly, pustular or vesicular. Commonly known as 'jock-itch' and often seen in those with tinea pedis. Itching is common feature. Tends to be persistent and recurring. Involvement of the scrotum is rare, unlike *Candida* infections in which it is common.
Tinea manuum (hand)	*T. rubrum* (rarely, zoophilic organisms are involved)	Typically appears as a unilateral, diffuse scaling of the palm. Can also affect dorsa of hand and if due to animal fungi more inflammatory lesions are present. Most common appearance is dry, scaly, sweatless palms, which can mimic eczema. Distinguishing feature is the unilateral nature of T. manuum, which is less likely with eczema and often nails show signs of fungal infection.
Tinea pedis (feet)	*T. rubrum* *T. interdigitale* *E. floccosum*	Very common in adults, especially men. Three distinct forms are commonly seen: 1. Interdigital toe webs become fissured, macerated and itchy. 2. Vesicular patches affect soles and sides of feet. Can be widespread, leading to large blisters, which are usually itchy. 3. Dry scaly changes extending over whole plantar surface and extending up the sides of the feet, producing a demarcated line ('moccasin pattern'). Can spread to dorsal surfaces and is often treated as eczema or psoriasis. Nail infection often accompanies this type.
Tinea unguium (nails)	*T. rubrum* *T. interdigitale*	Toe nails are most commonly affected and usually occurs with chronic and recurrent tinea pedis infection. Children are rarely affected. The nails separate from the nail-bed, the nail plate thickens and becomes crumbly and yellow-brown. Once fungal infections attack nails, it is very difficult to treat without systemic therapy.

Table 7.10 Predisposing factors for *Candida albicans* infection.

- Moist and opposing skin folds.
- Obesity.
- Diabetes mellitus.
- Anaemia.
- Broad-spectrum antibiotic therapy.
- Immunosuppression.
- Pregnancy.
- Poor hygiene.
- Humidity.

Table 7.11 Cutaneous *Candida albicans* and *Malassezia* infections.

Disease	Clinical features
Intertrigo	Affecting skin folds, presents as a moist, glazed, macerated appearance. Commonly found below the breasts, in axillary or inguinal folds. Can also be found in finger webs in those working in wet conditions.
Nappy area candida	Infants are susceptible to rashes and infection and *Candida* is a common secondary invader.
Paronychia	Affecting the nails, chronic paronychia is often seen in those working in wet conditions. Initially the protective cuticle is lost, allowing *Candida* to invade the space provided. The resulting inflammation leads to the proximal nail fold becoming boggy and swollen. The nail plate becomes irregular and discoloured.
Perianal	May occur alone or concurrently with genital infection or infection of the groin and scrotum.
Pityriasis versicolor	Caused by *M. globosa* which is found in high numbers in areas with increased sebaceous activity. Factors like heat, humidity, pregnancy, malnutrition, burns, immunosuppression and oral contraceptives, cause the yeast to convert to its mycelial form which leads to tinea versicolor. Common during years of increased sebaceous activity (i.e. adolescence). Lesions are highly characteristic and start as multiple, small, round white, pink or brown macules which gradually enlarge. Most commonly affects the trunk but can spread to arms, neck, legs and back. Lesions are not usually itchy unless inflammation is present.

clinical trials, there is compelling evidence for the validity of developing essential oil based prophylaxis and treatments either used alone, or alongside conventional antifungal treatments.

One study designed to provide base-line data for use in a clinical trial focused on the use of *Lavandula angustifolia* (lavender) and *Melaleuca alternifolia* (tea tree) oils in tinea infections.[43] Findings identified that synergistic activity impacted on the antifungal activity of the oils. Tested individually, both oils demonstrated antimycotic activity against *T. rubrum* and *T. mentagrophytes*. At 25% dilution they demonstrated fungicidal effects against *T. rubrum* and combinations of either 10% lavender and 20% tea tree or 10% tea tree and 20% lavender demonstrated the same fungicidal effects. However, against the more resistant *T. mentagrophytes,* 90% tea tree was required for fungicidal effects and a 100% concentration of lavender produced simply fungistatic effects. Synergistic activity was clearly identified when against *T. mentagrophytes,* 20% lavender with 40% tea tree, or 70% lavender with 10% tea tree produced fungicidal effects and 100% growth inhibition after 28 days.

Although it is sometimes claimed that the synergistic action of essential oils is simply the additive effect of combining chemicals with similar actions, analysis provided by this study suggests the contrary. In the blends with synergistic activity, the levels of alcohols and sesquiterpenes were similar, indicating these chemical groups to be responsible for the antifungal activity. For lavender alone, similar levels of alcohols and sesquiterpenes were present when 100% inhibition of *T. rubrum* was demonstrated, likewise at day seven against *T. mentagrophytes.* However, at day 14, undiluted lavender failed to be fungicidal. Something other than a direct additive effect must be responsible for the fungicidal activity of the blends, when it is noted that higher levels of alcohols and sesquiterpenes were present in the single essential oils than with the synergistic blends. As well as synergistic activity occurring within and between oils, it is also worth noting that antagonism may also occur, reducing their efficacy. For example, research shows that the antimicrobial activity of terpinen-4-ol in tea tree is lowered by the presence of non-oxygenated terpenes.[29]

Melaleuca alternifolia is perhaps the most widely researched essential oil with numerous studies from around the world providing reliable evidence for its antifungal efficacy against yeasts and a range of dermatophytes.[25,29,32,44–48] Despite a substantial evidence base to support its inclusion in future clinical trials, and the huge potential it offers for providing cheap, safe, effective alternatives to existing treatments, recent concerns have been raised by the European Commission's Scientific Committee on Consumer Products (SCCP) about the safety of tea tree oil.[49] Expert responses have vigorously stressed the overwhelming safety of the oil in topical use and the need to balance the benefits offered against the alleged adverse effects for a small minority of users.[50] It seems sensible to evaluate any therapy by looking at the proven benefits in light of its degree of risk, while accepting that no treatments are completely risk-free.

In the presence of increasing concerns over resistant infections and efforts to reduce transmission of nosocomial infections in clinical settings, the efficacy of tea tree formulations in hygienic hand washing has been confirmed.[51] Research suggests that the repeated use of hand-washing agents containing tea tree oil avoids the dermatological problems associated with many commonly used antiseptic agents.[52] Furthermore, as tea tree has greater activity against transient flora than commensals,[39] it underlines the importance of conducting more clinical trials to realise the full potential of this remarkable oil.

Much research exists which confirms that, in addition to tea tree, a range of essential oils possess significant antifungal activity and Table 7.12 provides an overview of those indicated for aromadermatological care which demonstrate in vitro activity. Although caution is required to maintain the correct, safe dosage of some of these oils, effective formulations can be produced with good skin-tolerability for long-term use. As in the case of bacterial infections, sub-

Table 7.12 Essential oils with proven antifungal activity against a range of dermatophytes. In conventional dermatology practice, it is not usual to identify the species of dermatophyte involved in infection.

Organism	Essential oil
Trichophyton species	*Citrus limonum*[58]
	Cymbopogon citratus[59–61]
	Foeniculum vulgare[55]
	Lavandula angustifolia[43]
	Lavandula officinalis[18]
	Melaleuca alternifolia[43,46,62]
	Melissa officinalis[18]
	Ocimum basilicum[53]
	Ocimum gratissimum[53,54]
	Pelargonium graveolens[57]
	Rosmarinus officinalis[18]
	Thymus vulgaris[53]
	Vetiveria zizanioides[56]
Epidermophyton species	*Citrus limonum*[58]
	Cymbopogon citratus[61]
	Foeniculum vulgare[55]
	Melaleuca alternifolia[46,47]
	Mentha spicata[63]
Microsporum species	*Citrus limonum*[58]
	Cymbopogon citratus[59–61]
	Foeniculum vulgare[55]
	Melaleuca alternifolia[46,47]
	Mentha spicata[63]
	Ocimum basilicum[53,64]
	Ocimum gratissimum[53]
	Satureja montana[65]
	Thymus vulgaris[53,65]
	Vetiveria zizanioides[56]
Malassezia species	*Melaleuca alternifolia*[62,67]
	Origanum vulgare ssp. hirtum[66]
Candida albicans	*Backhousia citriodora*[23]
	Citrus aurantium fol.[25]
	Coriandrum sativum[25]
	Cymbopogon citratus[25,60]
	Cymbopogon martini[25]
	Foeniculum vulgare[25,55]
	Lavandula angustifolia[25]
	Melaleuca alternifolia[25,45,47,62,69]
	Melaleuca quinquenervia[25]
	Melissa officinalis[18,68]
	Mentha piperita[25]
	Mentha spicata[25]
	Ocimum basilicum[25,53]
	Ocimum gratissimum[53,54]
	Origanum vulgare[25]
	Origanum majorana[25]
	Pelargonium graveolens[25]
	Pogostemon pathouli[25]
	Salvia officinalis[25]
	Santalum album[25]
	Syzygium aromaticum[25]
	Thymus vulgaris[25,53,64]
	Vetiveria zizanioides[25,56]

therapeutic dosages must be avoided and the same ratio of dermo-reactive oils maintained for safety.

Mediums

Fungi require humidity to thrive. This is especially notable with *Candida* species, hence their rapid colonisation of body folds and moist areas. Therefore, the choice of base medium is of equal therapeutic importance to the selection of essential oils if we are to avoid trapping heat and increasing local humidity. Any base medium with a high percentage of lipids – for example beeswax, cholesterol, fatty acids, fatty alcohols and ceramides – should be avoided as, like petroleum jelly, they have an occlusive effect. Rather than ointments, essential oils are best applied in a lotion, gel or cream base. Remembering that user compliance is a major factor in how effective treatment is, we should not only select the best medium for the location being treated but also consider the aesthetics.

- *Gels*: form a good base for most applications and are ideal for scalp treatments. However, if the scalp is very dry, vegetable oils are required to nourish the tissues and improve the overall health of the scalp. This is especially important once the infection has cleared.
- *Lotions*: like gels these have a slightly drying effect on the skin and make ideal mediums for treating fungal infections. They are generally well accepted.
- *Powders*: indicated in intertrigo and tinea infections causing maceration. It is important that the texture of the powder remains as fine as possible and that 'caking' does not occur as this will produce an abrasive medium rather than one which absorbs moisture and keeps body folds and clefts dry.

Holistic advice

It is often necessary to treat for sustained periods of time as symptoms often disappear without achieving full mycological cure, only to reappear once treatment has stopped. There are a number of measures that can be adopted to improve the chances of success and to prevent recurrence of infection.

- Reduce humidity as much as possible, exposing affected areas to air.
- Minimise the wearing of occlusive footwear in tinea pedis infections.
- Dry hands and feet carefully, especially interdigitally.
- Wear cotton gloves under rubber gloves in wet working conditions, changing them frequently.
- Improve general hygiene, changing footwear regularly and using foot-baths.
- Use essential oil based pre-wash soaks for clothing and wash at temperatures above 55 degrees.
- Try to separate body folds in intertriginous infections, for example by using absorbent cotton cloths under breasts.
- Avoid close contact with animal bedding.
- Spores may remain viable for months on furniture, clothing and brushes and cleaning these with essential oil wipes helps prevent re-infection.

In the case of nail infections it may take a year of twice-daily applications to be effective and in most infections a minimum of one month of treatment will be required. A number of factors will affect treatment outcomes:

- infection history: chronic conditions can be extremely resistant to treatment
- general health status of the individual
- compliance with treatment regime: the aesthetics of formulations is crucial in maintaining this and can make or break a treatment
- presence of environmental factors, e.g. pets, communal showering, working conditions
- personal hygiene
- suitability of essential oil selection for each case
- whether concurrent conventional medication is being used.

Antiviral aromatherapy

Viruses are not believed to be part of normal skin flora but do cause many of the common skin lesions seen by aromatherapists, for example warts, herpes and molluscum contagiosum. The structure and biology of viruses makes them distinct from all other pathogenic organisms. Without a host cell, viruses cannot carry out their life-sustaining functions or reproduce. They cannot synthesise proteins, because they lack ribosomes so use the ribosomes of the host cell to translate viral messenger RNA into viral proteins. They parasitise the host cell for energy, basic building materials and all other metabolic functions. All viruses contain nucleic acid, either DNA or RNA (but not both), and a protein coat, the capsid, which encases the nucleic core. A lipid envelope and protein molecules also enclose some viruses. This lipoprotein bilayer contains material derived from the membrane of the host cell as well as proteoglycans of viral origin.

Viruses are classified into families and genera based on the following structural considerations:

1 type and size of their nucleic acid
2 size and shape of the capsid
3 whether they possess a lipid envelope surrounding the nucleocapsid.

Viral skin lesions commonly seen in aromatherapy practice are caused by DNA-enveloped viruses and are given in Table 7.13. They enter through breaks in the skin and since there is no circulation of blood or lymphatics in the epidermis the virus has no means of transport, resulting in it replicating there; in order to spread further it needs to infect the well-vascularised dermis. Genital lesions caused by HSV-2 and anogenital warts, caused by the human papilloma virus, are beyond the scope of this book and require medical care. Detailed aromatic treatment of warts affecting children can be found in Chapter 8.

Antiviral treatment

The intracellular parasitic nature of viruses makes it difficult to find a treatment that directly attacks the virion (virus particles outside the host cell) or its replication without causing adverse effects to the infected cells. Table 7.14 lists the types of chemotherapeutic agents considered for viral infections.

Virucides may cause direct inactivation in a single step and can be used to prevent the transmission of viral infections. Their use is often limited as they

Table 7.13 Common viral skin diseases.

Disease	Virus	Comments
Herpes simplex Cold sores Cutaneous herpes Genital herpes	DNA enveloped HSV-1 HSV-2	The virus is ubiquitous and carriers continue to shed particles in their bodily fluids. The route of infection is through mucous membranes or abraded skin. The virus replicates within epithelial cells causing bouts of vesication. Two types of virus are involved: Type 1 is usually facial or non-genital and Type 2 are commonly genital. Type 1 primary infection mainly occurs in childhood and is usually asymptomatic.[70,71] Subsequent lesions present as a group of painful blisters of a uniform size and can be confused with impetigo as both form a crust. Recurrence is a hallmark of HSV infection, occurring in similar sites, as the virus remains in the body in the latent form. Tingling and burning is quickly followed by erythema and clusters of vesicles. Crusting occurs within 24–48 hours with the episode lasting approximately 12 days.
Herpes zoster Chickenpox Shingles	DNA enveloped Varicella-zoster virus (VZV)	Varicella or chickenpox is highly contagious, being transmitted via the respiratory route or vesicular fluid. VZV lies dormant in the sensory root ganglion of the spinal cord following an episode of chickenpox and when reactivated VZV replicates and migrates along the nerve to the skin where it induces shingles lesions and pain. Some people with shingles have no history of chickenpox, acquiring the infection via the transplacental route.[70] Shingles presents with pain before lesions appear, followed by burning and itching. Vesicles differ from HSV in that they vary in size and are umbilicated. Scarring results if inflammation is intense. Post-herpetic neuralgia is a major complication of shingles which can last sometime after eruptions have disappeared. Patients with shingles can transmit the virus to others in whom it will cause chickenpox.
Warts Common warts Plantar warts Mosaic warts Flat warts	Enveloped DNA Papovavirus Human papilloma virus (HPV)	Commonly occur in children and adolescents. Infections occur when wart virus in the skin comes into contact with breaches in the mucous membranes or skin. There are more than 100 HPVs which infect epithelial cells causing a variety of lesions by inducing hyperplasia and hyperkeratitis. The hands and feet are common sites of infection; those on the plantar surface are commonly called verrucae. The wart regresses in a period of months but viral DNA remains in basal epithelial cells and can reactivate. Skin warts rarely undergo malignant change but genital warts may do so.

Table 7.13 (*cont.*)

Disease	Virus	Comments
Molluscum contagiosum	Enveloped DNA Poxvirus	Common infection in children, rarely adults. Multiple, waxy, dome-shaped papules, 1–5 mm in size. Commonly found on the face, neck and trunk. Squeezing of the lesion releases a creamy material. Spread may be via direct contact or indirectly through clothing, towels, etc. Lesions spontaneously resolve in 6–9 months but can persist for longer. Prolonged infection frequently occurs in those with impaired skin barrier function, for example atopic dermatitis.

must inhibit virus-specific events while not damaging the host cell and this is difficult to achieve. They typically have a restricted spectrum of activity.

Antiviral activity can be classified as:

- preventing attachment to the host cell
- inhibiting reproduction or growth – such agents are not effective in elimination of non-replicating or latent virus.

Recovery from viral infections requires an intact immunologic response from the host. Response to antiviral therapy may be delayed in individuals with a suppressed immune system and reactivation of latent viruses is a likely event.

Activity of essential and vegetable oils and their components

From the limited research currently available, some essential oils have been shown to inactivate intact virions. It is suggested that this occurs directly by a specific interaction with the viral envelope. Such oils exert a direct virucidal effect prior to adsorption but show no antiviral activity after penetration into the host cell. *Melaleuca alternifolia* (tea tree), *Mentha piperita* (peppermint), *Origanum majorana* (marjoram), *Eucalyptus globulus* (blue gum eucalyptus), *Ravensara aromatica* (ravintsara), *Lavandula latifolia* (spike lavender), *Citrus limonum* (lemon), *Rosmarinus officinalis* (rosemary) and *Cymbopogon citratus* (lemongrass) have been shown to completely inhibit the growth of HSV-1 in vitro at a concentration of 1%.[72] Lemongrass demonstrated the strongest antiviral activity with complete inhibition at 0.1%. The authors conclude that the antiherpetic activity of the oils is due to direct interaction with the virions by binding to the viral envelopes. The oils were shown to have no direct inhibiting effect on host cell adhesion, penetration or replication and therefore do not offer full cure of HSV-1 infection, but can suppress and prevent infectivity prior to attachment to

Table 7.14 Chemotherapeutic agents for viral infections.

- Virucides – agents that inactivate intact viruses.
- Antivirals – agents that inhibit viral replication at cellular level.
- Immunomodulators – agents that augment the host response to infection.

the host cell. Essential oils with proven virucidal activity against HSV-1 are listed in Table 7.15 and Table 7.16 lists essential oil isolates.

Hypericin, a polycyclic anthrone, responsible for the deep red colour in the infused oil *Hypericum perforatum* (St John's wort), inactivates enveloped viruses, in particular HSV-1.[79] In line with other research in this area, Tang *et al.*[79] found hypericin in vivo to be virucidal if incubated with the virus prior to infection but ineffective when concurrently administered to the host. The monoterpenoid alcohol isoborneol and its stereoisomer borneol have demonstrated virucidal activity against HSV-1, albeit in relatively high concentrations (1%) by interactions with lipids present in the cell envelope.[77] Isoborneol, but not borneol, was shown to possess dual antiviral activity by specific inhibition of viral glycosylation and hence viral replication at a concentration of 0.06%, which is not toxic to human cells. Use of oils containing isoborneol such as *Picea mariana* (typically containing 0.05% isoborneol) and *Rosmarinus pyramidalis* (rosemary) (typically containing 0.24%) should be considered when formulating for inhibition of the HSV lifecycle, although there is no research at present on the antiviral activity of the complete oils. To date there are no other essential oil isolates or essential oils that have demonstrated dual antiviral activity against enveloped DNA viruses.

Ideally when formulating for any viral skin infection, antiviral agents with different mechanisms of action are chosen. However, based upon current evidence, as all oils and isolates discussed, apart from isoborneol, act by interaction

Table 7.15 Essential oils with virucidal activity against HSV-1.

Citrus limonum[72]
Cymbopogon citratus[72]
Eucalyptus globulus[72,73]
Lavandula latifolia[72]
Melaleuca alternifolia[72,73]
Melaleuca ericifolia[74]
Melaleuca leucadendron[74]
Mentha piperita[72,75]
Origanum majorana[72]
Ravensara aromatica[72]
Rosmarinus officinalis[72]
Santalum album[76]

Table 7.16 Essential oil isolates with virucidal activity against HSV-1.

isoborneol[77]
borneol[77]
eugenol[76]
neral/geranial[72]
terpinen-4-ol[73,74,78]
α-terpineol[73]
1,8 cineole[73,74]

Table 7.17 Suggested essential oils for the treatment of HPV infections.[81]

Essential oil	Active chemical component
Eucalyptus polybractea ct cryptone	cryptone
Eugenia caryophyllata	eugenol
Melaleuca quinquenervia	α terpineol, 1,8 cineole
Melaleuca alternifolia	terpinen-4-ol
Origanum compactum	thymol/carvacrol
Salvia officinalis	thujone
Trachyspermum ammi	thymol

with the lipid envelope this may not be achievable. Where essential oils certainly have therapeutic value is in combination with allopathic medicines, as this synergy potentially increases antiviral potency, reduces the risk of resistant viruses emerging and lowers the required doses of toxic components.

The activity of eugenol is slight when compared to the pharmaceutical agent acyclovir. However, Benencia et al.[80] demonstrated a synergistic inhibition of HSV-1 replication in vitro when used concomitantly. Acyclovir inhibits DNA replication while eugenol disables the viral lipid envelope. *Mentha piperita* (peppermint) has been shown to be virucidal against an acyclovir-resistant strain of HSV-1 at non-cytotoxic concentrations and could prove useful in recurrent herpes infection[75] if used in combination with antiviral pharmaceuticals.

Baudoux et al.[81] acknowledge the scant research concerning the efficacy of essential oils, specifically against the human papilloma virus (HPV). Extrapolating from research with other viruses, together with their clinical experience, they propose a selection of oils with therapeutic interest (*see* Table 7.17). The safety implications when using some of these are reviewed in Chapters 2, 3 and 8.

The effects of massage

Recurrent viral infections or reactivation of HSV is associated with a deficient host immune response. In these cases, response to antiviral therapy may be delayed and drug resistance to viruses greater. Stress, anxiety and depression are all thought to overactivate the hypothalamic pituitary axis (HPA) resulting in the production of cortisol and neuropeptides that suppress the immune system, in particular Natural Killer (NK) cells, which provide protection against tumours and lyse virus infected cells.[82,83] Several studies have measured the effect of massage on NK cell counts. Diego et al.[84] found twice-weekly massage therapy in depressed HIV-positive adolescents improved immune function with an increased production of NK cell numbers being reported. This finding is supported by a recent study of breast cancer patients following thrice-weekly massage:[85] improved immune and neuroendocrine functions were demonstrated with raised levels of NK cells and lymphocytes.

In summary, for optimal effect using aromatic interventions a full repertoire of massage, inhalation and baths should be employed, with the clear aim of modulating the host immune response. This is especially important with resistant viral skin lesions, to augment cell-mediated immunity and viral inhibition thus providing a safe integrated care option.

Aromatic support in the treatment of herpes zoster (shingles and chickenpox)

Varicella, or chickenpox, is highly contagious and affects the majority of children before adolescence.[70] When it affects adults and immunocompromised patients they experience a prolonged course, with more extensive eruptions and a greater risk of complications. After it has caused chickenpox the virus remains latent in the dorsal root ganglia. Shingles results from its reactivation. Shingles affects all ages with the incidence increasing with age as T-cell immunity to the virus lessens. Stress, immunosuppression, fatigue and radiation therapy are all associated with reactivation of the latent virus. Before shingles lesions become apparent, pain, itching, burning, tenderness, headaches, fever and malaise may be present for several days. The eruption begins with painful clusters of red, swollen vesicles that spread to part or all of a dermatome and continue to appear over a week or so. Vesicles rupture or umbilicate before crusting over. For the weak and elderly, inflammation can be severe and secondary infection may occur, delaying healing.

In mild cases, treatment includes rest, analgesia and the topical application of cooling preparations. If seen within 48 hours of onset, oral pharmaceuticals can promote resolution, reduce viral shedding time and possibly lessen post-herpetic neuralgia.[71] Serious complications can occur, especially in the immunocompromised, and aromatic interventions alone are not appropriate in these cases.

Treatment options

Treatment for both shingles and chickenpox is kept simple and focused on relief of symptoms in mild cases. Cool compresses of essential oil–hydrosol mixtures are applied to vesicles regularly throughout the day for topical relief. Additionally, an atomiser spray of the same preparation can be provided for regular use as required. Essential oils are first mixed with a suitable dispersant (e.g. Solubol) before adding to the hydrosol preparation. Oils with anti-inflammatory and analgesic activity are selected. Useful essential oils and hydrosols include:

- *Achillea millefolium*
- *Chamaemelum nobile*
- *Cymbopogon martini*
- *Lavandula angustifolia*
- *Mentha piperita*
- *Melaleuca alternifolia.*

Bathing facilitates whole-body immersion in essential oil-containing warm water, ensuring all lesions are attended to, providing maximum relief. Bathing is especially soothing for a fractious, irritable child with chickenpox and can really help to minimise the itching and accompanying scratching. Essential oils selected from those above are dispersed in a suitable medium before adding to the water.

Following the application of sprays, compresses or bathing, an oily lotion can be applied to the lesions to provide further relief and aid in resolution. *Hypericum perforatum* (St John's wort) infused oil offers analgesic activity and should be incorporated into the preparation. Tissue healing can be further promoted once the initial inflammatory phase is over by making full use of vegetable oil-rich preparations containing *Rosa rubiginosa* (rosehip), *Simmondsia chinensis* (jojoba) and *Persea gratissima* (avocado). The prolonged use of *Hypericum perforatum* may help to reduce any post-herpetic neuralgia from developing in the case of shingles.

References

1 Graham-Brown R, Bourke JF. *Mosby's Color Atlas and Text of Dermatology*. London: Mosby; 1998.
2 Winter G. A bug's life. *Nursing Standard*. 2005; **19**: 16–18.
3 Koning, S, van Suijlekom-Smit LWA, Nouwen JL *et al*. Fusidic acid cream in the treatment of impetigo in general practice: double blind randomised placebo controlled trial. *BMJ*. 2002; **324**: 203–6.
4 Koning S, Verhagen AP, van Suijlekom-Smit LWA *et al*. Interventions for impetigo. *The Cochrane Database of Systematic Reviews*. 2003: Issue 2. Art. No.: CD003261.pub2.
5 Nelson RRS. In-vitro activities of five plant essential oils against methicillin-resistant *Staphylococcus aureus* and vancomycin-resistant *Enterococcus faecium*. *J Antimicrob Chemother*. 1997; **40**: 305–6.
6 Bassett IB, Pannowitz DL, Barnetson RS. A comparative study of tea-tree oil versus benzoylperoxide in the treatment of acne. *Medical J of Australia*. 1990; **153**: 455–8.
7 Caelli M, Porteous J, Carson CF *et al*. Tea tree oil as an alternative topical decolonisation agent for methicillin-resistant *Staphylococcus aureus*. *J Hosp Infect*. 2000; **46**: 236–7.
8 www.hpa.org.uk/infections/topics_az/staphylo/MRSA_Guidelines_final_(revised)_aug98.pdf (accessed 20.06.05).
9 Dryden MS, Dailly S, Crouch M. A randomised, controlled trial of tea tree topical preparations versus a standard topical regimen for the clearance of MRSA colonization. *J Hosp Infect*. 2004; **56**: 283–6.
10 Edwards-Jones V, Buck R, Shawcross SG *et al*. The effect of essential oils on methicillin-resistant *Staphylococcus aureus* using a dressing model. *Burns*. 2004; **30**: 772–7.
11 Elsom GKF, Hide D. Susceptibility of methicillin-resistance *Staphylococcus aureus* to tea tree oil and mupirocin. *J Antimicrob Chemother*. 1999; **43**: 427–8.
12 Carson CF, Cookson BD, Farrelly HD *et al*. Susceptibility of methicillin-resistant *Staphylococcus aureus* to the essential oil of *Melaleuca alternifolia*. *J Antimicrob Chemother*. 1995; **35**: 421–4.
13 May J, Chan CH, King A. Time-kill studies of tea tree oils on clinical isolates. *J Antimicrob Chemother*. 2000; **45**: 639–43.
14 Nostro A, Blanco AR, Cannatelli MA *et al*. Susceptibility of methicillin-resistant staphylococci to oregano essential oil, carvacrol and thymol. *FEMS Microbiol Lett*. 2004; **230**: 191–5.
15 Opalchenova G, Obreshkova D. Comparative studies on the activity of basil L. – against multidrug resistant clinical isolates of the genera *Staphylococcus, Enterococcus* and *Pseudomonas* by using different test methods. *J of Microbiol Methods*. 2003; **54**: 105–10.
16 Skocibusic M, Bezic N. Phytochemical analysis and in vitro antimicrobial activity of two Satureja species essential oils. *Phyto Res*. 2004; **18**: 967–70.
17 Coung ND, Xuyen TT, Motl O *et al*. Antibacterial properties of Vietnamese cajuput oil. *JEOR*. 1994; **6**: 63–7.
18 Larrondo JV, Agut M, Calvo-Torras MA. Antimicrobial activity of essences from labiates. *Microbios*. 1995; **82**: 171–2.
19 Carson CF, Hammer, KA, Riley TV. In vitro activity of the essential oil of *Melaleuca alternifolia* against *Streptococcus ssp*. *J Antimicrob Chemother*. 1996; **37**(6): 1177–81.
20 Kandil O, Radwan NM, Hassan AB *et al*. Extracts and fractions of *Thymus capitatus* exhibit antimicrobial activities. *J Ethnopharmacol*. 1994; **44**(1): 19–24.
21 Raman A, Weir U, Bloomfield SF. Antimicrobial effects of tea tree oil, and its major

components on *Staphylococcus aureus, Staphylococcus epidermidis* and *Propionibacterium acnes. Lett Appl Microbiol.* 1995; **21**(4): 242–5.

22 Carson CF, Riley TV. Susceptibility of *Propionibacterium acnes* to the essential oil of *Melaleuca alternifolia. Lett Appl Microbiol.* 1994; **19**(1): 24–5.

23 Hayes AJ, Markovic B. Toxicity of Australian essential oil *Backhousia citriodora* (lemon myrtle). Part 1. Antimicrobial activity and in vitro cytotoxicity. *Food Chem Toxicol.* 2002; **40**: 535–43.

24 Inouye S, Yamaguchi H, Takizawa T. Screening of the antibacterial effects of a variety of essential oils on respiratory tract pathogens, using the modified dilution assay method. *J Infect Chemother.* 2001; 7: 251–4.

25 Hammer KA, Carson CF, Riley TV. Antimicrobial activity of essential oils and other plant extracts. *J Appl Microbiol.* 1999; **86**: 985–90.

26 Orafidiya LO, Oyedele AO, Shittu AO *et al*. The formulation of an effective topical antibacterial product containing *Ocimum gratissimum* leaf essential oil. *Int J Aromatherapy.* 2002; **12**(1): 16–21.

27 Dorman HJD, Deans SG. Antimicrobial agents from plants: antibacterial activity of plant volatile oils. *J Appl Microbiol.* 2000; **88**: 306–16.

28 Gangrade SK, Shrivastava RD, Sharma OP *et al*. Evaluation of some essential oils for antibacterial properties. *Indian Perfumer.* 1990; **34**(3): 204–8.

29 Cox SD, Mann CM, Markham JL. Interactions between components of the essential oil of *Melaleuca alternifolia. J Appl Microbiol.* 2001; **91**: 492–7.

30 Mann CM, Cox SD, Markham JL. The outer membrane of *Pseudomonas aeruginosa* NCTC 6749 contributes to its tolerance to the essential oil of *Melaleuca alternifolia* (tea tree oil). *Letts in Appl Microbiol.* 2000; **30**: 294–7.

31 Carson CF, Mee BJ, Riley TV. Mechanism of action of *Melaleuca alternifolia* (tea tree) oil on *Staphylococcus aureus* determined by time-kill, lysis, leakage and salt tolerance assays and electron microscopy. *Antimicrob Agents Chemother.* 2002; **46**(6): 1914–20.

32 Cox SD, Mann CM, Markham JL *et al*. The mode of antimicrobial action of the essential oil of *Melaleuca alternifolia* (tea tree oil). *J Appl Microbiol.* 2000; **88**: 170–5.

33 Brem-Stecher BF, Johnson EA. Sensitization of *Staphylococcus aureus* and *Escherichia coli* to antibiotics by the sesquiterpenoids nerolidol, farnesol, bisabolol and apritone. *Antimicrob Agents Chemother.* 2003; **47**(10): 3357–60.

34 Sikkema J, de Bont JAM, Poolman B. Interactions of cyclic hydrocarbons with biological membranes. *J Biol Chemistry.* 1994; **269**: 8022–8; cited in Cox SD, Mann CM, Markham JL *et al*. The mode of antimicrobial action of the essential oil of *Melaleuca alternifolia* (tea tree oil). *J Appl Microbiol.* 2000; **88**: 170–5.

35 Nelson RRS. Selection of resistance to the essential oil of *Melaleuca alternifolia* in *Staphylococcus aureus. J Antimicrob Chemother.* 2000; **45**: 549–50.

36 Sagdic, O, Ozcan, M. Antibacterial activity of spice hydrosols. *Food Control.* 2003; **14**: 141–3.

37 Sagdic, O. Sensitivity of four pathogenic bacteria to Turkish thyme and oregano hydrosols. *Lebensmittel-Wissenschaft und-Technologie.* 2003; **36**(5): 467–73.

38 Jeannot V, Chahboun J, Russel D *et al. Origanum compactum* Bentham: composition of the hydrolat aromatic fraction, comparison with the essential oil and its interest in aromatherapy. *Int J Aromatherapy.* 2003; **13**(2/3): 90–4.

39 Hammer KA, Carson CF, Riley TV. Susceptibility of transient and commensal skin flora to the essential oil of *Melaleuca alternifolia* (tea tree oil). *Amer J Infect Control.* 1996; **24**(3): 186–9.

40 Gueho E, Meyer SA. A re-evaluation of the genus *Malassezia. Antonie Van Leeuwenhoek.* 1989; **55**(3): 245–51.

41 Anon. *Mycoses Newsletter.* 2004; **9**(1): 1–25.

42 Inamadar AC, Palit A. The genus Malassezia and human disease. *Indian J Dermatol Venereol Leprol.* 2003; **69**(4): 265–70.

43 Cassella S, Cassella J, Smith I. Synergistic antifungal activity of tea tree (*Melaleuca alternifolia*) and lavender (*Lavandula angustifolia*) essential oils against dermatophytes infection. *Int J Aromatherapy*. 2002; **12**(1): 2–15.

44 Carson CF, Riley TV, Cookson BD. Efficacy and safety of tea tree oil as a topical antimicrobial agent. *J Hosp Infection*. 1998; **40**: 175–8.

45 Oliva B, Piccirilli E, Ceddia T. Antimycotic activity of *Melaleuca alternifolia* essential oil and its major components. *Lett Appl Microbiol*. 2003; **37**: 185–7.

46 Hammer KA, Carson CF, Riley TV. *In vitro* activity of *Melaleuca alternifolia* (tea tree) oil against dermatophytes and other filamentous fungi. *J Antimicrob Chemoth*. 2002; **50**: 195–9.

47 Hammer KA, Carson CF, Riley TV. Antifungal activity of the components of *Melaleuca alternifolia* (tea tree) oil. *J Appl Microbiol*. 2003; **95**: 853–60.

48 Mondello F, De Bernardis F, Girolamo A *et al*. *In vitro* and *in vivo* activity of tea tree oil against azole-susceptible and resistant human pathogenic yeasts. *J Antimicrob Chemoth*. 2003; **51**: 1223–9.

49 http://europa.eu.int/comm/health/ph_risk/committees/04_sccp/docs/sccp_o_018.pdf (accessed 10.10.05).

50 www.rirdc.gov.au/programs/tto.html (accessed 20.01.06).

51 Messager S, Hammer KA, Carson CF *et al*. Effectiveness of hand-cleansing formulations containing tea tree oil assessed *ex vivo* on human skin and *in vivo* with volunteers using European standard EN 1499. *J Hosp Infect*. 2005; **59**: 220–8.

52 Carson CF, Riley TV. Toxicity of the essential oil of *Melaleuca alternifolia* or tea tree oil. *J Toxicol Clin Toxicol*. 1995; **33**: 193–5.

53 Amvam Zollo PH, Tchoumbougnang F, Menut C *et al*. Aromatic plants of tropical Africa. Part XXXII. Chemical composition and antifungal activity of thirteen essential oils from aromatic plants of Cameroon. *Flav Fragr J*. 1998; **13**: 107–14

54 Ndounga M, Ouamba JM. Antibacterial and antifungal activities of essential oils of *Ocimum gratissimum* and *O. basilicum* from Congo. *Fitoterapia*. 1997; **68**(2): 190–1.

55 Patra M, Shahi SK, Midgely G *et al*. Utilization of essential oils as natural antifungal against nail-infective fungi. *Flav Fragr J*. 2002; **17**: 91–4.

56 Chaumont JP, Bardey I. The *in vitro* antifungal activities of seven essential oils. *Fitoterapia*. 1989; **60**(3): 263–6.

57 Shin S, Lim S. Antifungal effects of herbal essential oils alone and in combination with ketoconazole against *Trichophyton ssp*. *J Appl Microbiol*. 2004; **97**: 1289–96.

58 Misra N, Batra S, Mishra D. Fungitoxic properties of the essential oil of *Citrus limonum* (L.) Burm. against a few dermatophytes. *Mycoses*. 1988; **31**(7): 380–2.

59 Onawunmi GO. Evaluation of the antifungal activity of lemongrass oil. *Int J Crude Drug Res*. 1989; **27**(2): 121–6.

60 Onawunmi GO. Evaluation of the antimicrobial activity of citral. *Lett Appl Microbiol*. 1989; **9**: 105–8.

61 Wannisorn B, Jarikasem S, Soontorntanasart T. Antifungal activity of lemongrass oil and lemongrass oil cream. *Phyto Res*. 1996; **10**(7): 551–4.

62 Nenoff P, Haustein U-F, Brandt W. Antifungal activity of the essential oil of *Melaleuca alternifolia* (tea tree oil) against pathogenic fungi *in vitro*. *Skin Pharmacol*. 1996; **9**: 388–94.

63 Pandey KP, Shahi SK, Singh R *et al*. Antifungal efficacy of *Taxodium* and *Mentha* oils against some human pathogenic fungi. *Flav Fragr J*. 2002; **17**: 443–4.

64 Pina-Vaz C, Goncalves Rodrigues A, Pinto E *et al*. Antifungal activity of *Thymus oils* and their major compounds. *JEADV*. 2004; **18**: 73–8.

65 Perrucci S, Mancianti F, Cioni PL *et al*. *In vitro* antifungal activity of essential oils against some isolates of *Microsporum canis* and *Microsporum gypseum*. *Planta Medica*. 1994; **60**(2): 184–6.

66 Adam K, Sivropoulou A, Kokkini S *et al*. Antifungal activities of *Origanum vulgare*

subsp. *hirtum, Mentha spicata, Lavandula angustifolia* and *Salvia fruticosa* essential oils against human pathogenic fungi. *J Agric Food Chem*. 1998; **46**: 1739–45.

67 Hammer KA, Carson CF, Riley TV. In vitro susceptibility of *Malassezia furfur* to the essential oil *Melaleuca alternifolia*. *J Med Vet Mycology*.1997; **35**: 375–7.

68 Larrondo JV, Calvo MA. Effect of essential oils on *Candida albicans*: a scanning electron microscope study. *Biomedical Lett*. 1991; **46**(184): 269–72.

69 Hammer KA, Carson CF, Riley TV. *In vitro* activity of essential oils, in particular *Melaleuca alternifolia* (tea tree) oil and tea tree oil products against *Candida ssp*. *J Antimicrob Chemother*. 1998; **42**: 591–5.

70 Habif TP. *Clinical Dermatology*. 4th ed. Edinburgh: Mosby; 2004.

71 Gawkrodger DJ. *Dermatology, An Illustrated Colour Text*. 3rd ed. Edinburgh: Churchill Livingstone; 2002.

72 Minami M, Kita M, Nakaya T *et al*. The inhibitory effect of essential oils on Herpes simplex virus type-1 replication *in vitro*. *Microbiol Immunol*. 2003; **47**(9): 681–4.

73 Schnitzler P, Schon K, Reichling J. Antiviral activity of Australian tea tree and eucalyptus oil against herpes simplex virus in cell culture. *Die Pharmazie*. 2001; **56**: 343–7.

74 Farag RS, Shalaby AS, El-Baroty GA *et al*. Chemical and biological evaluation of the essential oils of different *Melaleuca* species. *Phytother Res*. 2004; **18**: 30–5.

75 Schuhmacher A, Reichling J, Schnitzler P. Virucidal effect of peppermint oil on the enveloped viruses herpes simplex virus type 1 and type 2 *in vitro*. *Phytomedicine*. 2003; **10**(6/7): 504–10.

76 Benencia F, Courreges MC. Antiviral activity of sandalwood oil against herpes simplex viruses-1 and -2. *Phytomedicine*. 1999; **6**: 119–23.

77 Armaka M, Papanikolaou E, Sivropoulou A *et al*. Antiviral properties of isoborneol, a potent inhibitor of herpes simplex virus type 1. *Antiviral Res*. 1999; **43**: 79–92.

78 Cox SD, Mann CM, Markham JL. Interactions between components of the essential oil of *Melaleuca alternifolia*. *J Appl Microbiol*. 2001; **91**: 492–7.

79 Tang J, Colacino JM, Larsen SH *et al*. Virucidal activity of hypericin against enveloped and non-enveloped DNA and RNA viruses. *Antiviral Res*. 1990; **13**: 313–26.

80 Benencia, F, Courreges MC. In vitro and in vivo activity of eugenol on human herpes virus. *Phytother Res*. 2000; **14**: 495–500.

81 Baudoux D, Zhiri A. Aromatherapy alternatives for gynaecological pathologies: recurrent vaginal Candida and infection caused by the human papilloma virus (HPV). *Int J Clinical Aromatherapy*. 2005; **2**: 34–9.

82 Whiteside TL, Herberman RB. The role of natural killer cells in human disease. *Clin Immunol Immunopathol*. 1989; **52**: 1–23.

83 Locke S, Kraus L, Leserman J *et al*. Life change stress, psychiatric symptoms and natural killer cell activity. *Psychosom Med*. 1984; **46**: 441–53.

84 Diego M, Field T, Hernandez-Reif M *et al*. HIV positive adolescents showed improved immune function following massage therapy. *Int J Neuroscience*. 2001; **106**: 35–45.

85 Hernandez-Reif M, Ironson G, Field T *et al*. Breast cancer patients have improved immune and neuroendocrine functions following massage. *J Psychosomatic Res*. 2004; **57**: 45–52.

Chapter 8

Childhood skin complaints

Introduction

Skin diseases are relatively common in childhood and the prevalence of conditions such as atopic dermatitis, a chronic inflammatory skin disease, has shown an increasing tendency to occur over the last few decades.[1,2] Immediately after birth the skin has to perform vital functions, such as thermoregulation, desquamation and protection against damage from external factors such as UV radiation and micro-organisms that it was not exposed to in utero. The skin of a newborn differs from that of adult skin in several ways and infants and young children are at increased risk of skin damage, toxicity from topically applied products and infection; they are especially susceptible to contagious skin diseases caused by viruses, fungi or bacteria. Transient, mild rashes are common with the true cause frequently not being discovered. There are a number of conditions such as atopic dermatitis, allergic contact dermatitis and irritant contact dermatitis, which result in severe skin eruptions with accompanying barrier breakdown enhancing susceptibility to irritation and sensitisation.

The use of CAM in paediatrics

The use of complementary and alternative medicine (CAM) by patients with skin disease, especially in those with chronic inflammatory conditions such as atopic dermatitis and psoriasis, continues to rise.[3] Complete clinical cure for such conditions remains unattainable and may account for why complementary treatments are sought. Further insight into the reasons for individuals using CAM is provided by findings from a survey in 2001 into why parents particularly chose CAM for their children.[4] Reasons included:

- word-of-mouth recommendation
- dissatisfaction with conventional medicine
- fear of side effects from conventional medicine
- greater personal attention
- having a child with a chronic condition.

A study into the use of complementary medicine in children with atopic dermatitis in secondary care showed the majority of patients used CAM on the recommendation of family and friends because conventional approaches did not sufficiently improve their skin condition.[3] Short- or long-term topical corticosteroid treatments are frequently prescribed and, while such therapy is very effective for reducing inflammation and itching, it is not curative and many parents are concerned about their local and potential systemic side effects (*see*

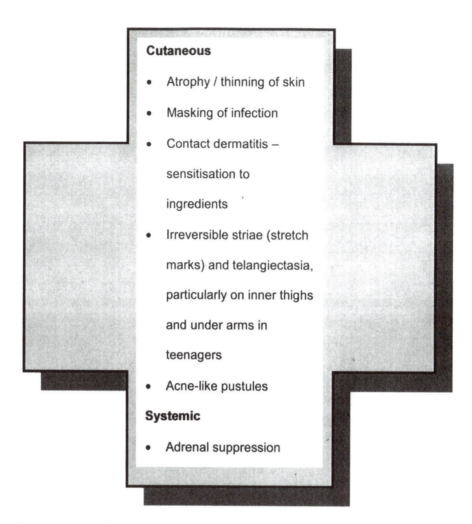

Figure 8.1 Side effects associated with topical corticosteroids.

Figure 8.1). Parents of children with this condition are notably turning to complementary medicine for health promotion as well as for treatment of the condition itself (ibid.).

Rational, informed adults are entitled to use any form of therapy, including CAM, to treat themselves. However, special issues arise when parents choose CAM treatments for their children[5] with some authors raising the issue of whether CAM should be used by children at all.[6] The use of aromatherapy for paediatric skin conditions falls within the same legal framework in the UK as other therapeutic interventions. The 1989 Children Act requires consent to treatment and the duty of parents and guardians is to ensure that children in their care receive appropriate treatment for any illness or condition they have. This has implications for therapists if they are aware that a known and effective orthodox treatment for the child's skin condition has been rejected in favour of relying solely and inappropriately on aromatherapy.

It is not the aim of this chapter to enable the reader to diagnose paediatric skin conditions or to promote the replacement of effective orthodox treatments. Rather, it is to illustrate that as a number of the conditions detailed here respond well to adjunctive aromatherapy care, ultimately this can lead to a reduction in the use of topical steroids and antibiotics and the promotion of health and well-being of the child.

Skin barrier functions in the neonate and young infant

Skin development

The skin is derived from two embryological sources, the mesoderm and ectoderm. Initially the embryo is covered in a single layer of ectodermal cells. At four to five weeks gestation the ectoderm is covered by the periderm, another single layer of cells. The peridermal layers proliferate and by the eighth week of gestation an intermediate layer is formed between the ectoderm and the periderm. It is in this intermediate layer that the stratum corneum is formed, being responsible for the barrier function of the skin. As the stratum corneum matures into stratified layers, the peridermal cells regress, slough and float around in the amniotic fluid, and become part of the vernix caseosa. Although the epidermis and dermis are correctly arranged by the end of the fourth month, the stratum corneum is thin and porous and the subcutaneous fat is poorly developed. It is not until the third trimester that foetal skin contains mature horny, granular and spinous layers together with a mature lipid bilayer and substantial subcutaneous fat. Premature infants therefore have an imperfect and compromised skin barrier, which is approximately two and a half times more permeable than adult skin.[7]

Transepidermal water loss (TEWL), a measure of skin barrier function, increases proportionally with immaturity, with TEWL in a 24-week gestational age infant being 10 times greater than a full-term infant.[8] By comparison, the full-term neonate has a well-developed epidermis, similar to the adult with respect to stratum corneum thickness and lipid composition.[9] The protective lipid film, which at birth is very similar to that of the adult, changes after a few weeks: the secretion of sebum, rich in waxes, diminishes and is replaced by lipids such as membrane cholesterol. At puberty, the secretion of sebum restarts, leading to more efficient skin surface protection.

Increased susceptibility to irritants

Despite similarities with adult skin, studies have shown epidermal and dermal development to be incomplete at birth[10] with the skin undergoing a process of maturation and adaptation during the first three months of life.[11,12] The skin of full-term newborns is known to be relatively susceptible to irritants, which cannot be attributed to a reduction in skin barrier function according to findings from TEWL studies.[13,14] Other variables such as pH and stratum corneum hydration may be involved: skin surface pH values in newborns are significantly higher in all body sites than those in adult skin, but stabilise to adult values within the first month.[12] Exposure to alkaline soaps and detergents is thought to inhibit stabilisation and irritate the protective acid mantle. There are also significant changes in the metabolic capacity of infants, whether full or pre-term, and adult levels of cutaneous enzyme activity are not observed until at least two months or even 6–12 months of age, which may additionally account for the susceptibility to irritants.[15]

Percutaneous absorption

Different considerations are needed for children and infants compared with adults when applying topical essential oil formulas. There are significant variations in absorption along with the potential for resultant systemic toxicity or damage to the epidermal barrier. Notably, the majority of reported percutaneous drug toxicity cases have happened in newborns although cases in infants and children have also occurred.[16] The ratio of skin surface to body weight is highest at birth and declines progressively during infancy. Therefore, whereas the proportion of the applied substance absorbed through the skin is equal, in the infant the total amount absorbed per kilogram will be higher than the adult. Other factors to take into account when applying anything to the skin of infants include their immature drug metabolism systems, the disruption or immaturity of the epidermal barrier and finally the properties of what is being applied.

Skin cleansing in children

Good skin hygiene requires effective cleansing to remove dirt, oil, environmental pollutants and bacteria from the skin while preserving its barrier function. Washing with water will not remove fat-soluble impurities; these require emulsification by detergents or surfactants to produce fine droplets that can then be removed by water. Detergents act by suppressing the surface tension that allows fatty deposits to remain on the skin surface. The greater the suppression of surface tension, the increased risk of damage to the epidermal structure.

The natural exploration and play of young children inevitably exposes them to micro-organisms, dirt and minor accidents that require cleansing. Several common childhood skin disorders such as atopic dermatitis and nappy rash are linked to varying degrees of barrier dysfunction and good skin hygiene practice is essential in the management of these disorders. When selecting suitable mediums for skin cleansing, remembering the distinctive properties of infants' skin that predispose it to irritancy, dryness and itchiness is vital.

Bathing

Special consideration should be given to the bathing of newborns, which in the past has proved controversial. It is now generally agreed that healthy full-term newborns can be bathed almost immediately after birth,[17] following the guidelines in Table 8.1.

The duration of the bath is short since overhydrated skin is more fragile, with the superficial skin cells becoming thicker, losing cellular cohesion, thus lowering the threshold at which friction can cause damage.[17] Bubble bath products are frequently used with older infants and are intended to replace soap and make bathing more agreeable. However, even when specially formulated for children, these can dry and irritate the skin, particularly when used at too great a concentration or too frequently.

Table 8.1 Guidelines for newborn bathing (adapted from Gelmetti, 2001).[17]

- Vernix caseosa should not be removed suddenly.
- Wash with water alone.
- Maintain bath temperature between 34°C and 36°C.
- Bathe for less than five minutes.
- On separation of umbilical cord use a mild detergent (neutral or mildly acidic pH).
- Apply detergent directly to the skin with the hands and rinse with fresh water.
- Avoid use of shampoos.
- Dry baby with cotton or linen towels, avoid vigorous rubbing and pay attention to skin folds.

Bath water is an excellent medium through which to administer essential oils to children, either for relaxation, the management of skin problems or simply skin cleansing. Essential oils do not disperse in water unless first mixed with a non-polar solvent such as vegetable oils, or to some extent full-cream milk (*see* Figure 8.2). Ethanol (alcohol), being both a polar and non-polar solvent, will dissolve oils and also dissolve in water. However, since alcohol has a drying effect on the skin, dispersion in lipid emollients is preferable but it is imperative that the child is observed at all times since the bath will become slippery. Dispersion in colour and fragrance-free shampoo bases is particularly popular with younger children as they provide bubbles in which to play.

Too much of a good thing?

The routine use of adding essential oils to children's baths is frequently advocated in popular aromatherapy literature. Unfortunately the potential risk for sensitisation or irritation is rarely addressed and too frequently oils that are recommended contain known sensitisers or components that are included in the fragrance mix patch test used in dermatology clinics. Exposure to fragrance allergens in cosmetic products starting at an early age may cause sensitisation, resulting in clinical contact dermatitis, and fragrances are cited as a common cause of contact sensitisation in children with atopic dermatitis.[18] Since the quantity and frequency of exposure to known fragrance allergens increases the

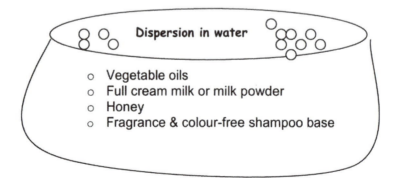

Figure 8.2 Mediums used for essential oil dispersion in water.

Table 8.2 Essential oils indicated for general skin hygiene, suitable for inclusion in baths for children over the age of two.

Boswellia carteri
Chamaemelum nobile
Citrus aurantium var. amara fol.
Citrus reticulata
Citrus sinensis
Lavandula angustifolia
Matricaria recutita
Melaleuca alternifolia
Melaleuca quinquenervia
Santalum album

risk of sensitisation and later elicitation, the repeated, routine use of a limited number of essential oils or a favoured blend is to be discouraged. Table 8.2 gives essential oils suitable for inclusion in baths as part of skin hygiene maintenance in children aged over two.

Hydrosols and skin cleansing

Hydrosols offer an excellent substitute or complement to essential oil usage in baths, since being distilled plant waters they do not require dissolution in a suitable solvent; their use reduces the potential for irritation and sensitisation and will not adversely affect plastic baths.[19,20] Suggestions for hydrosol use during bathing with infants and children include *Lavandula angustifolia* (lavender), *Chamaemelum nobile* (Roman chamomile), *Matricaria recutita* (German chamomile), *Rosa damascena* (rose) and *Citrus aurantium* flos. (neroli). In addition to bathing, hydrosols can be used with gauze or cotton wool as gentle cleansing wipes, as first-aid sprays on minor scratches and grazes and in hair rinses.

Dermatitis or eczema?

The term dermatitis is synonymous with eczema and describes a variety of non-infectious conditions characterised by sore, red, itchy skin. Allergic contact dermatitis, irritant contact dermatitis, and atopic dermatitis are the most common forms affecting children (*see* Table 8.3).

Any clinical variant of dermatitis may be acute, sub-acute or chronic and it is necessary to identify these three phases or stages in the dermatitis reaction, as they require different approaches to treatment (*see* Figure 8.3). At any one time, an individual may be experiencing a combination of stages. The symptom common to all three phases is itch or pruritus, causing children to rub the skin, which causes flare of the eruption with excoriation of the skin that subsequently becomes infected.

Table 8.3 Common forms of dermatitis affecting children.

Atopic dermatitis (AD) – a chronic relapsing skin disease, mainly occurs on flexural surfaces. Familial hypersensitivity of the skin to environmental triggers with increased production of IgE and xerosis, associated with asthma, allergic rhinitis and/or hayfever.

Irritant contact dermatitis (ICD) – for example nappy (diaper) dermatitis where the presence of moisture, friction, urine and faeces makes the skin susceptible to injury.

Allergic contact dermatitis (ACD) – an acquired delayed-type hypersensitivity reaction mediated by sensitised T lymphocytes. Most common contact allergens in infants include nickel, rubber components, and components of topical medications and cleansing products.

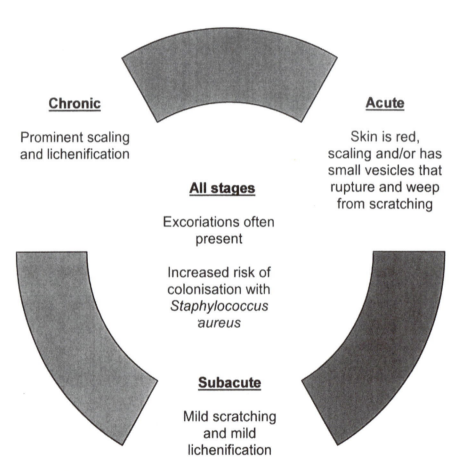

Chronic

Prominent scaling and lichenification

All stages

Excoriations often present

Increased risk of colonisation with *Staphylococcus aureus*

Acute

Skin is red, scaling and/or has small vesicles that rupture and weep from scratching

Subacute

Mild scratching and mild lichenification

Figure 8.3 The three stages of dermatitis.

Atopic dermatitis

Lichenification or thickening of the skin with exaggeration of skin lines is considered a trophic response to chronic rubbing and a typical clinical finding in atopic dermatitis. The distribution and type of lesions in sufferers of atopic dermatitis vary at different stages of childhood. Babies usually have facial involvement and patchy, red, vesicular and weeping lesions on the limbs or trunk. As the child ages, the pattern changes: facial lesions improve with lesions mainly affecting the inner surfaces of the limbs and flexural areas, skin becomes dry and the plaques show lichenification (*see* Figure 8.4). Figure 8.5 describes the interactions of the central features of atopic dermatitis.

There is strong evidence that genetic factors are important in the predisposition to atopic dermatitis, with maternal atopy causing a greater risk of atopic disease in the offspring than paternal atopy.[21] The increase in prevalence of the disease over the last few decades strongly suggests environmental factors in determining disease expression which may include: increased industrialisation and pollution, changes in the home environment such as insulation materials, synthetic fabrics, bed linen and wall-to-wall carpeting,[22,23] all of which may contribute to antigen exposure triggering disease. Provocation factors include aeroallergens (house dust mite, pollen), foods, microbes, contact allergens and irritants, climatic influences and stress.

Clinical considerations

Predisposition of infants' skin to irritancy, dryness and itchiness provides a challenging clinical dilemma when using aromatherapy as any breakdown of the skin barrier accelerates essential oil permeation and the risk of irritation and sensitisation.[24] Although it may be difficult for some aromatherapists to clinically assess the distinct problems posed by using essential oils and other natural raw materials, acknowledgment that these products have the potential to cause irritant contact dermatitis, allergic contact dermatitis and a flare of atopic dermatitis, encourages the innovative development of correct, informed treatment approaches.

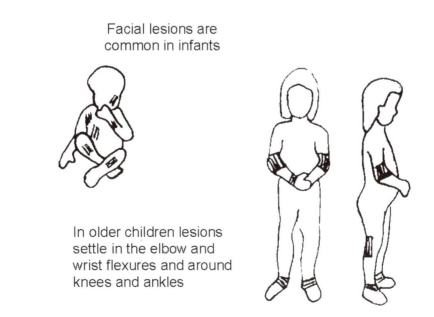

Facial lesions are common in infants

In older children lesions settle in the elbow and wrist flexures and around knees and ankles

Figure 8.4 The changing pattern of atopic dermatitis in babies and older children.

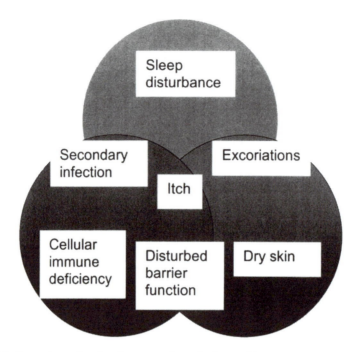

Figure 8.5 Central overlapping features of atopic dermatitis.

Important aromatherapeutic considerations when treating conditions with impaired skin barrier function are outlined in Figure 8.6. In line with advice given by essential oil specialists any essential oils containing known sensitisers should be avoided in children with dermatitis as well as doses of potentially irritant oils tempered considerably.[25,26] In children with skin disease, where essential oil formulas may be poorly tolerated, alternatives include the use of simple anti-inflammatory carrier or infused oils. *Calendula officinalis* (calendula) and *Hypericum perforatum* (St John's wort) infused oils are worthy of inclusion in formulas for their tissue-regenerating[27] and anti-inflammatory properties.[28] However, while judicious application of the latter is considered safe for children, excessive use may cause skin allergy[29] and lead to an increased susceptibility to the photosensitising properties of hypericin when applied to lesional skin.[30] Calendula CO_2 extract contains significantly greater concentrations of the active anti-inflammatory and healing triterpene monools, diols and their esters as compared with the typical infused oil[31] and up to 10% concentration can be applied even on young infants.[32] The infused oil is recommended for poorly healing skin tissue by the German Commission E, and has no known contra-indications.[28]

Allergies and nut and seed oils

The potential for nut and seed based carrier oils to cause type 1 sensitisation to nuts provides further treatment dilemmas. According to research by Lack *et al.*[33] the use of skin creams containing peanut oil to treat nappy rash, dermatitis and other inflammatory skin conditions in babies, may lead to peanut allergy in

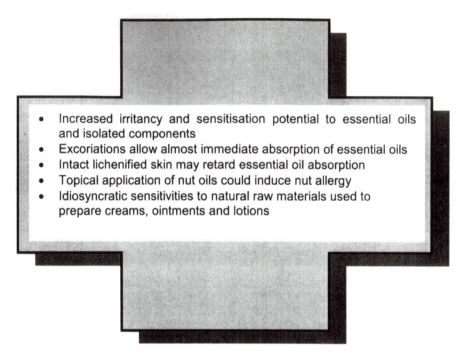

- Increased irritancy and sensitisation potential to essential oils and isolated components
- Excoriations allow almost immediate absorption of essential oils
- Intact lichenified skin may retard essential oil absorption
- Topical application of nut oils could induce nut allergy
- Idiosyncratic sensitivities to natural raw materials used to prepare creams, ointments and lotions

Figure 8.6 The altered skin barrier function in AD requires consideration of these factors for the topical application of aromatic preparations.

childhood. Children who had skin rashes over their joints and skin creases had more than a two-fold increased risk of peanut allergy, while in those whose rashes were oozing or crusting, the odds ratio increased to over five, indicating that exposure through inflamed skin is a cause of sensitisation. Sesame seed oil in cosmetics is known to induce hypersensitivity reactions[34] and severe allergic reactions to sesame are becoming increasingly frequent.[35] Since best aromatherapy practice uses unrefined, cold-pressed carrier oils that are more antigenic than refined oils, it is recommended that for babies and children with any form of dermatitis or inflamed skin condition, nut and seed carrier oils are avoided. Table 8.4 gives suitable alternatives.

Addressing the symptoms

Adopting a treatment approach, which is centred on an integrated, holistic model involving various therapy options, allows a truly individualised and effective programme to develop. Treatment strategies that take full account of disease severity and extent, along with the child's particular symptom picture, form the ideal approach.

Itching

Itching interferes with sleep, rest and concentration, which can all affect growth and learning. In the infant, since motor co-ordination is immature, itchiness is often shown by general restlessness and irritability. The sensation of itch is more

Table 8.4 Alternatives to nut and seed oil.

Borago officinalis
Calendula officinalis (infused)*
Carthamus tinctorius
Cocos nucifera
Hypericum perforatum (infused) *
Oenothera biennis
Simmondsia chinensis
Vitis vinifera

* These should not be used if infused in a nut oil.

frequently reported at night and it is suggested that children with atopic dermatitis can lose an average of two hours' sleep per night.[36] Sleep loss can lead to increases in daytime drowsiness, as can some oral antihistamines often prescribed to deal with the vicious 'itch–scratch–dermatitis–itch' cycle. However, the efficacy of antihistamines in this area is contested[37] since the underlying immune response is cell-mediated immunity in which symptoms are not mediated by histamine but lymphocyte secretions such as IL-4 and IL-5; nevertheless sedative antihistamines do promote sleep.

Lavandula angustifolia (lavender),[38] *Matricaria recutita* (German chamomile)[39] and *Melaleuca alternifolia* (tea tree)[40,41] essential oils have demonstrated antihistamine activity and in conditions that are mediated by histamine, such as irritation reactions, urticaria or hives, these oils can be effective at reducing inflammation. However, the question of whether they are useful in the specific control of itch currently remains unanswered as there is some evidence to suggest the contrary. For example, while *Melaleuca alternifolia* (tea tree) reduces histamine-induced skin inflammation, it has been shown to have no effect on the severity of itching.[41]

The use of sedative essential oils in the bath before sleep could reduce the need for oral antihistamines. Bathing has been shown to enhance the quality of sleep in young people, with body movements during the first three hours of sleep being less frequent.[42] The addition of sedative essential oils dispersed in an emollient vegetable oil to tepid-warm bath water not only promotes sleep but also moisturises the skin and may act as a reminder to parents to apply an emollient, essential first-line treatment for dryness and pruritus. The importance of varying oil selection and reducing dosages in order to prevent the development of allergic dermatitis needs to be remembered.

In children where bathing causes increased itching and irritation, direct inhalation of oils or vaporising is an option. Essential oils with sedative activity suitable for use in this area are listed in Table 8.5.

General approaches to control pruritus include formulating with anti-inflammatory oils and using cooling mediums such as gels, lotions, cool compresses or hydrosol sprays. There have been no reports of hydrosol-induced allergic reactions and as well as their use in bathing, they can be used to prepare compresses or be included in the water phase when formulating gels, creams and lotions. Used neat, liberal applications of *Achillea millefolium* (yarrow), *Lavandula angustifolia* (lavender) and *Hamamelis virginiana* (witch hazel) hydrosols are cited as alleviating itching, pain and peeling.[19] Hamamelis hydrosol has

Table 8.5 Essential oils with sedative properties, both proven and experiential.

Anthemis nobilis[43]
Citrus aurantium ssp. aurantium flos. *(neroli)*[44,45]
Citrus sinensis (orange)
Commiphora myrrha var. molmol (myrrh)
Lavandula angustifolia (lavender)[46-48]
Matricaria recutita (German chamomile)[49]
Origanum majorana (marjoram)
Santalum album (sandalwood)[50]
Valeriana officinalis (valerian)[51]

been shown to promote wound healing via anti-inflammatory effects and is widely used in skin-care products for the treatment of irritation and atopic dermatitis.[28,52,53] As they are prone to bacterial contamination, hydrosols must be shown to be free from contamination if used on broken skin.

Incorporating hydrosols into the wet wrap dressings that are often used in the orthodox treatment of atopic dermatitis to control itch is simple and effective. Following bathing an emollient or corticosteroid is applied to the skin and then covered with two layers of tubular dressing with the inner layer pre-soaked in warm water – this can be replaced with hydrosol-soaked dressing to provide additional therapeutic effects – and the outer layer applied dry. The evaporation of fluid from the bandages cools the skin, providing relief.

Inflammation

The acute stage of dermatitis is highly inflammatory and frequently exudative. Similar inflammatory mediators (prostaglandins, cytokines and leucotrienes) are common to all subtypes of dermatitis. There are three ways that essential oils have been shown to exert anti-inflammatory effects:

- through inhibition of the enzyme 5-lipoxygenase and hence leucotriene synthesis[54]
- through prostaglandin inhibition[55]
- through the stabilisation of mast cells[56] (*see* Table 8.6).

The treatment of exudative dermatitis starts with a compress prepared using anti-inflammatory oils and hydrosols. Wet compresses provide an anti-inflammatory effect and gentle debridement of crusts and serum. Repeated wetting and drying of the area eventually dries the lesion and the application of compresses is then stopped. Creams and lotions containing anti-inflammatory oils are then applied to provide a cooling, moisturising and emollient effect.

Infection

Due to constant scratching and hence excoriation of the skin, a major complication of dermatitis is secondary infection often caused by *Staphylococcus aureus*, which also acts as a 'superantigen', activating lymphocytes which further perturb an already disturbed immune response. Even clinically uninfected skin can harbour colony counts of *S. aureus* of infection-magnitude.[58] Antibacterial oils with proven activity against *S. aureus* such as *Leptospermum scoparium*

Table 8.6 Anti-inflammatory
essential oils indicated for use
in childhood dermatitis.

Chamaemelum nobile
Boswellia carterii
Cedrus deodara[56]
Commiphora myrrha[54]
Helichrysum italicum[54]
Lavandula angustifolia
Matricaria recutita[54,57]
Pogostemon cablin[54]
Santalum album[54]

(manuka),[59] *Melaleuca alternifolia* (tea tree),[60] *Melaleuca viridiflora* (niaouli),[61] *Santalum album* (sandalwood)[62] and *Vetiveria zizanoidies* (vetiver)[62,63] can be added to baths, creams and lotions to control colony counts when used at inhibitory concentrations. A honey-coloured crusting is regarded as a clinically significant impetigo and treatment options for this are found in Chapter 7.

Xerosis (dry skin)

As loss of integrity of the lipid barrier in the stratum corneum is a central factor in the development of dermatitis, it is very important that emollients and moisturisers are used for its restoration. Emollient products include creams, ointments, lotions and bath oils, all of which prevent the evaporation of water from the skin, thus mimicking the barrier effects of the deficient lipids and preventing penetration of irritants and allergens.

Generally, greasier oil-based products are the most efficacious but are often disliked by children and there is some trade-off required between efficacy and acceptability. Some over-the-counter emollient products contain potential allergens that can exacerbate dermatitis: creams and lotions usually contain preservatives such as benzyl alcohol and the hydroxybenzoates (parabens) or the surfactant sodium lauryl sulphate, which is notably found in aqueous cream. Alternatively, natural materials such as beeswax, cocoa butter, shea butter and vegetable carrier oils can be individually formulated to address allergen sensitisation and meet the cosmetic acceptability for each individual child.

The disturbed epidermal barrier function in atopic dermatitis is linked to altered metabolism of unsaturated fatty acids. Transformation of linoleic acid into gamma linolenic acid is impaired; this not only results in reduced barrier function but also a decreased production of arachidonic metabolites (prostaglandin E_1). As a result, there is decreased differentiation of suppressor T lymphocytes, allowing helper T cells and IgE production of B cells to dominate. Clinical studies to correct the deficiency using *Oenothera biennis* (evening primrose) and *Borago officinalis* (borage) oils, which contain the fatty acid gamma linolenic acid, have produced contradictory results. Some authors describe an improved epidermal barrier and amelioration of symptoms.[64,65] Work by Schliemann-Willers *et al.*[66] demonstrated that topical application of oils with higher linoleic acid and lower oleic acid contents positively influenced epidermal lipids in experimentally induced irritant contact dermatitis. Others, however, point to low efficacy with no statistically significant advantage over placebo.[67,68] Since topical application of these oils is well tolerated and some individuals have been shown to benefit, their inclusion in emollient formulations seems appropriate.

Sample cream preparation for childhood dermatitis

Cream base containing 20% *Calendula officinalis* infused oil.*
Essential oils:

- *Boswellia carterii* 30%
- *Matricaria recutita* 20%
- *Melaleuca alternifolia* 25%
- *Santalum album* 25%.

The concentration that is added to the base will be dependent upon a number of factors including: age of child, body surface area to which it is applied and skin integrity/lichenification. From experience for children under three years, 1.5–2% concentrations on lesions covering less than three-fifths of the body have proven effective in practice and with older children 3% concentrations have been used successfully.

Massage therapy

Children who suffer with atopic dermatitis have been shown to exhibit emotional disturbances, leading to behavioural problems.[69] The severity of atopic dermatitis has been correlated with depression, stress and anxiety, which all potentially cause negative effects on the immune system. Massage and tactile contact between a mother and child can reduce anxiety levels in children and improve clinical symptoms such as redness, scaling, lichenification and pruritus[70] as well as being vital in the developing parent–child relationship.[71]

Anderson *et al.*[72] investigated the use of essential oils and massage on children with atopic dermatitis who were unresponsive to orthodox treatment. Daytime irritation and night-time disturbances were reduced in those who received massage alone and massage with essential oils selected by their mothers. Unfortunately, during two subsequent eight-week treatment periods, symptoms deteriorated in those receiving essential oils. The authors concluded that adverse effects of repeated usage could overturn any short-term beneficial results, while the positive results from the massage were in part due to the emollient properties of the massage oil. On reviewing the oils selected by the mothers, this deterioration could potentially have been avoided by the inclusion of appropriate anti-inflammatory and skin-healing oils in the massage medium.

Exacerbation of atopic dermatitis

Irritants may be more important than allergens in causing skin inflammation in atopic dermatitis.[73] Low humidity, excessive use of soaps and hard water all increase the vulnerability to sensitisation and direct chemical irritation. House dust mites are the most important indoor allergen and can worsen atopic dermatitis via both inhalation and skin contact. The inclusion of essential oils

---

* Must not be infused in a nut oil.

in the washing of clothing and bedding can alleviate the need for washing above 55°C, a temperature necessary to achieve acaricidal effects. Essential oils found to be effective acaricides include eucalyptus, citronella, tea tree and spearmint.[74,75]

Although allergy to perfume is an increasing problem in adolescents and adults, sensitisation to perfume is unlikely in early infancy;[76] however, patch testing for fragrance mix commonly produces irritation reactions.[77] This tendency towards irritation in atopic dermatitis, along with disrupted skin barrier function, presents real therapeutic challenges. Patch testing is therefore an important and necessary safety procedure and guidelines are given in Chapter 3.

Nappy dermatitis

Common nappy (diaper) dermatitis, or 'nappy rash', is a prototypical example of irritant contact dermatitis affecting infants. Its prevalence is the same between sexes and races[78] with the peak incidence occurring around 9–12 months of age.[79] Contributory factors in its development include:

- overhydration of the skin
- maceration
- prolonged contact with urine and faeces
- friction
- topical preparations
- more than three diarrhoeal stools per day.

Areas that are in greatest contact with the nappy are typically affected with an erythematous scaly area often with papulovesicular lesions, fissures and erosions. The eruption may be patchy or confluent, with the skin folds usually being spared (*see* Figure 8.7).

Increased moisture in the area impairs the barrier function of the skin, subsequently increasing permeability of irritants and bacteria (and essential oils). Friction between the skin and nappy further damages the stratum corneum. Normal skin has an acidic pH, but the presence of urine and faecal urease increases the pH in this area. This change in pH enhances the activity of faecal proteases and lipases, which, together with prolonged occlusion, also contributes to the severe erythema and barrier disruption.[80] There is a clear association between the characteristic irritation of nappy dermatitis and the increased presence of digestive enzymes and bile salts in the faeces, as there is a correlation between the numbers of daily bowel movements and frequency of nappy dermatitis. Furthermore, breastfed infants have been shown to be less likely to develop moderate to severe forms of the condition compared to formula-fed infants due to lower stool pH and faecal enzymes.[79]

There is evidence to suggest that microbes do not play a direct role in causing the condition[81,82] but when there is damage to the skin barrier the potential for the development of a secondary bacterial or fungal infection increases. When nappy dermatitis has been present for more than 72 hours *Candida albicans* is likely to be cultured; a significant increase in the number of organisms has been found in children who developed nappy dermatitis following amoxicillin treatment for otitis media.[83]

A variety of primary skin conditions may manifest in the nappy area including seborrheic dermatitis, psoriasis, intertrigo, candidiasis, irritant and allergic contact dermatitis, although true allergic contact dermatitis is thought to be rare in

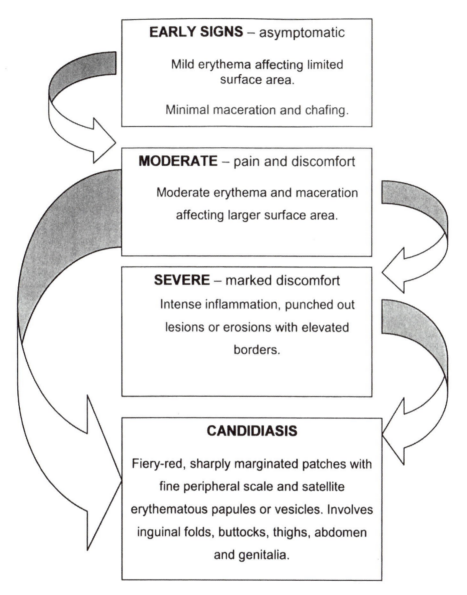

Figure 8.7 Signs and symptoms of nappy dermatitis.

infants due to immaturity of the immune system.[84] There are reports that rubber components in nappies may cause contact dermatitis on the outer buttocks and hips, referred to as 'Lucky Luke' since the inflammatory pattern is reminiscent of a cowboy's holster.[85,86]

Treatment options
Treatments for nappy dermatitis target the exacerbating factors: minimising exposure to urine, faeces, moisture and friction in the area. Educating parents and caregivers is essential for successful aromatic care, which can reduce the need for topical corticosteroid, antifungal or antibiotic medication.

Nappies

As the condition is strongly influenced by both the length of time a nappy is worn as well as its type, ideally it should be changed immediately following urination or defecation. According to Wolf *et al.*[87] in neonates it should be changed every hour and every three to four hours throughout infancy. Exposure to potential irritants may be minimised by exposing the skin to air whenever possible. The airtight occlusion from plastic or rubber pants, which were once used to cover cloth nappies, prevents the evaporation of water from the skin and results in increased hydration of the skin. Modern disposable nappies contain an absorbent gelling material (AGM), which is capable of absorbing at least 80 times their weight in liquid. Use of these is associated with reduced severity and frequency of dermatitis in comparison to home-laundered cloth nappies.[88] For children with mild and infrequent outbreaks, the choice of nappy is less significant and is often based on practicality, cost or environmental issues.

Aromatic cleansing

The use of harsh soaps or alcohol-impregnated wipes to cleanse the nappy area can further damage the barrier properties of the skin. Baby wipes that contain preservatives or fragrances are best avoided when the skin is broken as they are potential sensitisers.[89] Gentle rinsing with warm water and a minimal amount of mild soap, followed by patting the area dry, provides a simple, effective approach. Patting rather than rubbing keeps irritation to a minimum. If the area is eroded, gentle irrigation using soothing hydrosols such as *Chamaemelum nobile* (Roman chamomile) or *Lavandula angustifolia* (lavender) may be done using a plastic squeeze bottle or by squeezing a cloth soaked in the hydrosol. To remove dried faeces or pastes use either vegetable oils such as *Simmondsia chinensis* (jojoba) on a cotton ball or the simple nappy cleanse formula:

Nappy cleanse:

- 3 parts *Carthamus tinctoris* L. (safflower oil)
- 1 part *Hamamelis virginiana* (witch hazel hydrosol).

Use to cleanse the nappy area as necessary.

Barrier preparations, creams and lotions

Barrier preparations are useful for both the prevention and treatment of the condition. Ointments and pastes are generally more effective than creams and lotions in protecting the skin from irritants and micro-organisms. Zinc oxide ointment is ideal, having the following properties:

- antiseptic and astringent
- low risk for allergic or contact dermatitis
- significant role in wound healing.

Essential oils can be added to zinc oxide ointment or an emollient ointment can be prepared using natural lipid materials and vegetable oils. Since the absorption of essential oils in the nappy area is enhanced by occlusion and hydration of the skin, the concentration of essential oils in barrier preparations for frequent applications should not exceed 0.2% in children of three to nine months; if the skin is eroded, dosages are further reduced. Above nine months, dosage can

Table 8.7 Essential oils, hydrosols and vegetable oils with soothing, anti-inflammatory, tissue-healing or antifungal properties which make them ideal for use in preparations to treat and prevent nappy dermatitis. Sample formulations for barrier preparations and treatment.

Essential oils	Hydrosols
Matricaria recutita[54,57]	Lavandula angustifolia
Chamaemelum nobile	Chamaemelum nobile
Citrus reticulata	Matricaria recutita
Lavandula angustifolia	Hamamelis virginiana[28]
Boswellia carteri	For candidiasis:
Santalum album[54]	Melissa officinalis
Pogostemon cablin[54]	Thymus vulgaris ct linalol

Vegetable and infused oils	Candida-sensitive essential oils
Calendula officinalis[27,28]	Citrus aurantium fol.[62]
Hypericum perforatum[27,28]	Lavandula angustifolia[62]
Daucus carota	Melaleuca alternifolia[62,90]
Persea gratissima	Melaleuca quinquenervia[62]
Rosa rubiginosa	Origanum majorana[62]
Simmondsia chinensis	Pogostemon cablin[62]
	Santalum album[62]
	Vetiveria zizanoides[62,91]

Sample nappy barrier ointment	Nappy rash cream
Ointment containing: • beeswax • cocoa butter • Simmondsia chinensis liquid wax • Persea gratissima unrefined oil. Apply after nappy change.	Treatment of erythema without infection: • Lavandula angustifolia 5 drops • Matricaria recutita 3 drops • Citrus reticulata 6 drops • Rosa damascena 1 drop. In 100 g cream base containing 10% Calendula officinalis infused oil. Apply as necessary after each nappy change. If no improvement after three days seek medical advice as infection likely.

increase to 0.5%. Formulations require variation in oil selection to prevent the development of allergic contact dermatitis, and recommended essential and vegetable oils, plus hydrosols, are listed in Table 8.7. Acute and exudative eruptions are best treated with lotions and compresses for their soothing, cooling and drying effects.

Antifungal and antibacterial aromatherapy
If candidiasis is suspected or the condition has been present for more than 72 hours, the inclusion of essential oils effective against *Candida albicans* is required. For children over one year cream formulations containing non-irritant and non-sensitising antifungal oils (*see* Table 8.7) at a maximum concentration of 2% should be applied twice a day. If no improvement of the condition occurs after

three days or the condition worsens, treatment should cease and medical care given. Otherwise treatment should continue for one week after the eruption has cleared.

The presence of pustules may indicate a secondary bacterial infection requiring medical diagnosis and treatment. Adjunctive antibacterial essential oil therapy may lessen the duration of treatment necessary to eradicate the infection. *Lavandula angustifolia* (lavender), *Leptospermum scoparium* (manuka), *Melaleuca alternifolia* (tea tree), and *Thymus vulgaris* ct linalol (thyme ct linalol), which show broad-spectrum antibacterial activity (*see* Chapter 7), can be added to bath water or used when cleansing the area prior to the application of prescribed topical antibiotics.

Common viral warts

Warts are caused by infection of the epidermis with the human papilloma virus (HPV). Different HPV types selectively infect either the cornified stratified squamous epithelium of the skin or uncornified mucous membranes. The appearance of the wart is not only influenced by the viral type but also environmental and host factors. As anogenital warts require medical investigation and treatment, they are not included here.

Unusual in infancy and early childhood, there appears to be no gender difference in wart prevalence, which affects approximately 4 to 5% of school children and adolescents at any one time.[92] The appearances of common forms of warts affecting children are described in Table 8.8. Warts are spread either by direct contact from person to person or indirectly from surfaces; indirect transmission is favoured in the swimming pool environment when skin is macerated and in contact with roughened surfaces.[93]

In healthy children, warts resolve spontaneously as the immune system responds to the infection. Two-thirds of common warts in children can be expected to resolve within a two-year period without any treatment.[94] It is not known whether cell immunity is responsible for regression or whether destruction of wart-infected cells releases the virus, inducing the immune response. Remission is frequently heralded by capillary thrombosis causing punctate blackening of the wart. There is no specific antiviral treatment against HPV and medical treatment is still unable to offer a safe, painless and permanently effective cure.[93,95]

Essential oils and warts

Since HPV cannot currently be reproduced within a laboratory setting, experimental research is limited. The efficacy of essential oils specifically in relation to HPV is anecdotal and based upon empirical evidence. Existing antiviral research on other viruses may give some indication of potentially effective oils, but it must be recognised that drawing direct links solely from such evidence has its limitations. Used together with an understanding of therapeutic efficacy of oils closely based upon chemical criteria for their activity, along with case reports, this provides further insight into how essential oils may be used.

Many of those suggested contain dermocaustic phenols such as thymol in *Trachyspermum ammi* (ajowan), carvacrol in *Origanum compactum* (oregano) or eugenol in *Eugenia caryophyllata* (clove bud).[96] The application of such irritating oils to the surface of the wart, while at the same time avoiding the surrounding unaffected soft tissue, can be especially difficult in young children but this may be overcome by following procedures outlined below.

Essential oils containing the monoterpene ketone thujone have long been used in traditional herbal medicine to treat corns, warts and venereal warts.[97,98] In vitro research confirms that thujone possesses virucidal activity.[99] There are two isomers of thujone, α-thujone and β-thujone with α-thujone demonstrating greater toxicity with the potential to cause damage to the central nervous system and induce seizures.[100,101] *Thuja occidentalis* (cedarleaf, thuja) essential oil contains around 60% α-thujone and is considered too toxic for use in aromatherapy. However, it is reported by Opdyke[102] to be non-toxic when applied externally. The thujone content of *Salvia officinalis* (common sage) is less than that of *Tanacetum vulgare* (tansy) and *Thuja occidentalis* (cedarleaf, thuja), but is still considered equally as toxic by some. The German Commission E Monographs state that sage essential oil is contraindicated in pregnancy and prolonged use may cause epileptiform convulsions.[28]

In the case of a wart, only a very small fraction of the skin's surface is involved and essential oil flux through the hyperkeratinised and acanthotic wart will be slowed. *Salvia officinialis* (common sage) is well tolerated on the skin and can be safely considered for the treatment of warts in older children and adolescents. Baudoux and Zhiri[96] suggest *Salvia officinalis* as potentially one of the most effective essential oils for the treatment of HPV along with *Eucalyptus polybractea* ct cryptone (blue mallee eucalyptus) (*see* Table 8.9).

An unpublished study comparing the effectiveness of two home treatments, *Melaleuca alternifolia* (tea tree) and salicyclic acid (salactol), on the resolution rates of single plantar warts over a 12-week period demonstrated no significant difference.[103] However, *Melaleuca alternifolia* was shown to significantly reduce pain levels associated with plantar warts.

Table 8.8 Appearance of warts common in childhood.

Clinical name	Appearance	HPV type
Common warts	Irregular rough keratotic papules occurring commonly on the hands. More often multiple than single. Rarely painful.	1,2,4,5,7
Plantar warts	Rough keratotic surface, which protrudes slightly from skin surrounded by a horny collar. Distinguished from corns by presence of bleeding capillary loops. Often painful.	1,2,4,5,7
Plane warts	Multiple, smooth, flat-topped, skin-coloured or brown papules, 2–4 mm, found on face and brow and backs of hands. Not painful but inflammation occurs just before spontaneous remission due to an immunological reaction.	3,10
Mosaic warts	Rough marginated plaques resulting from the coalescence of common and plantar warts. Frequently found on the soles of feet but also seen on palms and around fingernails. Rarely painful.	2

Treatment procedure

The problems inherent in applying dermocaustic essential oils to warts while avoiding the surrounding tissue on small children are clear. They can, however, be overcome by following these procedures:

- Cut a hole in a piece of zinc oxide plaster that is just large enough for the wart to pass through before applying neat oil or formulation.
- Alternatively surround the edges of the wart with petroleum jelly to prevent essential oil contact with the healthy skin.
- Occlude the surface with a suitable non-allergenic dressing or film of petroleum jelly to enhance oil penetration into the hyperkeratinised stratum corneum.
- At least once-daily application is required, which may need to be continued for several months.
- Light rubbing with a pumice stone prior to oil application will encourage penetration. However, avoid the aggressive use of pumice as this can lead to secondary infection; warts cannot be pumiced away.
- Treatment needs starting as soon as warts first appear since the response rate of wart treatments decreases as their duration increases.[104]

Sample wart preparation
Essential oils:

- *Thuja occidentalis* 3 ml
- *Citrus limon* 1 ml
- *Lavandula angustifolia* 1 ml
- *Matricaria recutita* 1 ml.

Apply one drop twice daily to wart surface, avoiding contact with healthy skin.

Molluscum contagiosum

Molluscum contagiosum is a common contagious viral disease primarily affecting children and young adults with a peak age of onset in developed countries being

Table 8.9 Although research evidence is scarce for the use of essential oils in the specific treatment of warts, the chemical profiles of oils listed here suggest keen therapeutic interest.

Cinnamomum camphora ct cineole
Cinnamomum camphora ct linalol
Cymbopogon martini
Eucalyptus polybractea ct cryptone
Eugenia caryophyllata
Melaleuca quinquenervia
Melaleuca alternifolia
Origanum compactum
Rosmarinus officinalis ct verbenone
Salvia officinalis

in school-aged children.[105] It is caused by the molluscum contagiosum virus (MCV), a pox virus which only infects squamous epithelia.[106] Its pathogenesis is unclear since it cannot be grown in the laboratory and there is no animal model. The typical lesion is a small firm umbilicated papule with a smooth waxy or pearly surface. The base is sometimes erythematous and varies in size from 1 mm to 1 cm. The average child has between 10 and 20 lesions, which generally clear spontaneously in the immunocompetent in 12 to 30 months,[107] but can leave pock-marked scarring. The limbs, trunk and face are frequently affected. Skin-to-skin transmission is thought to be the main method of spread, with autoinoculation and scratching spreading lesions and causing secondary infections. The use of swimming pools and increased risk of infection are widely documented.[105,108,109]

Parents are generally concerned with the physical issues associated with infection such as scarring, itching, pain and the chance of spread to peers.[105] Since it is a self-limiting infection, the general recommended advice is to leave untreated and await spontaneous resolution. Allopathic treatments often rely on tissue destruction, causing pain, irritation and an increased risk of infection and scarring.

What can aromatherapy offer?

The use of aromatherapy can potentially:

- speed up the resolution of molluscum contagiosum
- reduce the risk of scarring and promote skin healing
- control itching so lessening scratching
- address secondary infection.

Anecdotal reports suggesting *Backhousia citriodora* (lemon myrtle) is effective against molluscum contagiosum have recently been supported by a study in children where 10% (v/v) *Backhousia citriodora* was applied to individual lesions at bedtime.[110] At the end of 21 days, nine of the 16 children treated showed a 90% reduction in the number of lesions compared to none of the 16 children who received treatment with only the vehicle. Redness around the base of some of the lesions was the only adverse effect reported.

The authors suggest that the moderate efficacious activity of the oil may be due to direct inhibition of viral propagation rather than non-specific tissue destruction. Citral is the main component in Australian lemon myrtle (85%) but it was not established whether this is the active component responsible for molluscum contagiosum inhibition. Its use and dosage needs to be considered together with research demonstrating skin sensitisation and cytotoxic activity caused by citral to human fibroblast cell lines when used at high concentrations.[111] The authors conclude it should not be used topically at concentrations greater than 1%. Formulating or blending with oils rich in d-limonene and α-pinene may potentially reduce or 'quench' the sensitising potential of *Backhousia citriodora*.[112] *See* Chapters 2 and 3 for a fuller discussion of this.

In a case report, Harris[113] describes the successful rapid resolution of molluscum lesions in an eight-year-old boy using *Melissa officinalis* (lemon balm), *Cinnamomum camphora* ct 1,8 cineole (ravensare) and *Melaleuca quinquenervia* ct 1,8 cineole (niaouli) which have claimed or actual activity against enveloped viruses (MCV being an enveloped virus). *Thymus vulgaris* ct thymol (thyme) was also included to provide antioxidant and immunostimulant properties. To prevent scarring and aid skin regeneration the essential oils were diluted in *Calophyllum inophyllum* (tamanu), *Hypericum perforatum* (St John's wort) and *Rosa mosqueta* (rosehip seed) oils.

Head lice

Head lice (*Pediculosis humanus capitis)* infestation is a common perennial problem in primary school-aged children (4–11 year olds), with girls suffering more often than boys since they generally have greater head-to-head contact while they play and chat. Figure 8.8 describes the three stages that occur in the life cycle of *Pediculosis humanus capitis*. Most parents and carers of young children know about head lice, yet there are still many myths surrounding them (*see* Table 8.10).

A child may not immediately show the characteristic itching that accompanies infestation and it may take a number of weeks before they become aware.[114] In cases where the skin has become excoriated through scratching, infestation can be further complicated by impetigo. A diagnosis of head lice can only be made if a living, moving louse is found.

The role of combing

Wet combing is more effective than dry combing for the detection and removal of lice, since the adult louse is immobilised by moisture whereas it moves quickly through dry hair.[115] Combing is promoted as a means of treatment ('Bug Busting') by the UK charity Community Hygiene Concern. Using a fine-toothed comb, combing should begin at the top of the head with the comb touching the scalp and drawn slowly through the hair to the ends. Lice are most often found behind the ears and at the back of the neck since they find food, moisture, warmth and shelter there. Traditionally, conditioner has been used to make combing easier but this can foam at the comb surface making lice detection more difficult. Ian Burgess, former Director of the Medical Entomology Centre, Cambridge, advises against the use of conditioners containing components such as panthenol and surfactants since they may lead to adverse reactions in addition to foaming. He suggests using olive oil, a useful scalp emollient, or grape seed oil, which he suggests has some insecticidal activity.[116]

A recent study by Hill *et al*.[117] compared the effectiveness of the Bug Buster Kit, comprising specially designed combs, with a single treatment of over-the-counter aqueous formulations of pediculicides containing malathion or permethrin. Wet combing was significantly more effective than the normal unsupervised use of the pediculicides. The results of this study are controversial since medical advice regarding the use of these insecticides is two doses, six days apart, despite this being an unlicensed use. Although wet combing is successful for detection purposes, the Bug Buster Kit only provided a cure rate of 57%.[117]

Aromatherapeutic interventions

Recommending that wet combing may need to be continued for up to two hours at a time and carried out four times over a period of at least two weeks,[116] despite

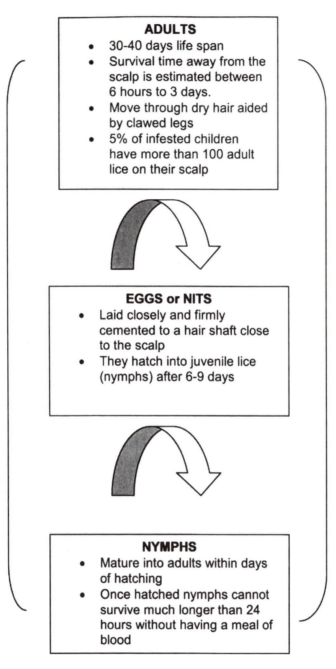

Figure 8.8 The life cycle of head lice.

being 'harm free', is not an easy task on a wriggling toddler. The impracticability of this advice, together with the development of resistance to current pediculicides and concerns over their safety,[118] has contributed to a search for 'natural' head lice remedies, including the use of essential oils. Frequently many medical journals and publications, despite acknowledging increasing interest, quickly

Table 8.10 Head lice – dispelling the myths.

- Adult lice do not hop, jump or fly. Prolonged head-to-head contact (over 30 seconds) is required for infestation to occur.
- Lice do not prefer dirty to clean hair. A healthy clean scalp provides a good blood supply on which to feed.
- Most often, fewer than 10 adult lice are found on the head.
- Having nits (egg cases) does not mean live lice are present.
- Using an insecticide does not stop a child getting head lice.

dismiss their usefulness, expressing concern that there is no conclusive evidence to support their effectiveness or toxicity.[119,120] While it is true that there are no double-blind, placebo-controlled clinical trials there is certainly evidence of pediculicidal and niticidal activity for some vegetable and essential oils,[121–124] which can be used to progress work in this area.

Suffocating vegetable oils

Olive, soya, sunflower and corn oils are reported as having the ability to kill a significant number of lice by suffocation of the lice spiracles if applied in liberal quantities for more than 12 hours.[125] Olive oil, although not able to kill 100% of eggs, has been shown to reduce egg hatch, probably by sealing the eggshell opening, thereby depriving the egg of oxygen.[126] It appears to be extremely difficult to drown lice on a host since they must be unable to breathe for at least eight hours continuously before mortality occurs (ibid.). Although keeping oily products on the hair for prolonged periods is not easy, if it can be encouraged, their use does lubricate the hair and scalp thereby facilitating combing and removal of lice and eggs. For such oily remedies to be an effective method of lice eradication, multiple treatments together with a great deal of combing are, however, required.[119]

The use of neem seed oil (*Azadirachta indica*) in healthcare products for the treatment of head lice is receiving increasing attention from parents looking for safe alternatives to the potentially toxic organo-phosphate and pyrethroid insecticides currently offered as front-line therapy. An effective pesticide and insect repellent,[127] neem oil has traditionally been used to treat a variety of skin, nail and scalp complaints. The primary active ingredient of the oil is azadirachtin, a potent natural insect antifeedant and growth regulator. It does not immediately kill but disrupts the growth and life cycle of the insect. The UK marketplace now supports many neem-based formulations for the eradication of head lice, many of which also contain essential oils: examples include Nitty Gritty™, NeemCare avoidance™ and Nice 'n' Clear ™.

Essential oils as pediculicides

Table 8.11 lists essential oils reported to be pediculicidal or niticidal.

Melaleuca alternifolia at 5% concentration has also been shown to be an effective acaricide in vitro against *Sarcoptes scabiei var. hominis* (scabies mite); terpinen-4-ol was identified as the primary active component.[133] The regular application of tea tree shampoo or conditioner for the prevention of head lice is frequently advocated by the media but overuse should be discouraged as this has

Table 8.11 Essential oils possessing pediculicidal and/or niticidal activity. Although some are unsuitable for topical use, especially with children, they are given to illustrate potential avenues for further research into natural alternatives to pesticides.

Pediculicidal	Niticidal
Cinnamomum zeylanicum[123,131]	*Eugenia caryophyllata* gem. and fol.[128]
Eucalyptus globulus[130]	*Eucalyptus globulus*[130]
Lippia multiflora[124]	*Cinnamomum zeylanicum* cort.[131]
Melaleuca alternifolia[123]	
Myristica fragrans[123]	
Myrtus communis[121,129]	
Origanum vulgare[123]	
Pinus sylvestris[123]	
Rosmarinus officinalis[123,129]	
Thymus vulgaris[123]	
Anise[132]	
Cade[129]	
Cardamom[129]	
Clove bud[129]	
Marjoram[129]	
Rosewood[129]	
Sage[129]	
Ylang ylang[132]	

not been shown to be an effective deterrent and there are increasing reports of sensitisation to the oil.[134]

Alcohol-based pharmacological lotions that have a contact time of 12 hours are reported as being more effective than aqueous formulations or shampoos. These products may not be in contact with the hair long enough and may be diluted too much during use to be effective.[135] Veal[123] showed that essential oils dissolved in alcohol produced greater mortality to lice and lice eggs if exposed overnight compared to when water was used as the solvent. Ethanol not only penetrates the insect cuticle faster than water but also aids dissolution of the glue attaching eggs to the hair shaft and degreases the skin aiding oil absorption. Interestingly the application of an oil/vinegar/essential oil rinse, following the alcohol-oil based treatment, appeared to greatly increase the effectiveness of the oils. The author suggests that it is the second application of the oils that makes the rinse effective, rather than the vinegar. A recent study by Takano-Lee *et al.*[126] confirms vinegar to be ineffective at killing live female lice or preventing eggs from hatching.

Inhalation of alcoholic fumes can be problematic for asthmatics and very young children. Advice from the Medical Entomology Centre in Cambridge, depending on the severity of asthma, is that alcohol lotions can be used as long as they are applied at least two hours before going to bed, close to the scalp and in the open air. For those that do not want to use alcohol-based products, combing is a better option.[116]

Phenols, phenolic ethers, ketones, oxides and aldehydes are most likely to be responsible for the pediculicidal and niticidal activity of essential oils (*see* Table 8.12).[123,124,131] It should, however, be noted that complete oils containing

Table 8.12 Essential oil components with demonstrated pediculicidal activity.

eugenol[124,128]	(–)-fenchone[124]
myrtenol[124]	(–)-menthol[124]
1,8 cineole[121,129]	limonene[124]
methyl salicylate[128]	citronellal[124]
α- and β-pinene[121,129]	
pinocarveol[129]	
γ-terpinene[129]	
α-terpineol[129]	
benzaldehyde[131]	
cinnamaldehyde[131]	
linalol[121,124,131]	
salicylaldehyde[131]	

concentrations of individual components that demonstrate activity may be ineffective on lice. This has been identified in *Rosmarinus officinalis*, an oil relatively rich in 1,8 cineole and also containing moderate levels of α-pinene.[123] The activity of the complete oil may on the other hand demonstrate greater inhibition than the isolated component, for example the acaricidal activity of *Melaleuca alternifolia* oil is greater than terpinen-4-ol alone.[133]

It is worth noting that like many current over-the-counter pediculicides, effective essential oils carry safety concerns. Formulations using essential oils require close attention regarding dose and chemistry to produce safe but potent pediculicidal effects. More information on essential oil safety can be found in Chapter 3.

Veal[123] suggests the mechanism by which essential oils exert their pediculicidal activity is through inhibition of acetylcholinesterase, like most commercial insecticides, which results in overstimulation of the nervous system. Yang *et al.*[131] suggest the mode of delivery of essential oils is most likely to be by vapour action via the respiratory system of the lice. *Cinnamomum zeylanicum* cort. (cinnamon bark) oil, and other oils which are considered unsafe for topical application, could potentially act as fumigants for treating objects. However, some authors believe there is a lack of evidence that transmission of head lice occurs via shared articles such as hats and combs since few lice fall off the head and those that do are likely near death.[125]

Practical advice for managing head lice infestations

- Early detection using a fine-toothed plastic comb reduces the time of treatment.
- Close contacts during the period preceding infestation should be examined and only treated if there is physical evidence of living lice.
- Wet combing as a physical method of lice elimination should be considered for asthmatics, the very young and pregnant women. This should take place every third or fourth day over a two-week period.
- Treatment is unlikely to be successful after only one application of essential oil formulation since it is unlikely that 100% of eggs will be killed. A second application one week later is advised to kill any lice hatched from the remaining eggs.

References

1 Williams H. On the definition and epidemiology of atopic dermatitis. *Dermatol Clin.* 1995; **13**(3): 649–57.

2 Wuthrick B. Clinical aspects, epidemiology, and prognosis of atopic dermatitis. *Ann Allergy Asthma Immunol.* 1999; **83**: 464–70.

3 Johnston GA, Bilbao RM, Graham-Brown RAC. The use of complementary medicine in children with atopic dermatitis in secondary care in Leicester. *Brit J Dermatol.* 2003: **149**: 566–71.

4 Simpson H, Roman K. Complementary medicine use in children: extent and reasons. A population-base study. *Brit J Gen Pract.* 2001; **51**(472): 914–16.

5 Mantle F. *Complementary and Alternative Medicine for Child and Adolescent Care.* Edinburgh: Butterworth Heinemann; 2004.

6 Spigelblatt L. Alternative medicine: a paediatric conundrum. *Contemp Pediatr.* 1997; **14**(8): 51–61.

7 Fischer LB. In vitro permeability of infant skin. In: Bronaugh RL, Maibach HI, editors. *Percutanoeus Absorption.* New York: Marcel Dekker; 1985.

8 Hammarlund KM, Sedin G. Transepidermal water loss in newborn infants III. Relation to gestational age. *Semin Neonatol.* 2000; **5**: 281–7.

9 Harpin VA. Barrier properties of the newborn infant's skin. *J Pediatr.* 1982; **102**: 419–25.

10 Evans NJ, Rutter N. Development of the epidermis in the newborn. *Biol Neonate.* 1986; **49**: 74–80.

11 Visscher MO, Chatterjee R, Munson KA *et al.* Changes in diapered and non diapered infant skin over the first month of life. *Paed Dermatol.* 2000; **17**: 45–51.

12 Hoeger PH, Enzmann CC. Skin physiology of the neonate and young infant: a prospective study of functional skin parameters during early infancy. *Paed Dermatol.* 2002; **19**(3): 256–62.

13 Willhelm KP, Cua AB, Maibach HI. Skin ageing effect on transepidermal water loss, stratum corneum hydration, skin surface pH and casual sebum content. *Arch Dermatol.* 1991; **127**: 1806–9.

14 Rougier A, Lotte C, Concuff TP. Relationship between skin permeability and corneocyte size according to anatomic site, age and sex in man. *J Soc Cosmet Chem.* 1988; **39**: 15–26.

15 Plunkett LM, Turnbull D, Rodricks JV. Differences between children and adults affecting exposure assessment. In: Guzelian PS, Henry CJ, Olin SS, editors. *Similarities Between Children and Adults, Implications for Risk Assessment.* Washington DC: International Life Sciences Institute Press; 1995. p. 79–94.

16 Marcini AJ. Skin. *Paediatrics.* 2004; **113**(4): 114–19.

17 Gelmetti C. Skin cleansing in children. *J Eur Acad Dermatol and Venereol.* 2001; **15**(Suppl. 1): 12–15.

18 Rastogi SC, Johansen D, Menne T *et al.* Contents of fragrance allergens in children's cosmetics and cosmetic-toys. *Contact Derm.* 1999; **41**: 84–8.

19 Catty S. *Hydrosols: the next aromatherapy.* Vermont: Healing Arts Press; 2001.

20 Price L, Price S. *Understanding Hydrolats: the specific hydrosols for aromatherapy.* Edinburgh: Churchill Livingstone; 2004.

21 Schultz Larsen F. Genetic epidemiology of atopic dermatitis. In: Williams HC, editor. *Atopic Dermatitis.* Cambridge: Cambridge University Press; 2000. p. 113–24.

22 McNally NJ, Williams HC, Phillips DR. Atopic eczema and the home environment. *Br J Dermatol.* 2001; **145**: 730–6.

23 Williams HC. Epidemiology of atopic dermatitis. *Clin Exp Dermatol.* 2000; **25**: 522–9.

24 Buck P. Skin barrier function: effect of age, race and inflammatory disease. *Int J Aromatherapy.* 2004; **14**: 70–6.

25 Burfield T, Sheppard Hanger S. *Essential Safety: sensitisation revisited again.* Atlantic Institute of Aromatherapy. www.atlanticinstitute.com/es_spring2000.html (accessed 20.09.05).

26 Guba R. Toxicity myths – the actual risks of essential oil use. *Int J Aromatherapy.* 2000; **10**(1/2): 37–49.

27 Lavagna SM, Secci D, Chimenti P *et al.* Efficacy of hypericum and calendula oils in the epithelial reconstruction of surgical wounds in childbirth with caesarean section. *Il Farmaco.* 2001; **56**: 451–3.

28 Blumenthal M, editor. *The Complete German Commission E Monographs.* Austin, Texas: American Botanical Council; 1998.

29 Price L. *Carrier Oils for Aromatherapy and Massage.* Stratford-upon-Avon: Riverhead; 1999.

30 Schempp CM, Ludtke R, Winghofer B *et al.* Effect of topical application of Hypericum perforatum extract (St John's wort) on skin sensitivity to solar simulated radiation. *Photodermatol Photoimmunol Photomed.* 2000; **16**: 125–8.

31 Guba R. The modern alchemy of carbon dioxide extraction. *Int J Aromatherapy.* 2002; **12**(3): 120–6.

32 Quirin, K, Gerard, D. New aspects on calendula CO_2 extract as a cosmetic ingredient. *Cosmetics Toiletries.* 1999; **112**(4): 55–8.

33 Lack G, Fox D, Northstone K *et al.* Factors associated with the development of peanut allergy in childhood. *N Eng J Med.* 2003; **348**: 977–85.

34 Pecquet C, Leynadier F, Saiag P. Immediate hypersensitivity to sesame in foods and cosmetics. *Contact Derm.* 1998; **39**: 313.

35 Levy Y, Danon YL. Allergy to sesame seed in infants. *Allergy.* 2001; **56**: 193–4.

36 Reid P, Lewis-Jones MS. Sleep difficulties and their management in pre-schoolers with atopic eczema. *Clin Exp Dermatol.* 1995; **20**: 38–41.

37 Klein PA, Clark RA. An evidence based review of the efficacy of antihistamines in relieving pruritus in atopic dermatitis. *Arch Dermatol.* 1999; **135**(12): 1522–5.

38 Kim HM, Cho SH. Lavender oil inhibits immediate-type allergic reaction in mice and rats. *J Pharm Pharmacol.* 1999; **51**(2): 221–6.

39 Miller TM, Wittstock U, Lindequist U. Effects of some components of the essential oil of chamomile, *Chamomilla recutita*, on histamine release from rat mast cells. *Planta Med.* 1996; **62**(1): 60–1.

40 Khalil Z, Pearce AL, Satkunanathan N. Regulation of wheal and flare by tea tree oil: complementary human and rodent studies. *J Invest Dermatol.* 2004; **123**: 683–90.

41 Koh KJ, Pearce AL, Marshman G. Tea tree oil reduces histamine induced skin inflammation. *Br J Dermatol.* 2002; **147**: 1212–17.

42 Khanda K, Tochihara Y, Ohnaka T. Bathing before sleep in the young and in the elderly. *Eur J Appl Physiol Occup Physiol.* 1999; **80**: 71–5.

43 Rossi T, Melegari M, Bianchi A. Sedative, anti-inflammatory and anti-diuretic effects induced in rats by essential oil varieties of *Anthemis nobilis:* a comparative study. *Pharmacol Res Commun.* 1998; **20**(Suppl. 5): 71–4.

44 Buchbauer G, Jirovetz L, Jager W *et al.* Fragrance compounds and essential oils with sedative effects upon inhalation. *J Pharm Sci.* 1993; **82**(6): 660–4.

45 Miyake Y, Nakagawa M, Asakuru Y. Effects of odours on humans (1): effects on sleep latency. *Chem Senses.* 1991; **16**(2): 183.

46 Hardy M, Kirk-Smith MD, Stretch DD. Replacement of drug treatment for insomnia by ambient odour. *Lancet.* 1995; **346**: 701.

47 Karamat E, Ilmberger J, Buchbauer G. Excitatory and sedative effects of essential oil on human reaction time performance. *Chem Senses.* 1992; **17**: 847.

48 Buchbauer G, Jirovetz L, Jager W. Aromatherapy evidence for sedative effects of the essential oil of lavender after inhalation. *Z Naturforsch C.* 1991; **46**(11–12): 1067–102.

49 Viola H, Waowaski C, Levi de Stein M *et al.* Apigenin, a component of *Matricaria recutita* flowers, is a benzodiazepine receptor-ligand with anxiolytic effects. *Planta Med.* 1995; **61**(3): 213–16.

50 Hongratanaworakit T, Heuberger E, Buchbauer G. Evaluation of the effects of east Indian sandalwood oil and α-santalol on humans after trans dermal absorption. *Planta Med.* 2004; **70**: 3–7.

51 Houghton PJ. The scientific basis for the reputed activity of valerian. *J Pharm Pharmacol.* 1999; **51**: 505–12.

52 Korting HC, Schafer-Korting M, Hart H *et al.* Anti-inflammatory activity of Hamamelis distillate applied topically to the skin. Influence of dose vehicle and dose. *Eur J Clin Pharmacol.* 1993; **44**: 315–18.

53 Korting HC, Schafer-Korting M, Klovekorn W *et al.* Comparative efficacy of Hamamelis distillate and hydrocortisone cream in atopic eczema. *Eur J Clin Pharmacol.* 1995; **48**: 461–5.

54 Baylac S, Racine P. Inhibition of 5-lipoxygenase by essential oils and other natural fragrant extracts. *Int J Aromatherapy.* 2003; **13**(2/3): 138–42.

55 Krishnamoorthy G, Kavimani S, Loganathan C *et al.* Anti-inflammatory activity of the essential oil of *Cymbopogon martini. Ind J Pharm Sci.* 1998; **60**(2): 114–16.

56 Shinde UA, Kulkarni KR, Phadke AS *et al.* Mast cell stabilising and lipoxygenase inhibitory activity of *Cedrus deodara* (Roxb.) Loud. Wood oil. *Ind J Exp Biol.* 1999; **37**: 258–61.

57 Safayhi H, Sabieraj J, Sailer ER *et al.* Chamazulene: an antioxidant type inhibitor of leucotriene B4. *Planta Med.* 1994; **60**: 410–13.

58 Leicht S, Hanggi M. Atopic dermatitis: how to incorporate advances in management. *Postgrad Med.* 2001; **109**: 111–31.

59 Porter NG, Wilkins AL. Chemical, physical and antimicrobial properties of essential oils of *Leptospermum scoparium* and *Kunzea ericoides. Phytochemistry.* 1999; **50**(3): 407–15.

60 Nelson RRS. In vitro activities of five plant essential oils against methicillin-resistant *Staphylococcus aureus* and vancomycin-resistant *Enterococcus faecium. J Antimicrob Chemother.* 1997; **40**: 305–6.

61 Ramanoelina AR, Terrom GP, Bianchini JP *et al.* Antibacterial action of essential oils extracted from Madagascan plants. *Arch Inst Pasteur Madagascar.* 1987; **53**(1): 217–26.

62 Hammer KA, Carson CF, Riley TV. Antimicrobial activity of essential oils and other plant extracts. *J of Appl Microbiol.* 1999; **86**: 985–90.

63 Gangrade SK, Shrivastava RD, Sharma OP *et al.* Evaluation of some essential oils for antibacterial properties. *Indian Perfumer.* 1990; **34**(3): 204–8.

64 Gehring W, Bopp R, Ripkke F *et al.* Effect of a topically applied evening primrose oil on epidermal barrier function in atopic dermatitis as a function of vehicle. *Drug Res.* 1999; **49**: 635–42.

65 Andreassi M, Forleo P, Di Lorio A *et al.* Efficacy of γ-linoleic acid in the treatment of patients with atopic dermatitis. *J Int Med Res.* 1997; **25**: 266–74.

66 Schliemann-Willers S, Wigger-Alberti W, Kleesz P *et al.* Natural vegetable fats in the prevention of irritant contact dermatitis. *Contact Derm.* 2002; **46**: 6–12.

67 Worm M, Henz BM. Novel unconventional therapeutic approaches to atopic dermatitis. *Dermatology.* 2000; **201**: 191–5.

68 Borrek S, Hildebrandt A, Forster J. Gamma-linoleic-acid-rich borage seed oil capsules in children with atopic dermatitis: a placebo-controlled double blind study. *Klin Padiatr.* 1997; **209**: 100–4.

69 Daud L, Garralda M, David T. Psychological adjustment in pre-school children with atopic eczema. *Arch Dis Child.* 1993; **68**: 670–6.

70 Schachner L, Field T, Hernandez-Reif M *et al.* Atopic dermatitis symptoms decreased in children following massage therapy. *Paed Dermatol.* 1998; **15**(5): 390–5.

71 Titman P. The impact of skin disease on children and their families. In: Walker C, Papadopoulos L, editors. *Psychodermatology*. Cambridge: Cambridge University Press; 2005. p. 89–100.

72 Anderson C, Lis-Balchin M, Kirk-Smith M. Evaluation of massage with essential oils on childhood atopic dermatitis. *Phytother Res*. 2000; **14**: 452–6.

73 Williams HC. Atopic dermatitis. In: Williams HC, Strachan DP, editors. *The Challenge of Dermato-Epidemiology*. Boca Raton: CRC Press; 1997. p. 13–24.

74 Tovey ER, McDonald LG. A simple washing procedure with eucalyptus oil for controlling house dust mites and their allergens in clothing and bedding. *J Allergy Clin Immunol*. 1997; **100**(4): 464–6.

75 Mcdonald LG, Tovey E. The effectiveness of benzyl benzoate and some essential oils as laundry additives for killing dust mites. *J Allergy Clin Immunol*. 1993; **92**: 771–2.

76 Johnke H, Norberh LA, Vach W *et al*. Reactivity to patch tests with nickel sulphate and fragrance mix in infants. *Contact Derm*. 2004; **51**: 141–7.

77 Carder RK. Hypersensitivity reactions in neonates and infants. *Dermatol Ther*. 2005; **18**: 160–75.

78 Ward DB, Fleischer AB, Feldman SR *et al*. Characterisation of diaper dermatitis in the United States. *Arch Pediatr Adolesc Med*. 2000; **154**: 943–6.

79 Jordan WE, Lawson KD, Franxman JJ *et al*. Diaper dermatitis: frequency and severity among a general infant population. *Pediatr Dermatol*. 1986; **3**: 198–207.

80 Andersen PH, Bucher AP, Saeed I *et al*. Faecal enzymes: in vivo human skin irritation. *Contact Derm*. 1994; **30**: 152–8.

81 Brookes DB, Hubbert RM, Sarkany I. Skin flora of infants with napkin rash. *Br J Dermatol*. 1971; **85**: 250–3.

82 Montes LF, Pittillo RF, Hunt D *et al*. Comparison of types of microorganisms between normal skin and diaper dermatitis. *Arch Dermatol*. 1971; **103**: 400–6.

83 Honig PJ, Gribetz B, Leyden JJ *et al*. Amoxicillin and diaper dermatitis. *J Am Acad Dermatol*. 1988; **19**: 275–9.

84 Shin HT. Diaper dermatitis that does not quit. *Dermatol Ther*. 2005; **18**: 124–35.

85 Roul S, Ducombs G, Leaute-Labreze C *et al*. 'Lucky Luke' contact dermatitis due to rubber components in diapers. *Contact Derm*. 1988; **38**: 363–4.

86 Larralde M, Raspa ML, Silvia H *et al*. Diaper dermatitis: a new clinical feature. *Pediatr Dermatol*. 2001; **18**(2): 167–8.

87 Wolf R, Wolf D, Tuzan B *et al*. Diaper dermatitis. *Clin Dermatol*. 2000; **18**: 657–60.

88 Campbell RL, Bartlett AV, Sarbaugh FC *et al*. Effects of diaper types on diaper dermatitis associated with diarrhoea and antibiotic use in children in day care centres. *Pediatr Dermatol*. 1988; **5**: 83–7.

89 Manzini BM, Ferdani G, Simonetti V *et al*. Contact sensitization in children. *Pediatr Dermatol*. 1998; **15**: 12–17.

90 Nenoff P, Haustein U-F, Brandt W. Antifungal activity of the essential oil of *Melaleuca alternifolia* (tea tree oil) against pathogenic fungi *in vitro*. *Skin Pharmacol*. 1996; **9**: 388–94.

91 Chaumont JP, Bardey I. The *in vitro* antifungal activities of seven essential oils. *Fitoterapia*. 1989; **60**(3): 263–6.

92 Williams HC, Potter A, Strachan D. The descriptive in British schoolchildren. *Br J Dermatol*. 1993; **128**: 504–11.

93 Sterling JC, Handfield-Jones S, Hudson PM. Guidelines for the management of cutaneous warts. *Br J Dermatol*. 2001; **144**: 4–11.

94 Massing AM, Estonia WL. Natural history of warts; a two year study. *Arch Dermatol*. 1963; **87**: 306–10.

95 Torello A. What's new in the treatment of viral warts in children. *Pediatr Dermatol*. 2002; **19**(3): 191–9.

96 Baudoux D, Zhiri A. Aromatherapy alternatives for gynaecological pathologies: recurrent vaginal *Candida* and infection caused by the human papilloma virus (HPV). *Int J Clinical Aromatherapy.* 2005; **2**(1): 34–9.

97 Albert-Puelo M. Mythobotany, pharmacology, chemistry of thujone containing plants and derivatives. *Econ Bot.* 1978; **32**(1): 65–74.

98 Dupont P. Cosmetic compositions for the treatment of corns and warts comprising of plant tinctures and essential oils. Pat. no. Fr 2710266 (Abstract AL23–017496X). 1995.

99 Sivropoulou A, Nikolaou C, Papanikolaou E *et al*. Antimicrobial, cytotoxic and antiviral activities of Salvia fructicosa essential oil. *J Agric Food Chem.* 1997; **45**(3): 197–201.

100 Hold KM, Sirismoa NS, Ikeda T *et al*. Alpha-thujone (the active component of absinthe): gamma-aminobutyric acid type A receptor modulation and metabolic detoxification. *Proc Natl Acad Sci USA.* 2000; **97**(9): 4417–18.

101 Burkhard PR, Burkhardt K, Haenggeli CA *et al*. Plant-induced seizures; reappearance of an old problem. *J Neurol.* 1999; **246**: 667–70.

102 Opdyke DLJ. Fragrance raw materials monographs. Cedar leaf oil. *Food Cosmet Toxicol.* 1974; **12**(Suppl.): 843–4.

103 James L. A random controlled trial to compare the effects of two home treatments: *Melaleuca alternifolia* and salicyclic acid (Salactol) on the resolution rates of verrucae pedis. BSc dissertation, University College Northampton. 2000.

104 Bunney MH, Benson C, Cubie HA. *Viral Warts: biology and treatment.* 2nd ed. Oxford: Oxford Medical Publishing; 1992.

105 Braue A, Ross G, Varigos G *et al*. Epidemiology and impact of childhood molluscum contagiosum: a case series and critical review of the literature. *Pediatr Dermatol.* 2005; **22**(4): 287–94.

106 Gottlieb SL, Myskowski PL. Molluscum contagiosum. *Int J Dermatol.* 1994; **33**: 453–61.

107 Husar K, Skerlev M. Molluscum contagiosum from infancy to maturity. *Clin Dermatol.* 2002; **20**: 170–2.

108 Castilla MT, Sanzo JM, Fuentes S. Molluscum contagiosum in children and its relationship to attendance at swimming pools: an epidemiological study. *Dermatology.* 1995; **191**: 165.

109 Choong KY, Roberts LJ. Molluscum contagiosum, swimming and bathing: a clinical analysis. *Australas J Dermatol.* 1999; **40**: 89–92.

110 Burke BE, Baillie JE, Olson RD. Essential oil of Australian lemon myrtle (*Backhousia citriodora*) in the treatment of molluscum contagiosum in children. *Biomed Pharmacother.* 2004; **58**: 245–7.

111 Hayes AJ, Markovic B. Toxicity of Australian essential oil *Backhousia citriodora* (Lemon myrtle). Part 1. Antimicrobial activity and in vitro cytotoxicity. *Food Chem Toxicol.* 2001; **40**: 535–43.

112 Opdyke DLJ. Inhibition of sensitization reactions induced by certain aldehydes. *Food Cosmet Toxicol.* 1976; **14**: 197–8.

113 Harris R. Case study Molluscum contagiosum. *Int J Aromatherapy.* 2004; **14**: 139–40.

114 Koch T, Brown M, Selim P *et al*. Towards the eradication of head lice: literature review and research agenda. *J Clin Nurs.* 2001; **10**: 364–71.

115 Burkhart CG, Burkhart CN, Burkhart KM. An assessment of topical and oral prescription and over-the-counter treatments for head lice. *J Am Acad Dermatol.* 1998; **38**(6 Pt 1): 979–82.

116 Burgess I. Pharmacy-based head lice management. *Pharm J.* 2001; **267**(7164): 317.

117 Hill N, Moor G, Cameron MM. Single blind, randomised comparative study of the Bug Buster kit and over the counter pediculicide treatments against head lice in the United Kingdom. *BMJ.* 2005; **331**: 384–7.

118 Willis J. Are head lice treatments poisoning our children? *Health Visitor.* 1999; **71**(1): 25–7.

119 Meinking TL. Infestations. *Curr Probl Dermatol.* 1999; **11**: 73–120.

120 Nash B. Treating head lice. *BMJ.* 2003; **326**: 1256–7.

121 Gauthier R, Agoumi A, Gourai M. Activite d'extraits de Myrtus communis contre. *Pediculus humanus capitis. Plantes Med Phytother.* 1989; **23**(2): 95–108.

122 Oladimeji FA, Orafidija OO, Ogunniyi TA. Pediculocidal and scabicidal properties of *Lippia multiflora* essential oil. *J Ethanopharmacol.* 2000; **72**: 305–11.

123 Veal L. The potential effectiveness of essential oils as a treatment for headlice, *Peiculus humanus capitis. Complement Ther Nurs Midwifery.* 1996; **2**: 97–101.

124 Lahlou M, Berrada R, Agoumi A. The potential effectiveness of essential oils in the control of human head lice in Morocco. *Int J Aromatherapy.* 2000; **10**(3/4): 108–23.

125 Mumcuoglu KY. Prevention and treatment of head lice in children. *Paediatr Drugs.* 1999; **1**(3): 211–18.

126 Takano-Lee M, Edman J, Mullens BA *et al.* Home remedies to control head lice: assessment of home remedies to control the human head louse, *Pediculus humanus capitis* (Anoplura: Pediculidae). *J Pediatr Nurs.* 2004; **19**(6): 393–8.

127 Blackwell A, Evans KA, Strong RH *et al.* Toward development of neem-based repellents against the Scottish Highland biting midge *Culicoides impunctatus. Med Vet Entomol.* 2004; **18**(4): 449–52.

128 Yang YC, Lee SH, Lee WJ *et al.* Ovicidal and adulticidal effects of *Eugenia carophyllata* bud and leaf oil compounds on *Pediculus capitis. J Agri Food Chem.* 2003; **51**: 4884–8.

129 Yang YC, Less HS, Clark JM *et al.* Insecticidal activity of plant essential oils against *Pediculus humanus cap* (Anoplura: Pediculidae). *J Med Entomol.* 2004; **42**: 699–704.

130 Yang YC, Choi HY, Choi WS. Ovicidal and adulticidal activity of *Eucalyptus globulus* leaf oil terpenoids against *Pediculus humanus capitis* (Anoplura: Pediculidae). *J Agric Good Chem.* 2004; **52**: 2507–11.

131 Yang YC, Lee HS, Lee SH. Ovicidal and adulticidal activities of *Cinnamomum zeylanicum* bark essential oil compounds and related compounds against *Pediculus humanus capitis* (Anoplura: Pediculicidae). *Int J Parasitology.* 2005; **35**: 1595–1600.

132 Mumcuoglu KY, Miller J, Zamir C. The in vivo pediculicidal efficacy of a natural remedy. *Isr Med Assoc.* 2002; **4**: 790–3.

133 Walton SF, McKinnon M, Pizzutto S *et al.* Acaricidal activity of *Melaleuca alternifolia* (tea tree) oil: in vitro sensitivity of *Sarcoptes scabiei var hominis* to terpinen-4-ol. *Arch Dermatol.* 2004; **140**: 563–5.

134 Carson CF, Riley TV. Safety, efficacy and provenance of tea tree (*Melaleuca alternifolia*) oil. *Contact Derm.* 2001; **45**: 65–7.

135 Hadfield-Law L. Head lice for A&E nurses. *Accid Emerg Nurs.* 2000; **8**: 84–7.

Chapter 9

Inflammatory disorders

Introduction

Skin inflammation characterises a number of common conditions. While infections and other disorders are invariably associated with varying degrees of inflammation, this chapter concentrates on psoriasis, eczema, urticaria and miliaria; disorders that are sometimes classified as eruptions.

Psoriasis

Although there is now a comprehensive body of research on the pathogenesis of psoriasis, a complete understanding of the disease remains elusive. Despite the availability of several treatment options, it is still a difficult condition to manage and treatment concentrates on minimising the severity and extent of symptoms. It is a common multifactorial chronic inflammatory hyperproliferative disease with variable clinical presentations, affecting approximately 1.5–3% of the population across ethnic groups, and men and women equally. Types of psoriasis commonly seen include:

- plaque psoriasis
- guttate psoriasis
- erythrodermic psoriasis
- pustular psoriasis
- flexural psoriasis.

Variations in the location of psoriasis are scalp, palms and soles, elbows, knees, base of spine and flexural areas. The typical picture is of areas of thickened, flaky, silvery white and reddened skin, which may itch and bleed. Nails may also be affected, in severe cases being completely destroyed, and if skin lesions are atypical, the pitting and thickening of nails can aid diagnosis. About 15% of people with psoriasis have joint inflammation that produces psoriatic arthritis. Table 9.1 presents the main clinical variants and Table 9.2 summarises the clinical features of the most common form, plaque psoriasis.

Pathogenesis

The exact pathogenesis of psoriasis remains unclear; however, understanding of the psoriatic process continues to expand. The disease picture features simultaneous hyperproliferation of the epidermis, vascular tissues and fibroblasts, an acute inflammatory reaction and an acceleration in the rate of dermal breakdown and repair. Epidermal transit time is much reduced, down from 28 to 4–8

Table 9.1 Clinical variants of psoriasis.

Plaque – Pink or red plaques which usually begin as small red papules that scale as their size increases. Plaques have a well-defined edge unlike the vague edge seen in eczema and tend to be symmetrical. Silvery scaling is characteristic.[3]

Guttate – Derived from the Latin word for 'raindrop', a reference to the small, drop-like lesions. Most commonly affects children and young adults, frequently triggered by bacterial infections, for example streptococcus. Each lesion is usually 0.2–1 cm diameter and round-oval in shape.[3]

Pustular – Can occur as part of a chronic, indolent form of psoriasis or as a more widespread, inflammatory condition. Pustules appear on the skin and may affect either small or large areas of the body. In the most severe form there is fever. Up to 95% of those affected are smokers.[3]

Erythrodermic – Widespread reddening and scaling of the skin accompanied by itching or pain. Can be precipitated by severe sunburn, use of oral steroids, severe emotional stress or illness.

Flexural – Affects the axillae, perineal creases and inframammary folds. Scale is absent or reduced, leaving shiny deep pink plaques. Most common in older and overweight patients.[3]

Scalp – A favoured site and may be the only area affected. Scale adheres to the hair, producing a dense-tight feeling scale that can cover extensive areas of the scalp.

Table 9.2 Clinical features of plaque psoriasis.

- Plaques are pink or red and scaly.
- Plaques coalesce, forming well-demarcated round-oval lesions.
- Surface scale is silvery white and can become very dense, especially on the scalp.
- Vigorous rubbing reveals pinpoint bleeding (Auspitz's sign).
- Plaque size varies considerably from millimetres to several centimetres.
- In intertriginous areas plaques may become macerated.
- Extent of body surface area affected varies considerably; it affects extensor surfaces more than flexor and usually spares the face.

days. Keratinocytes retain their nuclei, there is no granular layer and keratin accumulates in the horny layer. The vasculature in plaques shows abnormalities, with dilated capillaries populating the papillary dermis.

There appears to be an inherited predisposition to psoriasis, and several genetic loci associated with development of the disease have been identified.[1] Supporting evidence for genetic predisposition includes the following.

- There is a higher-than-average incidence of psoriasis in relatives of people with psoriasis. However, in some people with psoriasis there is no family history.
- There is an increased incidence of psoriasis in children when one or both parents has psoriasis.
- Twin studies show the concordance in identical twins to be 73%.[2] However, as in many other diseases with a genetic component, psoriasis involves multiple genes and gene mutations, as well as exogenous factors. It appears that the disease is only expressed after being triggered by other factors. Known triggers include dermatologic and systemic bacterial infections, stressful events, cold climate, sunlight, alcohol and physical trauma.

Koebner phenomemon is a feature of many cases of psoriasis and refers to the recorded incidence that, following a skin injury, psoriatic lesions appear around the site. It may result from antigen-presenting activation of T cells in the skin promoting the psoriatic changes by secreting certain cytokines in genetically predisposed individuals. It has been suggested that psoriasis is a T cell-mediated autoimmune disease[3] and psoriasis shares certain common features with other chronic T-cell-mediated diseases including Crohn's disease and rheumatoid arthritis.[4]

Inflammation is a major symptom of psoriasis and infiltration of the skin by activated T cells is regarded as a key factor in its development. Expanded, tortuous capillary loops within the papillary dermis, and extending close to the parakeratotic scale, are a distinctive feature of psoriatic skin and increased vascularisation precedes lesional development. This proliferation and expansion of blood vessels may contribute to plaque formation, by facilitating access of activated T cells to the skin.[5]

It has long been known that *Staphylococcus aureus* and streptococci infections aggravate psoriasis with the guttate form being closely associated with streptococcal throat infections. There is also evidence that sub-clinical streptococcal infection may be a contributory factor in chronic plaque psoriasis.[2] For some women, psoriasis will significantly improve during pregnancy and relapse in the post-partum period. This suggests a hormonal factor in the disease, which has yet to be fully elucidated.

Psychological impact

Psoriasis can have devastating psychosocial effects, with levels of depression and psychiatric distress among sufferers being significantly higher than among patients with hypertension, cancer, heart disease, diabetes and angina.[6] Emotional distress is aggravated by physical discomforts produced by the psoriasis such as pruritus, which has been associated with suicide.[7] The disfiguring nature of the condition can be overwhelmingly depressing for many sufferers. Depressive disease is a clinically important feature of psoriasis with related stress being associated with greater psychiatric morbidity (ibid.).

Adult psoriasis patients report increased levels of social touch deprivation – something directly associated with higher rates of depression than in non-stigmatised individuals. Several studies provide evidence that perceptions of stigmatisation are pronounced among psoriasis patients: for example one study reported that 26% of patients experienced people making an effort to avoid touching them because of their condition.[8]

The psychological impact is likely to be heightened when the onset of disease occurs early in life. Psychological problems can arise from feelings of social rejection, guilt, embarrassment for self and family, and loneliness. Sufferers may also deny themselves enjoyment of leisure activities. It has been suggested that psoriasis can limit career success because employers often fail to understand the nature of the disease. Psoriasis can lead to increased self-consciousness and affect how individuals approach new relationships and damage the stability of existing ones.[9]

Aromatherapy options

The primary aim is to control the extent and severity of the disease, thus limiting the damage to quality of life. Currently, a single effective conventional cure remains elusive. For chronic plaque psoriasis involving less than 20% of the body surface, initial therapy is topical; systemic therapies are employed for patients with unresponsive severe disease. Thus adjunctive topical use of aromatherapy preparations is indicated in less severe cases (*see* Figure 9.1). Various parameters are used to assess the clinical severity of the disease and corresponding treatments:

- sites affected
- extent of disease
- age and gender of patient
- previous treatment history
- general physical and psychological health of patient.

Psoriasis is particularly difficult to treat and not surprisingly the more severe the symptoms, the more difficult it is to provide effective treatment. Each case is assessed individually, including especially the psychological impact of the condition. The concomitant use of essential oils for both physical and psychological benefit is an important treatment strategy and Table 9.3 suggests oils frequently cited for addressing both aspects.

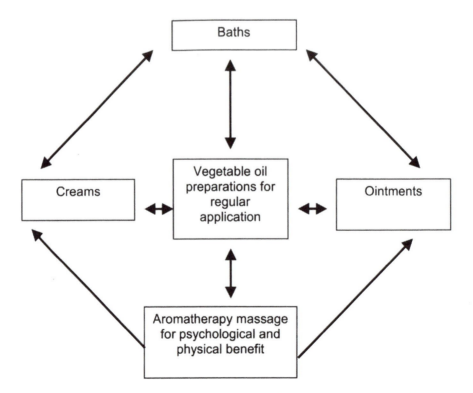

Figure 9.1 Using a sequence of inter-related, emollient-focused therapies offers maximum benefit in cases of mild–moderate psoriasis and dermatitis.

Table 9.3 Key essential oils for addressing the major psychological and physical symptoms of psoriasis.

Achillea millefolium
Boswellia carteri
Chamaemelum nobile
Cistus ladaniferus
Commiphora myrrha var. molmol
Cymbopogon martini
Helichrysum italicum
Lavandula angustifolia
Matricaria recutita
Pelargonium graveolens
Pogostemon cablin
Rosa centifolia
Santalum album

Encouraging a positive attitude is crucial in helping individuals come to terms with what may be a permanent condition and aesthetically pleasing preparations go some way to achieving this. If we consider the following words of a psoriasis patient describing the reality of using prescribed topical preparations it is clear that the aesthetic nature of aromatherapy offers something inherently valuable:

> Smearing on the evil smelling, sticky, staining stuff could take up to two or more hours a day, soaking in it another hour or so.[10]

Research into the efficacy of essential oils in psoriasis care is scarce; one of the few studies conducted to research the value of using aromatherapy concluded the following essential oils to be of use: bergamot, jasmine, geranium, lavender, melissa and sandalwood.[11] *Aloe vera* 0.5% cream resolved psoriatic plaques in 83.3% of patients in a double-blind, placebo-controlled study, compared with 6.6% placebo cure rate.[12] It was noted that patient compliance was excellent, with the cream being well tolerated, and there were no reports of hyper-sensitivity, dermatitis or adverse symptoms. Biopsy analysis of cured lesions showed a decrease in parakeratosis, epidermal acanthosis, thinning, and reduction of vascular dilatation and inflammatory infiltration. Formulating with essential oils and *Aloe vera* gel will maximise the effectiveness of each product, selecting oils from Table 9.3.

In one study[13] which looked at the prevalence of pruritus in patients with extensive psoriasis, it was found to be a feature in 84% of cases and in 77% of these it appeared on a daily basis, significantly affecting the quality of life for sufferers. Constant itching not only aggravates the psoriasis patient and their symptoms, it can severely add to the social impact of the disease. As well as using aromatherapy to alleviate itching, adopting these steps will offer further help.

- Keep skin cool – warmth aggravates pruritus.
- Take cool showers or tepid baths (maximum 30 minutes).
- Limit the use of soaps and cleansers.

- Keep skin moisturised, as dry skin tends to be more pruritic.
- Always moisturise following bathing.
- Wear light clothing (cotton and silk) for coolness and avoid scratchy pressure from wool and synthetic fibres.

Massage has been shown to decrease itching in post-burn patients[14] and therefore it is entirely possible this may also be achievable in cases of psoriasis. Furthermore, massage can help to counter-balance the stigmatisation so commonly experienced by sufferers. Bathing in tepid-warm water, to which essential oils and carrier oils are added, forms an essential part of the treatment plan, especially if large areas of the body are affected. Scales can be removed and itching reduced by soaking for approximately 20 minutes, followed by the liberal application of an appropriate moisturising formula. Table 9.4 provides a sample bath-soak formula.

Vegetable and infused oils

It is known that inhibition of keratinocyte proliferation can be achieved by inhibiting inflammatory mediators.[15] Many of the oils given in Table 9.3 are considered to have either proven or experiential value as topical anti-inflammatories and therefore may contribute to limiting keratinocyte proliferation. It has been demonstrated in vitro that gamma-linolenic acid (GLA) can significantly inhibit the generation of leucotriene B4, a major pro-inflammatory metabolite of arachidonic acid known to accumulate in the lesions of psoriasis.[16] This makes topical use of GLA-rich vegetable oils worthy of further research.

In the meantime, first-choice oils for aromatherapy formulations are *Borago officinalis* (borage) and *Oenothera biennis* (evening primrose). A randomised, prospective clinical trial provided good evidence that a vitamin B12 cream containing avocado oil could be an effective long-term topical treatment for psoriasis.[17] It is therefore possible that *Persea gratissima* oil within aromatherapy preparations offers credible efficacy. Other vegetable oils to consider include:

- *Simmondsia chinensis* (jojoba) for its anti-inflammatory, soothing qualities[18]
- *Calophyllum inophyllum* oil (tamanu), an excellent anti-inflammatory particularly valuable for scalp treatments but the strong odour requires careful balancing if aromatically pleasing preparations are to be achieved
- *Calendula officinalis* (calendula) used widely for its tissue-healing, anti-inflammatory effects.

In mild to moderate cases, clinical experience suggests that careful formulation of essential oils and carrier oils has a softening effect on the scaly layers, easing their removal. Ointment-based emollients are the best mediums for their hydrating, occlusive effects but their greasy feel can be problematic for some. Emollients should be applied as often as required but at least twice a day and always after bathing or showering.

Hydrosols

For symptomatic relief from itching, undiluted hydrosol sprays or cool compresses are ideal, with *Achillea millefolium* (yarrow), *Hamamelis virginiana* (witch hazel) and *Lavandula angustifolia* (lavender) being of particular value. Hydrosol sprays are especially useful for the scalp and can be the best way to encourage

Table 9.4 Sample formula for bath soak (e.g. psoriasis, dermatitis). Bathing provides an ideal medium for full body application of emollient oils. The temperature of the bath should be tepid-warm, not hot, as heat will exacerbate skin irritation and dryness.

Vegetable oils	Essential oils
Oenothera biennis 8.5 ml	Boswellia carteri 0.5 ml
Prunus dulcis 30 ml	Daucus carota 0.25 ml
Persea gratissima 10 ml	Lavandula angustifolia 0.5 ml
	Matricaria recutita 0.25 ml

This quantity is sufficient for approximately five baths. While soaking in the bath, the body can be gently self-massaged to aid absorption of oils and plaque removal and to minimise the chances of oily residue being left on the edges of the bath rather than on the body. Safety precautions regarding the slipperiness of the bath need to be provided.

compliance with treatment, as they are easy to use and provide quick relief. For some, other mediums are too greasy to be readily used on the scalp. One important point to note, however, is that hydrosols will not be effective at managing the dryness and scaling of psoriasis, so their use needs to be concurrent with emollient preparations.

Skin permeability

Skin permeability in psoriatic skin is increased due to the changes in epidermal structure and increased vascularisation. Differences between the clinical variants of psoriasis have been identified, with erythrodermic psoriatic skin showing more disruption to permeability barrier homeostasis than chronic plaque and pustular skin.[19] This affects essential oil dosages, particularly in light of the fact that any treatment regime is likely to involve the repeated, long-tem use of essential oils. Therefore, average concentration guidelines, using non-irritant, non-sensitising essential oils for psoriatic skin are:

- acute inflamed: 1–2%
- chronic, regular use: 2–5%.

It is recommended that formulas are regularly changed to maintain both therapeutic efficacy and safety.

Case example

A woman, 56 years old, presented with localised scalp psoriasis. The plaques were intensely itchy, especially at night. The following was prescribed for one month.

Vegetable oils	Essential oils
Calophyllum inophyllum 1 ml	Matricaria recutita 0.1 ml
Simmondsia chinensis 21 ml	Lavandula angustifolia 0.3 ml
Persea gratissima 3 ml	Helichrysum italicum 0.1 ml

A small amount of the oil was massaged into the local area at night and when possible during the day, although this was dependent upon daily activities and was not done regularly. After a few days there was a considerable reduction in itchiness and softening of plaques. After one month, all irritation had gone. Treatment continued for a further month and plaques resolved. Prophylactically, the vegetable oil mix alone is now used if any itchiness of the scalp is experienced, which occasionally occurs in the winter months and during periods of stress. There has been no return of psoriatic plaques.

Urticaria

The eruption of multiple wheals (hives) that are usually pruritic characterises urticaria. Wheals arise from the release from mast cells of histamine and other mediators that produce vasodilatation and increased vascular permeability. Angioedema is the same process involving the dermis and subcutis.[3] Individual wheals vary in size and shape and arise then disappear within a few hours, leaving no visible trace. In some, the process can last a few days, while in others it may last months or years, with periods of flare and remission.

Classification of urticaria

Urticaria is mediated through allergic and non-allergic mechanisms. Although the most important biologically active chemical involved is histamine, it is known that others are too. A variety of stimuli are responsible for the degranulation of mast cell granules and the release of histamine into the surrounding area. Several pathways, patterns and causes of urticaria are recognised.

- IgE-mediated (type I) hypersensitivity is involved in many acute reactions. The most commonly encountered antigenic substances are drugs (e.g. penicillin), foods (e.g. strawberries, shellfish), latex, nettle, inhaled pollens and moulds.
- Direct release of histamine from mast cells, in a non-immune manner; IgE is not involved. Aspirin, codeine and opiates are common causes.
- Chronic idiopathic attacks can last for weeks or years and specific triggers are rarely identified. Individual lesions last less than 24 hours but new lesions soon reappear. This is not a type I allergic response.
- Physical urticaria can be induced by cold, heat, water, sunlight or pressure.
- Cholinergic urticaria typically affects young adults following exercise or hot baths.

Aromatic management

A good history will help to identify possible triggers, which should be eliminated. As urticaria is typically pruritic (delayed-pressure urticaria is an exception), supportive aromatic care seeks to provide topical relief from itching. Cool hydrosol sprays or compresses are thus indicated. Select from *Achillea millefolium* (yarrow), *Hamamelis virginiana* (witch hazel), *Lavandula angustifolia* (lavender), *Matricaria recutita* (German chamomile), *Mentha piperita* (peppermint) or *Pelargonium graveolens* (geranium). They can be applied neat to wheals.

Histamine induces vascular changes through a number of mechanisms and when injected into the skin results in the 'triple response' of Lewis:

1 vasodilation
2 pruritus
3 wheal.

The two most important histamine receptors are H_1 and H_2 and activation of these leads to the symptoms described. In urticaria lasting longer than an hour, histamine is unlikely to be the sole cause.[20] The following essential oils have demonstrated antihistamine activity and can usefully be formulated into *Aloe vera* gel for topical relief:

- *Lavandula angustifolia* (lavender)[21]
- *Matricaria recutita* (German chamomile)[22]
- *Melaleuca alternifolia* (tea tree).[23,24]

Cedrus deodara (cedarwood) may also be helpful, as it has been shown to stabilise mast cells and inhibit leukotriene synthesis.[25] However, the question of whether any or all of these oils have a clinical benefit in specifically controlling the marked pruritus of urticaria awaits further confirmation as there is some evidence suggesting the contrary. For example, in one study, while *Melaleuca alternifolia* (tea tree) reduced histamine-induced skin inflammation, it had no significant effect on itching.[23] However, local anaesthetic effects may be achievable through the topical use of lavender and peppermint oil preparations, thereby contributing a degree of relief.[26,27]

Miliaria

Commonly known as heat rash, this is a common phenomenon affecting predisposed individuals during hot humid conditions or exercise. If occlusion of the skin occurs it leads to accumulation of sweat on the skin surface and overhydration of the stratum corneum. If conditions persist, excessive sweat continues to be produced but occlusion of the eccrine sweat ducts then leads to its accumulation within the skin. Three levels of occlusion occur, producing distinct forms.

- *Miliaria crystallina* – occlusion of the duct at the skin surface produces small non-itchy vesicles. There is little if any erythema. Most commonly seen in bed-ridden patients and infants. It is a self-limiting condition that resolves without complications.
- *Miliaria rubra* – the most common form, this is familiarly known as 'prickly heat'. Occlusion of the intraepidermal section of the duct results in chronic periductal inflammatory cell infiltrate in the papillary dermis and lower epidermis. Itchy papules and vesicles surrounded by a red halo or diffuse erythema appear. There is a characteristic stinging or prickling sensation rather than itching. Miliaria rubra also tends to resolve spontaneously when conditions are cooled. If prolonged heat exposure continues, heat exhaustion may result. Secondary infection is a possible complication.
- *Miliaria profunda* – deep-seated nodules develop as occlusion of the dermal section of the duct leads to sweat accumulating in the dermis. Lesions are asymptomatic. It can arise as a complication of repeated bouts of miliaria rubra and the resultant inability to sweat may predispose an individual to heat exhaustion.

Aromatic management

The treatment is essentially the same as for urticaria with an enhanced need to cool the area. Repeated, frequent applications of cool hydrosol compresses and heat avoidance are the best approaches. Prevention consists of reducing exposure to heat and humidity so that sweating is not induced. *Aloe vera* gel provides an ideal medium for application following the use of compresses, offering anti-inflammatory and topically cooling effects. Table 9.5 gives a sample essential oil formulation.

Dermatitis (eczema)

The term dermatitis covers a wide variety of non-infectious skin conditions characterised by red, sore and itchy skin. These include atopic dermatitis and irritant or allergic reactions to household substances. The causes can be broadly divided into contact factors (exogenous dermatitis) or constitutional (endogenous), which is often referred to as eczema. A convenient classification is outlined in Table 9.6. The various conditions share several clinical features. Acute forms are characterised by:

- papules, vesicles or blisters
- poorly defined erythema and swelling
- exudation and crusting
- itching and scaling.

Chronic forms display:

- dryness and painful fissures
- lichenification and excoriation.

Distinguishing between the different types of dermatitis can be difficult, but useful, in order to provide optimal care. These include the following.

- *Atopic dermatitis* – 65% of atopic dermatitis presents before the age of six months.[29] Diagnostic features include onset before two years old, itchy, dry skin, visual flexural eczema and a personal or family history (if under four years) of any atopic disease. The incidence in adults is less than that of psoriasis but it can have a chronic relapsing course. In adults lesions are thicker and have more lichenification. Hand involvement seems to be a marker of chronicity.
- *Irritant contact dermatitis* – acute states are often the result of a single exposure

Table 9.5 Sample formulation (5%) for relief of prickly heat or urticaria symptoms.

Essential oils:
Mentha piperita 0.5 ml
Lavandula angustifolia 2 ml
Helichrysum italicum 0.5 ml
Add *Aloe vera* gel to make a total of 60 ml and apply to affected skin three times daily immediately following the use of cool compresses, until symptoms clear.

---

to a substance, with lesions usually disappearing within days. Chronic forms develop as a result of cumulative exposure to irritants and, even following their removal, prolonged reactions may continue.

- *Allergic contact dermatitis* – this depends primarily on activation of allergen-specific T memory cells (delayed hypersensitivity).
- *Seborrheic dermatitis* – this is a chronic, inflammatory, scaly eruption usually affecting the scalp.
- *Discoid (nummular)* – an extremely itchy, vesicular or crusted dermatitis forming circular lesions which typically affect the limbs. Secondary bacterial infection is common.
- *Pompholyx* – is characterised by small multiple clear fluid-filled coalescent vesicles on the palms, fingers or soles. After a few days the vesicles weep and on drying cause painful fissures. It is often provoked by emotional stress, allergens or infection.
- *Venous (varicose; gravitational; stasis)* – chronic patchy dermatitis of the lower legs, associated with venous insufficiency. It commonly affects middle-aged or elderly females. Ulceration can develop.
- *Asteatotic (eczema craquelé)* – this is a dry eczema, has the appearance of paving stones and commonly occurs on the limbs and trunks of the elderly. Fissuring, itching and erythema characterise this form and it is associated with over-washing of patients in care facilities, dry environmental conditions and hypothyroidism.
- *Lichen simplex (neurodermatitis)* – this arises from repeated rubbing or scratching. Lesions are excoriated and become heavily lichenified. Itching is a major feature and extremely difficult to control.

Several of these forms are covered in detail elsewhere in the book.

Aromatic management

There are three stages of dermatitis: acute, sub-acute and chronic with each being part of a dynamic inflammatory process.[30] The stages evolve into one another, with scratching and rubbing inhibiting the healing process. A degree of itching is an inevitable feature of eczematous inflammation. Table 9.7 outlines the main clinical features and treatment for each stage.

Table 9.6 A simple classification of eczema.[3,28]

Type	Variant
Exogenous	Contact allergic
	Primary irritant
	Photoreaction
Endogenous	Atopic
	Seborrheic
	Discoid (nummular)
	Hand and foot: hyperkeratotic/fissured; vesicular (pompholyx)
	Venous (gravitational, stasis)
	Asteatotic (eczema craquelé)
	Lichen simplex (neurodermatitis)

Essential oils with anti-inflammatory and skin-healing activity combined with emollient vegetable oils, particularly those rich in GLA, form the mainstay of treatment. Approaches are similar to that for chronic plaque psoriasis (*see* Figure 9.1) but there is a difference in skin permeability between psoriatic skin and lichenified eczematous skin, characteristic of chronic dermatitis: intact lichenified skin may retard essential oil absorption.

Cool compresses

Cool hydrosol-soaked compresses will alleviate itching and inflammation in acute states, by the vasoconstriction produced by the evaporative processes. Occlusion of compresses will inhibit evaporation and should therefore be avoided. Vesicles are macerated and removal of the compress gently debrides the area, preventing serum and crust from accumulating.[30] Compresses are replaced after 20 minutes with fresh ones rather than re-soaking with hydrosol solution, which may lead to irritation from the accumulation of scale and crust. Once the acute inflammation has settled, compresses stop, as excessive wetting may lead to cracking and fissuring.

Emollients

Emollients are the first-line treatment for dermatitis and dry skin conditions. They soothe and hydrate dry, scaly skin and by increasing skin hydration this may have an anti-inflammatory, anti-pruritic effect through the inhibition of the pro-inflammatory cytokine interleukin-1alpha (IL-1a).[31] Emollients require frequent liberal application – four times a day or more – and therefore sufficient quantities need to be supplied. If applied sparingly or too infrequently emollients may appear ineffective. This reticence to use them may be due to the misconception that they are not 'active' or because they are unpleasant to use (ibid.). It is therefore important that the place of emollients in an overall treatment regimen is clearly explained to the client. The aesthetics of aromatic formulations considerably encourages application and the final choice of essential oils needs to reflect this.

Emollients are thought to restore the integrity of the skin barrier in two ways.

1 Formation of an oily barrier over the skin preventing evaporation of water.
2 They may penetrate deeper through the stratum corneum and mimic the effects of deficient lipids, preventing the penetration of allergens and irritants.

Table 9.7 Symptoms and treatment of dermatitis.

Stage	Symptoms	Treatment
Acute	Vesicles, blisters, intense erythema. Intense itch.	Cool hydrosol compresses. Emollients: lotions and cream formulations.
Sub-acute	Erythema, scaling, fissuring. Slight to moderate itch. Burning, stinging, pain.	Emollients: creams, lotions, bath preparations and ointments.
Chronic	Lichenification, excoriations, fissuring. Moderate to intense itch.	Emollients: creams, lotions, bath preparations and ointments.

Table 9.8 highlights practical considerations when using emollients.

Individuals using a combination of allopathic preparations such as topical corticosteroids and aromatherapeutic emollients (formulated with or without essential oils) should leave at least half an hour following the application of steroid before applying the emollient, to avoid dilution or spread to unaffected areas. It is important that the steroid is applied prior to the emollient. If the emollient formulation is particularly viscous it can be warmed in the hands to allow easier application. Where itching is problematic the emollient can be cooled in the fridge before application.

Case example
A woman, 30 years old, presented with atopic eczematous lesions on her neck. The lesions were intensely red, highly itchy and excoriated. Since childhood she had experienced regular flare-ups of atopic eczema and avoided dairy produce, gluten and fragranced products, all of which she suspected aggravated the condition. During the previous month, she had experienced personal stresses and was having building work done in the house which she felt had tipped the balance; she described the dust in the house as 'being like sandpaper' against her skin and her lesions were stinging and burning. An initial preparation containing a total of 2% *Matricaria recutita* and *Lavandula angustifolia* essential oils (1:1) in *Simmondsia chinensis* wax and *Calendula officinalis* infused oil (1:1) could not be tolerated and the decision was made to avoid essential oils in favour of a simple emollient cream.

Vegetable, infused oils, waxes and butters
Simmondisa chinensis 10 ml
Calendula officinalis 10 ml
Shea butter 3 g
Cocoa butter 3 g
Beeswax 3 g
Quantity sufficient for seven days.

Hydrosol
Hamamelis virginiana 20 ml

Table 9.8 Practical considerations when using emollients.

- Lotions, creams, ointments and bath oils all potentially achieve restoration of the skin barrier.
- Creams are preferred for day use with heavier ointments reserved for night-time use.
- Lotions are indicated for wet and weeping dermatitis.
- Flare-up can be prevented by continual application of emollients even when symptoms have resolved.
- Provide sufficient quantities for home use, together with smaller containers that can be carried throughout the day, thereby encouraging frequent application.
- Laundry – high temperatures are necessary to remove grease from clothing and bedding but biological powders and softeners are best avoided.
- Different emollients may be required for different body sites. For example ointment for limbs, lighter creams for the face.
- Applications need to follow the direction of the hair follicle to prevent folliculitis developing.

The cream was applied several times every day. Within 24 hours of starting treatment, the inflammation, burning, stinging and itching had noticeably subsided. Treatment was continued for one month, after which time all signs of erythema and discomfort had disappeared. Treatment continued for several weeks, with non-essential oil containing emollient creams to restore skin health.

Advice for avoiding irritant hand dermatitis

Hand dermatitis is very common and can interfere with daily activity, cause high levels of embarrassment and have social consequences. Several types of hand dermatitis occur: irritant, atopic, allergic, pompholyx and lichen simplex. Allergy, infection, scratching and stress complicate the picture.

As well as providing topical emollient, anti-inflammatory formulations, the following advice can be given.

- Avoid washing hands more than necessary and use tepid water.
- Use cotton towels for drying rather than paper towels.
- Avoid soaps, detergents, solvents and shampoos as far as is practical.
- Wear cotton-lined gloves when using household cleaners and doing any wet work.
- Avoid direct contact with anything that causes itching or burning (e.g. raw meat, tomatoes, potatoes, citrus fruits).
- Wear gloves in cold weather.
- Use emollients throughout the day and always after getting the hands wet.

References

1 Ortonne JP. Recent developments in the understanding of the pathogenesis of psoriasis. *Br J Dermatol.* 1999; (Suppl. 54): 1–4.
2 Stevenson O, Zaki I. Introduction to psoriasis. *Hospital Pharmacist.* 2002; **9**: 187–90.
3 Gawkrodger DJ. *Dermatology, An Illustrated Colour Text.* 3rd ed. Edinburgh: Churchill Livingstone; 2002.
4 Christophers E. The immunopathology of psoriasis. *Int Arch Allergy Immunol.* 1996; **110**(3): 199–206.
5 Hern S, Allen MH, Sousa AR *et al.* Immunohistochemical evaluation of psoriatic plaques following selective photothermolysis of the superficial capillaries. *Br J Dermatol.* 2001; **145**(1): 45–53.
6 Rapp SR, Feldman SR, Exum ML *et al.* Psoriasis causes as much disability as other major medical diseases. *J Am Acad Dermatol.* 1999; **41**(3): 401–7.
7 Gupta MA. Psychiatric comorbidity in dermatological disorders. In: Walker C, Papadopoulos L, editors. *Psychodermatology.* Cambridge: Cambridge University Press; 2005. p. 29–43.
8 Kent G. Stigmatisation and skin conditions. In: Walker C, Papadopoulos L, editors. *Psychodermatology.* Cambridge: Cambridge University Press; 2005. p. 44–56.
9 Anthis L. Skin disease and relationships. In: Walker C, Papadopoulos L, editors. *Psychodermatology.* Cambridge: Cambridge University Press; 2005. p. 72–88.
10 Thompson A. Coping with chronic skin conditions: factors important in explaining individual variation in adjustment. In: Walker C, Papadopoulos L, editors. *Psychodermatology.* Cambridge: Cambridge University Press; 2005. p. 57–71
11 Walsh D. Using aromatherapy in the management of psoriasis. *Nursing Standard.* 1996; **11**: 53–6.

12 Syed TA, Ahmad A, Holt AH *et al.* Management of psoriasis with *Aloe vera* extract in a hydrophilic cream: a placebo-controlled, double-blind study. *Trop Med Int Health.* 1996; **1**(4): 504–9.

13 Yosipovitch G, Goon A, Wee J *et al.* The prevalence and clinical characteristics of pruritus among patients with extensive psoriasis. *Br J Dermatol.* 2000; **143**(5): 969–73.

14 Field T. *Touch Therapy.* Edinburgh: Churchill Livingstone; 2000.

15 Mills S, Bone K. *Principles and Practice of Phytotherapy.* Edinburgh: Churchill Livingstone; 2000.

16 Ziboh VA. Implications of dietary oils and polyunsaturated fatty acids in the management of cutaneous disorders. *Arch Dermatol.* 1989; **125**: 241–5.

17 Stücker M, Memmel U, Hoffmann M *et al.* Vitamin B(12) cream containing avocado oil in the therapy of plaque psoriasis. *Dermatology.* 2001; **203**: 141–7.

18 Habashy RR, Abdel-Naim AB, Khalifa AE *et al.* Anti-inflammatory effects of jojoba liquid wax in experimental models. *Pharmacol Res.* 2004; **51**(2): 95–105.

19 Ghadially R, Reed JT, Elias PM. Stratum corneum structure and function correlates with phenotype in psoriasis. *J Invest Dermatol.* 1996; **107**: 558–64.

20 Charlesworth EN, Beltrani VS. Pruritic dermatoses: overview of etiology and therapy. *Am J Med.* 2002; **113**(9A): 25S–33S.

21 Kim HM, Cho SH. Lavender oil inhibits immediate-type allergic reaction in mice and rats. *J Pharm Pharmacol.* 1999; **51**(2): 221–6.

22 Miller TM, Wittstock U, Lindequist U. Effects of some components of the essential oil of chamomile, *Chamomilla recutita*, on histamine release from rat mast cells. *Planta Med.* 1996; **62**(1): 60–1.

23 Koh KJ, Pearce AL, Marshman G. Tea tree oil reduces histamine induced skin inflammation. *Br J Dermatol.* 2002; **147**: 1212–17.

24 Khalil Z, Pearce AL, Satkunanathan N. Regulation of wheal and flare by tea tree oil: complementary human and rodent studies. *J Invest Dermatol.* 2004; **123**: 683–90.

25 Shinde UA, Kulkarni KR, Phadke AS *et al.* Mast cell stabilising and lipoxygenase inhibitory activity of *Cedrus deodara* (Roxb.) Loud. Wood oil. *Ind J Exp Biol.* 1999; **37**: 258–61.

26 Ghelardini C, Galeotti N, Salvatore G *et al.* Local anaesthetic activity of the essential oil of *Lavandula angustifolia*. *Planta Med.* 1999; **65**: 700–3.

27 Galeotti N, Mannelli DC, Mazzanti A. Menthol: a natural analgesic compound. *Neurosci Lett.* 2002; **322**(3): 145–8.

28 Graham-Brown R, Bourke JF. *Mosby's Color Atlas and Text of Dermatology.* London: Mosby; 1998.

29 Friedmann PS. Allergy and the skin. II – Contact and atopic eczema. *BMJ.* 1998; **316**(7139): 1226–34.

30 Habif TP. *Clinical Dermatology.* 4th ed. Edinburgh: Mosby; 2004.

31 Clark C. Making the most of emollients. *Pharmaceutical J.* 2001; **266**: 227–9.

Chapter 10

Wound care

Introduction

Although wounds have many causes, the healing process remains an orderly though complex series of events that seek to repair the integrity of the damaged tissue. Irrespective of the causes of the damage, in an attempt to heal, proliferation and dividing of cells occurs, followed by the release of growth factors, formation of new blood vessels and a collagen matrix and finally repair. For some, certain intrinsic or extrinsic factors may alter this course and delay or prevent the healing process. In these cases, destructive processes override healing, and the wound becomes chronic.

The healing process

Although essentially the same process heals all wounds there are some that may not easily repair either because of their severity or because of the poor health status of the individual. Damage to the skin is classified according to depth of injury.

- Superficial – damage is confined to the epidermis and heals without scarring.
- Partial-thickness – the epidermis and the superficial dermis are penetrated. Healing occurs by regeneration of epithelial tissue (epithelialisation). Deeper dermal damage heals with scarring.
- Full-thickness – wounds involve epidermis, dermis and subcutaneous tissue as well as disruption of the blood vessels and possibly nerves. Healing leaves scarring.

Three separate but interdependent processes are triggered by the initial wound and involve both inhibitory and stimulatory activity of a host of chemical mediators.

Inflammatory phase – cleansing

Clotting and cleansing characterise the body's initial response to injury, resulting in haemostasis and inflammation. To prevent initial blood loss a temporary plug is formed by platelets becoming sticky, adhering to one another and to the collagen in the blood vessel walls. Vasoconstrictors, released by activated platelets, slow the flow of blood around the injury and, combined with plug formation, bleeding is restrained. Activated platelets continue to release clotting factors and growth factors, which are essential for healing to progress. The coagulation process is a complex chemical cascade where one reaction initiates another reaction, and so on. The last step in the clotting process produces fibrin, which is a strong, cross-linked protein that forms an integral part of the clot by weaving a mesh of long strands around platelets and blood cells, eventually producing a clot. Fibrin also holds the edges of the wound together; if left exposed, the surface of the clot dries, forming a scab.

After the initial blood loss is stopped, the wound undergoes cleansing: combined with the accumulation of neutrophils, monocytes and macrophages, chemotaxis by inflammatory mediators such as kinins and prostaglandins bring a host of cell types to the injury. The neutrophils and macrophages kill bacteria and aid in debridement; growth factors that are essential for healing are secreted by the macrophages. Blood flow increases as the initial phase of vasoconstriction is followed by a period of vasodilation mediated by histamine, prostaglandins, kinins and leukotrienes. The cardinal signs of inflammation appear: heat, redness, swelling and pain. The production of exudate containing neutrophils, monocytes, macrophages and proteins such as complement, antibodies, enzymes, albumin and growth factors continues throughout the healing process. The inflammatory cells debride injured tissue during the inflammatory phase and form the basis of pus. This inflammatory phase prepares the wound for the next phase of healing and therefore anything that limits inflammation, such as anti-inflammatory drugs, will slow the process. Chronic wounds remain in this inflammatory phase.

Proliferative phase – healing

Sometimes called the fibroblastic or collagen phase, the second stage of wound healing begins as early as 48 hours following injury and may be completed after 21 days. Two processes run in parallel at this time, dermal repair and epidermal regeneration, and involve epithelialisation, granulation and angiogenesis. Formation of granulation tissue, consisting of inflammatory cells, fibroblasts, and vascular tissue, in a matrix of fibronectin, collagen, glycosaminoglycans, and proteoglycans, is a central event during this proliferative phase.

The restoration of surface epithelium is precisely synchronised with the repair of the dermal layer through remarkable communication between diverse cell types. Following the end of the inflammatory phase, the formation of new tissue begins with the proliferation and migration of epithelial cells including fibroblasts and resident keratinocytes across the wound surface. A host of intercellular signals and molecules are involved in this migration and proliferation, with signals being initiated both by temporary populations of macrophages and neutrophils, as well as the fibroblasts and keratinocytes. Epithelial cells can only migrate over moist tissue not through dry scabs where it takes at least twice as long for epithelialisation to occur. Once the cells meet, they stop migration but continue to divide to restore normal epidermal tissue thickness. This new tissue is fragile and may easily be damaged by infection, abrasion or drying. Re-epithelialisation continues until the keratinocytes have covered the dermis and stratified, and a new basement membrane is formed. For superficial wounds, the epithelium spreads quickly, covering the entire surface within 10 to 14 days. For full-thickness injuries, epithelium can only migrate from the margins and may be insufficient for wound closure (*see* Figure 10.1).

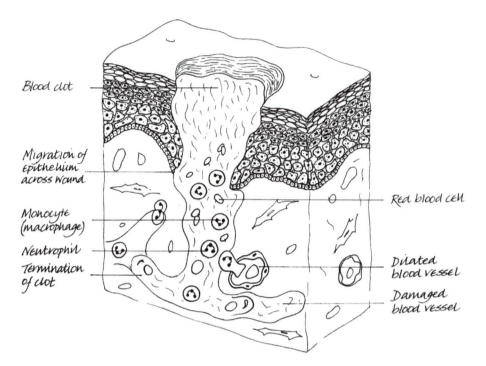

Blood clot

Migration of
epithelium
across wound

Monocyte
(macrophage)

Neutrophil

Termination
of clot

Red blood cell

Dilated
blood vessel

Damaged
blood vessel

Figure 10.1 Diagrammatic representation of a repairing wound.

At the same time as epithelialisation is happening, the basement membrane, which lies between the epidermis and dermis, is repairing via dermal fibroblasts and re-differentiation of components originating from the keratinocytes.[1] Having a complex composition and representing much more than a mere structural entity, the basement membrane plays an essential role in wound healing by providing molecular signals to synchronise repair between the epidermal and dermal layers (ibid.). In the dermis, growth factors regulate angiogenesis, allowing the area to be revascularised; once this is complete, angiogenic factors are inhibited and the growth of new blood vessels stops.

Fibroblasts, activated by platelet-derived growth factors and macrophages, enlarge and divide to produce a collagen network surrounding and strengthening the newly formed capillaries. The granulation tissue that is seen in wounds results from capillary and fibroblast proliferation. As collagen content increases, the wound site strengthens, a process that continues over several weeks. The restoration of dermal architecture by collagen fibres eventually enables wounds to have strength that is similar to that of unaffected skin. In the final stages of repair, the edges of the wound are drawn together by specialised fibroblasts (myofibroblasts) contracting under the influence of kinins.

Maturation phase – wound strengthening

The third and final stage of wound healing lasts the longest and may continue for several years. In this phase vascularisation lessens with excessive blood vessels being destroyed by enzymes, tight collagen cross-links are formed and collagen bundles realign along the direction of maximal stress to increase the tensile strength of the scar. Normal progressive collagen replacement yields a softer, less conspicuous scar but, in some cases, excessive amounts of collagen are produced, leading to hypertrophic or keloid scarring.

Delays in wound healing

Essentially, for a wound to heal, it must be moist with adequate supplies of nutrition and oxygen. Healing is influenced by a number of endogenous and exogenous factors and delays caused by any of these can lead to the formation of chronic wounds.

Endogenous factors affecting the healing process are:

- nutritional status of patient
- age
- general health status
- blood supply
- pharmacological agents.

Nutrition plays a vital role in healing, with vitamins A, B, C and E all influencing specific processes. Protein is necessary for wound contraction and the formation of collagen, fibroblasts and antibodies and an increased intake of amino acids, carbohydrates and lipids will satisfy the extra demands made during the healing process. Obesity adversely affects healing by compromising the blood supply due to fat tissue and at the other end of the spectrum emaciation or malnutrition leads to poor oxygen and nutrient supply. With increasing age, delays in wound healing are seen and part of this may be due to poor nutritional status, as well as concomitant disease. Diabetes, connective tissue disorders, malignancies, anaemia and jaundice all delay wound healing, as does immune suppression. Venous or arterial insufficiency is directly implicated in the development of leg ulcers. Medications that inhibit cell-mediated immune responses such as corticosteroids and other anti-inflammatories interfere with the healing process and cause delays.

Exogenous factors that influence wound healing are:

- moisture
- temperature
- oxygenation
- pH
- microbial colonisation and site cleanliness.

Epithelial cells cannot migrate in a dry environment so wounds heal best in a moist, warm one as this promotes angiogenesis and epithelialisation. However, excessive moisture leading to maceration impairs healing by encouraging bacterial and fungal proliferation and tissue damage. Wounds are generally low in oxygen and pH when nutritional status is poor or when a systemic infection is present. Since oxygen is necessary for fibroblasts to modify collagen and angiogenesis, a low-oxygen environment can cause a delay in wound healing. Vasoconstriction, caused by smoking for example, is associated with impaired healing partly because oxygen levels are reduced.

There is a clear distinction between microbial colonisation and infection: low bacterial colonisation is normal and so long as there is no infection present, wounds will heal. Studies have shown that wound contamination primarily arises from sites close to the wound and treatment needs to focus on minimising exposure to and growth of micro-organisms.[2] Particles arising from the treatment and healing processes, for example slough or dressing fibres, prolong the inflammatory stage by acting as foreign bodies and may inhibit the formation of granulation tissue. Cleansing wounds with appropriate mediums helps to prevent this.

Using aromatherapy to promote wound healing

There are several considerations to take into account when treating wounds with different therapeutic aims required during the healing process.

Different interventions for different wounds

Depending upon whether the wound is chronic or acute, the treatment needs will differ. Normal acute injuries are expected to heal with minimum intervention; it is when wounds become chronic that greater involvement is required.

First aid for acute wounds

In the case of acute injury, treatment must avoid inhibiting the inflammatory process for the first 36 hours, as it is through the inflammatory mediators that the cells necessary for healing are brought to the injury site. Essential oils with haemostatic effects will support the clotting process, helping to stop the initial bleeding. Research is lacking for the haemostatic activity of essential oils but the following oils are useful in practice and are often cited anecdotally:

- *Cistus ladaniferus*
- *Commiphora myrrha var. molmol*
- *Cupressus sempervirens*
- *Helichrysum italicum*
- *Pelargonium graveolens*
- *Rosa damascena*.

The haemostatic effect offered by these oils is not desirable in wounds where vasodilation assists wound cleansing, as only when a wound is red and clear of debris can progression into the proliferative phase of healing take place.

Cleansing an acute wound demands minimal intervention so as not to disturb the clotting process. If required, gentle irrigation with hydrosols should be sufficient but, just as with essential oils, the choice of hydrosol needs to take into account the nature of the wound and the stage of healing: *Cistus ladaniferus* (rock rose) and *Hamamelis virginiana* (witch hazel) are reputedly astringent,[3] thus tightening the blood vessels and preventing bleeding, an intervention indicated for clean cuts. In contrast the neutral pH of *Lavandula angustifolia* (lavender) lacks the astringent effect, making it a better choice in cases where the period of vasodilation facilitates wound cleansing and healing, for example irrigation of wounds containing foreign bodies and debris.

Furthermore it is sensible when using hydrosols to select those with demonstrated antimicrobial activity to minimise contamination of the site. *Satureja hortensis* (summer savory) is effective against *Staphylococcus aureus*[4] as are *Thymus vulgaris*, *Thymus serpyllum* (thyme) and species of oregano and marjoram (*Origanum onites*, *Oregano majorana*).[5]

Chronic wounds

Chronic wounds are most often associated with underlying or exogenous abnormalities that lead to tissue breakdown and ulceration, with venous leg ulcers, diabetic foot ulcers and decubitus ulcers (pressure sores) being examples of chronic wounds commonly seen in clinical practice. A number of factors are involved in slow-healing wounds, in particular the presence of infection, non-viable tissue, inadequate local tissue perfusion and unregulated inflammatory activity.[2] Treatment strategies therefore focus on clearing micro-organisms from colonised and infected sites and this is closely associated with the removal of non-viable tissue, the presence of which is conducive to microbial growth. Similarly where the microbial demands cannot be controlled by the host response, subsequent inflammation becomes a primary feature of chronic wounds and needs regulating as tissue breakdown, pain and malodour overrides the healing process. Maintaining or re-establishing blood flow to the wound site enables the delivery of immune cells, oxygen and nutrients and reduces the microbial load.[6]

Microbiological investigations indicate that in the majority of both acute and chronic wounds a polymicrobial situation exists, with *S. aureus* being the most significant pathogen.[2] It is suggested that it is the overall microbiology of a wound and its relationship with the host response that is more important to address than the presence and identification of specific microbes (ibid.). Suitable essential oils with broad-spectrum antimicrobial activity are given in Table 10.1. Many of these are also especially useful for assisting in controlling the pain of wound healing, a feature that is particularly associated with infected wounds.

The recommended concentration of essential oils is between 5 and 25% taking into account the chemical profiles of the selected oils as well as the degree of infection present. Although full corroborating evidence for essential oil dosages in this field is lacking, several case reports in the literature indicate this range to be effective in different wound types and clinical experience confirms this.[18–21]

Table 10.1 Essential oils with antimicrobial activity that can be used to control the microbial load in chronic wounds.

Ocimum basilicum[7]
Lavandula angustifolia[8,9]
Origanum vulgare[10]
Mentha piperita[11]
Satureja montana[12]
Melaleuca alternifolia[8,11,13–17]
Thymus vulgaris[11]

Wounds that are healthy and free from debris do not necessarily require routine cleansing. However, if devitalised tissue or debris is present, hydrosol irrigation of the site or the application of hydrosol-soaked sterile compresses prior to the application of a dressing is indicated. Those cited earlier for their anti-microbial activity are suitable, along with *Lavandula angustifolia* (lavender), *Achillea millefolium* (yarrow) and *Matricaria recutita* (German chamomile) for anti-inflammatory benefit.

The unregulated inflammatory environment of chronic wounds is a serious contributory factor to delays in healing time. The essential oils *Achillea millefolium* (yarrow), *Matricaria recutita* (German chamomile), *Lavandula angustifolia* (lavender), *Melaleuca alternifolia* (tea tree), *Cymbopogon martini* (palmarosa) and *Pogostemon cablin* (patchouli) are all indicated in preparations to control inflammation in wounds.

Matricaria chamomilla (German chamomile), which contains the important sesquiterpenol α-bisabolol, is widely recognised for its wound-healing activity and maintenance of tissue integrity.[22–24] α-bisabolol and α-terpineol have demonstrated significant in vivo cicatrisant activity, which is thought to be related to the 1-methylcyclohexane moiety and the tertiary hydroxyl group[25] (*see* Figure 10.2). Where wounds do not form granulation tissue (scar) easily, the inclusion of cicatrisant essential oils into formulations should be considered. The following are traditionally cited for their cicatrising activity: *Commiphora myrrha var. molmol* (myrrh), *Cistus ladaniferus* (rock rose), *Cymbopogon martini* (palmarosa), *Boswellia carterii* (frankincense), *Helichrysum italicum* (everlasting), *Lavandula angustifolia* (lavender) and *Santalum album* (sandalwood).

One final benefit of using essential oils in wound care is the control of malodour. The combined effectiveness of essential oil preparations is that, rather than merely using them to mask odours, they are actively employed to tackle the causes. (The causes always need identifying, for example infection, necrotic tissue and dressing.) On the other hand, it is possible that due to the close association found between smells and memory, for patients the aroma of the essential oils used in treatment may forever be linked with the experience of the wound, and careful management is required to avoid future distress.

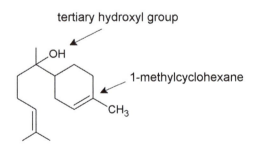

alpha-bisabolol

Figure 10.2 Alpha-bisabolol, a wound-healing component of *Matricaria chamomilla*.

Burn dressings and essential oils

A study, which highlights the potential for using essential oil impregnated dressings in the treatment of MRSA-infected wounds, compared the anti-bacterial properties of the vapours of a range of essential oils.[8] *Melaleuca alternifolia* (tea tree), *Pogostemon cablin* (patchouli), *Lavandula officinalis* (lavender), and *Pelargonium graveolens* (geranium) essential oils and Citricidal® (grapefruit seed extract) were tested against three strains of *S. aureus*, including two methicillin-resistant strains isolated from the wounds of burns patients. Although the findings relating to Citricidal® are of no relevance in view of the unreliability of this extract (*see* Chapter 4), those for the essential oils are promising in this context.

When the oils were in direct contact with the bacteria, inhibition of growth was seen, irrespective of the oil or bacterial strain. However, when tea tree was combined with the other oils, the susceptibility of the antibiotic-sensitive strain increased but decreased for the other strains, suggesting a dilution of tea tree's active components. When the vapour phases of the oils were looked at, the effects of single oils and combinations of oils markedly differed from those of direct contact: singly, only tea tree showed any inhibition and this was only present in the antibiotic-sensitive strain; combined patchouli and tea tree produced inhibition with all strains, but individually neither of these showed any effect on the MRSA strains in the vapour phase. The geranium–tea tree combination was most active against the antibiotic-sensitive strain.

Illustrative of how essential oils may be used in clinical practice, the researchers looked at the effects of the oil combinations in a dressing model. It was found that there was little difference in inhibitory effects when oils were placed in different layers of the dressing, leading to the suggestion that it should be possible to leave the inner dressing in place while changing or re-impregnating with oils the outermost layer, leaving the wound undisturbed. Although it was found that the inclusion of certain topical antimicrobial preparations interfered with the inhibitory effects of the oils, possibly by preventing vapour penetration, this could be overcome.

The findings from this study are of particular interest, as the observation that essential oils have different effects on different strains of the same bacterial species, and that combinations of essential oils produce greater antibacterial effects than single oils, confirm not only the chemical complexity of essential oils, but also how they work both synergistically and antagonistically.

Aloe vera and honey

As stated previously, in order to heal, a moist environment is needed and in wounds covered with occlusive dressings, epithelialisation has been shown to occur twice as fast and with less pain.[26] The use of gel formulations helps to rehydrate the wound site and maintain moisture at the dressing–wound interface, while also offering gentle debridement. In aromatic formulations, *Aloe vera* gel provides an ideal medium not only for these reasons but also for the specific benefit it has at the cellular level. However, although moisture is necessary, excessive fluid and the development of maceration needs to be prevented and honey has demonstrated efficacy in controlling oedema and microbial growth in several studies.

Aloe vera

Components of *Aloe vera* gel have been shown to significantly enhance kerati-nocyte proliferation and migration in wounds with the cell proliferation-stimu-latory activity shortening healing time.[27] Other work that looked specifically at the intercellular communication and proliferation of fibroblasts in diabetes mellitus skin demonstrated that aloe gel had a growth-promoting effect.[28] Interestingly this work identified that the diabetic fibroblasts were more sensitive to *Aloe vera* than non-diabetic ones, probably because of their different char-acteristics including the rate of proliferation, cell-to-cell communication and production of collagen.

Further evidence for the efficacy of *Aloe vera* at the cellular level identified that significant changes occurred in the content of components of the extracellular matrix when treated with the gel.[29] Glycosaminoglycans (GAGs) are the first components of the extracellular matrix to be synthesised during healing and are major components of the ground substance upon which elastin and collagen fibres are laid, therefore playing a vital role in healing. The key finding of this work was that *Aloe vera* gel significantly enhanced the synthesis of GAGs in healing wounds.

The anti-inflammatory activity of *Aloe vera* gel has been demonstrated in several studies[30,31] making it particularly useful in wound care when viewed in conjunction with the activities previously detailed. The use of gel formulations is not ideal however in wounds with excessive exudate as the gel may be too easily washed away.

Honey

Honey has been used for centuries in wound care and in recent years it has undergone a revival as research has shown how it can play an effective role in wound dressings, burns and ulcerated conditions. According to Peter Molan, a leading honey researcher at the University of Waikato, New Zealand, 'honey rapidly clears infection and promotes clean healthy granulation tissue'.[32] The high osmolarity of honey due to its high sugar content and its ability to generate hydrogen peroxide when diluted contribute greatly to its efficacy. (The proin-flammatory effect that in the past has been seen in hydrogen peroxide wound treatments is not seen in honey as the hydrogen peroxide levels generated are very low.)[32–34] Although many honeys inhibit microbial growth because of the generation of hydrogen peroxide there are specific phytochemicals in certain honeys that contribute to this effect: honey derived from *Leptospermum* species, for example manuka, generates no hydrogen peroxide[32] but demonstrates broad-spectrum antimicrobial activity.[35] A systematic review of randomised trials of honey wound dressings in 2001 concluded that, although studies were of limited quality, six out of seven studies showed honey to be superior to conventional treatments for wound healing, maintenance of sterility and clear-ance of infection.[36]

The proliferation of phagocytes, B- and T-lymphocytes in cell cultures is stimulated by honey at concentrations as low as 0.1%. Honey at a concentration of 1% also stimulates monocytes in cell cultures to release cytokines, tumor necrosis factor (TNF)-alpha, interleukin (IL)-1, and IL-6, which activate the host immune response in cases of infection. Autolytic debridement of wounds is

Table 10.2 Taken from the French aromatic model, this formula is cited by Baudoux and Zhiri[39] for the treatment of ulcerated skin conditions and illustrates how essential oils and honey may be combined.

Example formula

Essential oils:

Mentha piperita 0.3 ml
Laurus nobilis 0.5 ml
Lavandula latifolia spica 0.5 ml
Melaleuca alternifolia 1 ml

Add honey to make total quantity of 100 ml.
Apply twice daily until healing is complete.

assisted by the glucose content of honey and the acid pH (typically between pH 3 and 4) accelerating the activity of macrophages, so enhancing healing times.[37]

Examples of wounds that have been successfully treated with honey include minor abrasions, cuts, abscesses, large infected wounds, pressure sores and skin ulcers,[33] infected skin grafting donor sites[38] and burns.[37] Although no clinical trials have yet been published investigating the synergistic effects of essential oil and honey formulations, there is plenty of anecdotal evidence from the two traditions to suggest that the combination offers interesting avenues for much further research in wound treatments. Table 10.2 gives an example from the work of Baudoux and Zhiri[39] to illustrate how the combination may be used. Note that this formula forms part of a broader treatment regime that includes hydrosol and oil-based preparations.

Carrier oils

As well as hydrosols, honey and *Aloe vera*, aromatherapists can make excellent use of selected vegetable and infused oils as wound-healing mediums. The hydrophobic nature of the oils will prevent dessication of the wound, providing the essential moist environment for optimal healing to occur. Where inflammation is dominating the clinical picture, *Hypericum perforatum* (St John's wort) and *Calendula officinalis* (marigold) infused oils are indicated. Both have anti-inflammatory activity and efficacy in promoting wound healing[40] and appear on the German Commission E list of approved herbs for the external treatment of wounds and injuries. In the case of calendula, it is listed for poorly healing wounds as it has anti-inflammatory and granulatory action and *Hypericum* is cited for use in first-degree burns and for its anti-inflammatory activity.[41]

Looking at the traditional uses of *Calophyllum inophyllum* (tamanu) oil it shows interesting promise in wound healing, with reports from French medical literature citing its effectiveness in treating severe burns and even serious gangrenous conditions.[42] The anti-inflammatory activity of tamanu is partly due to the xanthones found in the oil and its significant antimicrobial and analgesic activity (ibid.) further strengthens its place in wound-healing preparations.

Rosa rubiginosa (rosehip seed) oil holds a well-established place in aromatherapy being particularly valued for its beneficial effects on scarring. The optimal therapeutic quality is obtained from cold pressing of plants grown in Chile, where much of the research has been conducted into its cicatrising effects. It has been suggested that the oil contains trans-retinoic acid, which would account for its healing activity; however, this has been disputed and research on other sources of the oil has not confirmed its presence.[43]

Vegetable oils can be used either as compresses or massaged lightly around the surrounding tissues of open wounds. Light massage is especially valuable in preventing the development of pressure sores in cases where the skin is fragile and inflamed but still unbroken. The beneficial effects of massage on skin blood flow is likely to play an important part in improving tissue-healing capacity, especially in ageing skin. In work that compared the application of Retin-A (a vitamin A derivative used to control hyperproliferative skin disorders, acne and to improve the appearance of photoaged skin) and petroleum jelly to the atrophic skin of the lower leg in elderly women, both agents increased resting blood flow.[44] As petroleum jelly is unlikely to have any effect on angiogenesis, the researchers suggested that the daily massage improved the skin's blood perfusion and lymph microcirculation. For those familiar with the clinical experience of massage, this research is not a surprising finding and it goes some way to confirming the value of regular massage in maintaining skin integrity and resilience.

Scarring

Skin scars are the normal, inevitable result of damage to the dermis and occur during the final phase of wound healing. Although normal, they can be unpleasant both aesthetically and physically, with accompanying itching, tenderness, pain and disfigurement as well as a host of psychological issues including stigmatisation being reported.[45] Normal scars are soft, not unduly red and do not restrict movement; if hair follicles are damaged, they lack hair. Pigmentation may not fully return but over a period of weeks and years, normal scars gradually fade, become flatter, softer and any pain that is present lessens.

Scar types

Scars range from a 'normal' fine line to widespread, atrophic or hypertrophic and keloid types. They tend to be most noticeable in the deltoid and sternal regions, and in adolescents and young adults compared with those seen in the very young and the elderly. Keloid scars are an excessive proliferation of connective tissue and are unique to humans. They have the following characteristics:

- present as raised, firm nodules or plaques
- protrude beyond the original wound and invade surrounding normal skin
- occur mainly on upper torso and ear lobes
- a keloid continues to grow and does not spontaneously regress
- the highest rates of incidence are among black Africans and in the second to fourth decades.

Similar to keloids, hypertrophic scars are raised, but they remain within the margins of the original wound and typically occur following burns. Like keloids, they are often red, inflamed and itchy. Unlike keloids, they regress over time and occur earlier after injury (within four weeks normally). Histologic differences exist between keloids and hypertrophic scars, with large collagen bundles characterising keloids. There is no routinely effective conventional treatment available and, in the case of keloids, surgical removal has a 50–80% risk of recurrence.[45] Intralesional steroid injections, cryotherapy, radiotherapy and compression therapy are the mainstay of treatment.

Widespread (stretched) scars are typically flat, pale, soft and asymptomatic and include common stretchmarks after pregnancy or significant weight gain. In these, damage to the dermis and subcutaneous tissues exist, but the epidermis is intact. Atrophic scars are small flat depressions and are commonly seen following chickenpox and acne. Scars that traverse joints or skin creases at right angles are prone to shortening, resulting in contractures occurring when the scar is immature. Scar contractures commonly follow burn injury, can restrict move-ment, and are typically disabling.

Scar management

Although evidence from clinical trials is scarce to support the empirical practice of using massage to improve the appearance of scars, it certainly has a long tradition of use. Massage works in a similar way to compression therapy, breaking up fibrous tissue and promoting blood flow, and as a non-invasive approach is worth considering. The application of vitamin E to scar tissue has gained popularity over the years due to its antioxidant activity. It is thought antioxidants enhance wound healing by reducing damage caused by the release of free radicals in the inflammatory phase. As vitamin E has been shown to prevent free radical induced changes in collagen and glycosaminoglycan bio-synthesis in vitro,[46] it follows that it may play a useful role in speeding up healing. However, results obtained from in vivo studies have not been encouraging, with few improvements being noted in human studies (ibid.).

Rosa rubiginosa (rosehip seed) oil is empirically valued for improving the appearance of scars. As previously stated this may be due to the presence of trans-retinoic acid that has been reported in some Chilean samples. Although work on samples from other sources has failed to identify its presence,[43] this is not the same as saying that the oil is ineffective on scarring. It may be that the effects traditionally reported arise from components other than trans-retinoic acid.

Chithra *et al.*,[29] in work looking at *Aloe vera* and healing, identified that both oral and topical use of the gel increased the levels of hyaluronic acid in wounds. Hyaluronic acid plays an important role in the early stages of healing, and may provide a more fluid and malleable matrix, facilitating greater cell mobility and early remodelling. In foetal fibroblast cultures, it has been shown to stimulate collagen synthesis and it is known that foetal wounds that heal without scarring contain 100% hyaluronic acid in the wound matrix. This makes *Aloe vera* a promising topical base, not only for application to open wounds, but also for massaging into newly healed tissue, to promote the formation of more stable, healthy scars.

References

1 Babu M, Wells A. Dermal-epidermal communication in wound healing. *Wounds*. 2001; **13**(5): 183–9.

2 Bowler PG. Wound pathophysiology, infection and therapeutic options. *Annals Med*. 2002; **34**: 419–27.

3 Catty S. *Hydrosols: the next aromatherapy*. Vermont: Healing Arts Press; 2001.

4 Sagdic O, Ozcan M. Antibacterial activity of spice hydrosols. *Food Control*. 2003; **14**: 141–3.

5 Sagdic O. Sensitivity of four pathogenic bacteria to Turkish thyme and oregano hydrosols. *Lebensmittel-Wissenschaft und-Technologie*. 2003; **36**(5): 467–73.

6 Bowler PG, Duerden BI, Armstrong DG. Wound microbiology and associated approaches to wound management. *Clin Microbiol Rev*. 2001; **14**(2): 244–69.

7 Opalchenova G, Obreshkova D. Comparative studies on the activity of basil L. – against multidrug resistant clinical isolates of the genera *Staphylococcus, Enterococcus* and *Pseudomonas* by using different test methods. *J Microbiol Methods*. 2003; **54**: 105–10.

8 Edwards-Jones V, Buck R, Shawcross SG *et al*. The effect of essential oils on methicillin-resistant *Staphylococcus aureus* using a dressing model. *Burns*. 2004; **30**: 772–7.

9 Inouye S, Yamaguchi H, Takizawa T. Screening of the antibacterial effects of a variety of essential oils on respiratory tract pathogens, using the modified dilution assay method. *J Infect Chemother*. 2001; **7**: 251–4.

10 Nostro A, Blanco, AR Cannatelli MA *et al*. Susceptibility of methicillin-resistant staphylococci to oregano essential oil, carvacrol and thymol. *FEMS Microbiol Lett*. 2004; **230**: 191–5.

11 Nelson RRS. In-vitro activities of five plant essential oils against methicillin-resistant *Staphylococcus aureus* and vancomycin-resistant *Enterococcus faecium*. *J Antimicrob Chemother*. 1997; **40**: 305–6.

12 Skocibusic M, Bezic N. Phytochemical analysis and in vitro antimicrobial activity of two Satureja species essential oils. *Phytother Res*. 2004; **18**: 967–70.

13 Caelli M, Porteous J, Carson CF *et al*. Tea tree oil as an alternative topical decolonisation agent for methicillin-resistant *Staphylococcus aureus*. *J Hosp Infect*. 2000; **46**: 236–7.

14 Dryden MS, Dailly S, Crouch M. A randomised, controlled trial of tea tree topical preparations versus a standard topical regimen for the clearance of MRSA colonization. *J Hosp Infect*. 2004; **56**: 283–6.

15 Elsom GKF, Hide D. Susceptibility of methicillin-resistance *Staphylococcus aureus* to tea tree oil and mupirocin. *J Antimicrob Chemother*. 1999; **43**: 427–8.

16 Carson CF, Cookson BD, Farrelly HD *et al*. Susceptibility of methicillin-resistant *Staphylococcus aureus* to the essential oil of *Melaleuca alternifolia*. *J Antimicrob Chemother*. 1995; **35**: 421–4.

17 May J, Chan CH, King A. Time-kill studies of tea tree oils on clinical isolates. *J Antimicrob Chemother*. 2000; **45**: 639–43.

18 Kerr J. The use of essential oils in healing wounds. *Int J Aromatherapy*. 2002; **12**(4): 202–6.

19 Hartman D, Coetzee JC. Two US practitioners' experience of using essential oils for wound care. *J Wound Care*. 2002; **11**(8): 317–20.

20 Guba R. Wound healing. *Int J Aromatherapy*. 1999; **9**(2): 67–74.

21 Buckle J. *Clinical Aromatherapy*. 2nd ed. Philadelphia: Churchill Livingstone; 2003.

22 Jakovlev V, Issac O, Thiemer K *et al*. Pharmacological investigations with compounds of chamomile. II. New investigations on the antiphlogistic effects of (–) alpha bisabolol and bisabolol oxides. *Planta Med*. 1979; **35**(2): 125–40.

23 Glowania HJ, Rawlin C, Svoboda M. Effect of chamomile on wound healing – a clinical double blind study. *Z Hautkr*. 1987; **62**(17): 1267–71.

24 Carl W, Emrich LS. Management of oral mucositis during radiation and systemic chemotherapy. *J Prosthet Dent*. 1991; **66**(3): 361–9.

25 Villegas LF, Marcalo A, Martin J *et al*. (+)-epi-alpha-bisabolol is the wound healing principle of *Peperomia galioides*: investigation of the in vivo wound healing activity of related terpenoids. *J Nat Prod*. 2001; **64**: 1357–9.

26 Cundell J, Donnelly J, Gill D *et al*. *Evidence-based Wound Management*. Belfast: Queen's University; 2002.

27 Choi SW, Son BW, Son YS *et al*. The wound healing effect of a glycoprotein fraction isolated from *Aloe vera*. *Br J Dermatol*. 2001; **145**: 535–45.

28 Abdullah KM, Abdullah A, Johnson ML *et al*. Effects of *Aloe vera* on gap junctional intercellular communication and proliferation of human diabetic and nondiabetic skin fibroblasts. *J Altern Complement Med*. 2003; **9**(5): 711–18.

29 Chithra P, Sajithlal GB, Chandrakasan G. Influence of *Aloe vera* on the glycosaminoglycans in the matrix of healing dermal wounds in rats. *J Ethnopharmacol*. 1998; **59**: 179–86.

30 Vázquez B, Avila G, Segura D *et al*. Anti-inflammatory activity of extracts from *Aloe vera* gel. *J Ethnopharmacol*. 1996; **55**: 69–75.

31 Reynolds T, Dweck AC. *Aloe vera* leaf gel: a review update. *J Ethnopharmacol*. 1999; **68**: 3–37.

32 Bonn D. Sweet solution to superbug infections? *Lancet*. 2003; **3**: 608.

33 Bang LM, Buntting C, Molan P. The effect of dilution on the rate of hydrogen peroxide in honey and its implications for wound healing. *J Altern Complement Med*. 2003; **9**(2): 267–73.

34 www.medlockmedical.com/mesitranlaunch/honeyeducation.htm (accessed 20.01.06).

35 Cooper RA, Molan PC, Harding KG. The sensitivity to honey of Gram-positive cocci of clinical significance isolated from wounds. *J Appl Microbiol*. 2002; **93**: 857–63.

36 Moore OA, Smith LA, Campbell F *et al*. Systematic review of the use of honey as a wound dressing. *BMC Complement Altern Med*. 2001; **1**: 2.

37 Bangroo AK, Ramji K, Smita C. Honey dressing in pediatric burns. *J Indian Assoc Pediatr Surg*. 2005; **10**(3): 172–5.

38 Misirlioglu A, Eroglu S, Karacaoglan N *et al*. Use of honey as an adjunct in the healing of split-thickness skin graft donor site. *Dermatol Surg*. 2003; **29**: 168–72.

39 Baudoux D, Zhiri A. *Les Cahiers Pratiques d'Aromathérapie Selon l'école Française*. Vol. 2. Luxembourg: Edition Inspir; 2003.

40 Lavagna SM, Secci D, Chimenti P *et al*. Efficacy of hypericum and calendula oils in the epithelial reconstruction of surgical wounds in childbirth with caesarean section. *Il Farmaco*. 2001; **56**: 451–2.

41 Blumenthal M, editor. *The Complete German Commission E Monographs*. Austin, Texas: American Botanical Council; 1998.

42 Kilham C. Tamanu oil: a tropical topical remedy. *HerbalGram*. 2004; **63**: 26–31.

43 Dweck AC. Formulating with natural ingredients. *Cosmetics Toiletries*. 2001; **116**(5): 57–60.

44 Strigini L, Ryan T. Wound healing in elderly human skin. *Clinics Dermatol*. 1996; **14**: 197–206.

45 Bayat A, McGrouther DA, Ferguson MWJ. Skin scarring. *BMJ*. 2003; **326**: 88–92.

46 Baumann LS, Spencer J. The effects of topical vitamin E on the cosmetic appearance of scars. *Dermatol Surg*. 1999; **25**: 311–15.

Chapter 11

Nails, hair and sebaceous glands

Introduction

By convention, the nails and hair follicles and their sebaceous glands are considered as 'appendages' or derivatives of the skin. All lie within the dermis or subcutis and connect with the surface. The nails are a remnant of the mammalian claw and consist of hardened plates of packed keratin. Some systemic diseases produce nail changes, but as these lie outside the aromatherapeutic range they are not included here.

Sebaceous glands are associated with hair follicles and are not found in non-hairy sites. They are formed from epidermis-derived cells and become active at puberty, producing sebum, the exact function of which is not yet fully understood. Recent work shows it is directly involved in epidermal structure and barrier maintenance and protection from ultraviolet radiation. It transports antioxidants to the skin surface and plays a role in skin-specific hormonal signalling.[1] Increased sebum secretion is known to be involved in the development of acne.

Disorders affecting the hair and sebaceous glands such as alopecia and acne can have devastating psychological consequences and effective treatments are increasingly recognised as being those which achieve improvement in psychiatric comorbidity as well as the physical symptoms[2] and here aromatherapy has much to offer as explored in Chapter 6. Unrealistic expectations of treatment need careful management as, for some of these conditions, symptom control is all that is achievable while cures remain elusive.

Acne

This is one of the most common skin diseases with the reported prevalence varying from 35 to 90% of adolescents with gender and age variations. The pathogenesis of acne is multifactorial with primary features being:

- increased sebum production
- proliferation of *Proprionibacterium acnes* in the pilosebaceous duct
- abnormal follicular keratinisation and plugging
- release of inflammatory mediators.

Genetic factors may contribute to the disorder, although precise mechanisms and influences are not fully elucidated. It may vary from mild with only a few comedones, papules and pustules to severe with highly inflammatory, nodulocystic, scarring lesions requiring medical treatment. Acne scars are permanent and distressing. Table 11.1 gives the clinical variants. The remainder of this section concentrates on the most common form, acne vulgaris.

Table 11.1 Variants of acne.

Form	Description
Acne excoriée	Most frequently seen in young girls and women. There are few primary acne lesions, the main ones are caused by picking and squeezing. A condition closely associated with body image pathologies and psychological dynamics that are very similar to those found in eating disorders.[2]
Acne conglobata	Nodulocystic acne lesions characterise this severe form, which heals with deep, sometimes keloidal scarring.
Drug induced	Corticosteroids, androgenic steroids, lithium and oral contraceptives may cause acneic eruptions. Lesions differ from acne vulgaris by being of uniform size and symmetric distribution on the neck, chest and back. Scarring is absent.
Infantile	More common in male infants. The changes are identical to common acne and unfortunately it is linked with severe acne in adolescence.
Acne fulminans	A rare form of nodulocystic acne accompanied by malaise, fever, joint pains and a high ESR. Requires prompt medical treatment.
Acne mechanica	Mechanical pressure leads to acneic lesions. Common causes include wearing orthopaedic braces, straps or violin playing.

Although principally a disorder affecting adolescents with the first signs commonly observed in early puberty, for some individuals, acne vulgaris can persist into middle age. It begins earlier in females than males, reflecting the earlier onset of puberty; however, in later teen years, the severity is worse in males than in females. This is in line with the relationship between androgenous hormones and sebum secretion as, in acneic skin, androgenic stimulation of the sebaceous glands leads to hyperseborrhoea and the characteristically shiny appearance of a greasy skin. However, this is not the same as saying that androgens cause acne as many factors appear to be involved in the process with a need for several to combine for acne to develop.

Changes in the pilosebaceous unit

The pilosebaceous unit consists of the hair shaft (pilo), the sebaceous gland and the infundibulum, or duct (pore), which leads to the skin surface. This is divided into the upper epidermal and the lower dermal parts. Stratum corneum lines the whole duct and the area closest to the skin surface normally sheds corneocytes, together with cells from the rest of the epidermis. However, in acneic skin, cells of the infundibulum become abnormally adherent and instead of being shed and discharged freely through the duct, they form a hyperkeratotic plug – a micro-comedo – in the canal.

Linoleic acid deficiency has been suggested as a causative factor in this process[3] and it is known that acneic skin contains much less linoleic acid than control subjects.[4] As microcomedones enlarge, these greasy plugs, made up of a mixture of keratin, sebum and bacteria, become the visually familiar early acneic lesions: open comedones form blackheads and closed ones whiteheads, which are the precursors of inflammatory acne lesions (*see* Figure 11.1).

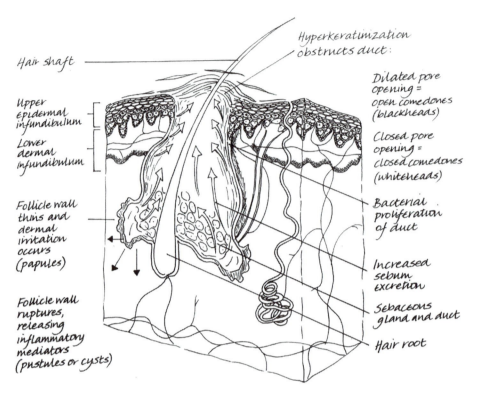

Figure 11.1 Pathogenesis of acne lesions.

Microbial proliferation and inflammation

Pre-pubertal skin is virtually free from *P. acnes* colonisation; however, following androgenic stimulation of the duct and the subsequent hyperseborrhoea, an ideal environment exists for bacterial proliferation. Progression to a second inflammatory stage is triggered by the release of pro-inflammatory mediators produced by both *P. acnes* and from corneocytes in the pilosebaceous duct. These inflammatory mediators penetrate the surrounding tissues leading to the formation of papules, nodules and pustules and eventual rupturing of the duct.[5] However, although *P. acnes* may induce inflammation, it is not entirely responsible. Involvement of endogenous inflammatory processes in the infundibulum requires therapy which targets this as well as reducing bacteria and sebum production.[6]

Aromatherapy treatment for mild acne

Essential oils

While cleansing helps to regulate the levels of oils on skin as well as reducing numbers of skin flora, it is incorrect to overemphasise the need for skin cleansing, as it can lead to irritation and dryness. Acne is not directly related to skin hygiene and inflammatory lesions may easily be worsened by aggressive external treatment. Therapy should centre instead on providing antibacterial, anti-inflammatory formulations which aid corneocyte shedding from the infundibulum.

There is currently limited research evidence for essential oil efficacy in acne treatments, with most existing research identifying the beneficial role of *Melaleuca alternifolia* (tea tree),[7] which is widely used in topical treatments. One study[8] showed results from a single-blind, randomised clinical trial on 124 patients, comparing the efficacy and skin tolerance of 5% tea tree gel with 5% benzoyl peroxide lotion in cases of mild to moderate acne. In both cases, there was a significant reduction in the number of inflamed and non-inflamed lesions, although the onset of tea tree's action was slower. Importantly, there were fewer side effects recorded by those using the tea tree gel.

In another study which compared the major components of tea tree oil, terpinen-4-ol, α-terpineol and α-pinene, all were found to be active against *P. acnes*, whereas 1,8 cineole was inactive. This study supported the use of tea tree oil in acne treatments, and demonstrated that terpinen-4-ol was not the sole active constituent of the oil.[9] Tea tree has been shown to have topical anti-inflammatory activity,[10,11] leading to it fulfilling the criteria for anti-inflammatory and antibacterial effects.

Backhousia citriodora (lemon myrtle) has greater activity than tea tree against a broad range of micro-organisms, including *P. acnes*.[12] With citral being the major component of the oil, this presents difficulties with regard to skin sensitisation (*see* Chapter 3). The addition of terpenes has been shown to prevent this occurring,[13] leading to the possibility of creating effective topical antimicrobials using lemon myrtle. As microbiological activity of tea tree is enhanced in lemon myrtle's presence, their synergistic use is indicated in acne treatment. One final caution that is required in the use of lemon myrtle oil is that at high concentrations it is toxic to skin fibroblasts and should not be included at greater than 1% in topical use.[12]

Essential oil from the leaves of *Ocimum gratissimum* (clove basil) was tested in a variety of bases and concentrations against benzoyl peroxide 10% lotion and a placebo in 126 subjects presenting with acne vulgaris.[14] The test products were significantly more effective in reducing lesions than the placebo, with the *Ocimum* preparations acting more quickly and effectively than the benzoyl peroxide. Adverse effects were minimal, with a mild tolerable burning sensation being reported, which reduced with continued application. The oil contains about 75% thymol and therefore requires careful use in topical therapy.

The study included patch testing the oil using a four-day repeated assault open patch test which assisted in determining the clinically effective concentration and most appropriate base: this was given as 2% *Ocimum* oil in a cetomacrogol (cream) hydrophilic base. It was suggested that 1% oil be used in those with sensitive skin. When the oil was in a petrolatum base the activity was lessened; this is unsurprising as the essential oil would have an affinity with the hydrophobic base and therefore be released more slowly.

Psychological factors

Assessing the severity of acne is an important part of the management of the condition. The severity is rated not only on how the acne appears visually but also on the psychological and social effects it has for the individual. It has been

Table 11.2 A selection of essential oils with anti-inflammatory activity on the skin that are traditionally valued for their effects on the psyche.

Researched anti-inflammatory activity	Traditional use
Anthemis nobilis[17,18]	Achillea millefolium
Cedrus deodara[19]	Boswellia carterii
Chamomilla recutita[22]	Rosa damascena
Commiphora myrrha[20]	
Cymbopogon martini[21]	
Helichrysum italicum[20]	
Lavandula angustifolia[25]	
Matricaria recutita[20]	
Melaleuca alternifolia[23,24]	
Pelargonium graveolens[26]	
Pogostemon cablin[20]	
Santalum album[20]	

shown that the older the sufferer, the greater the psychological distress, regardless of the severity of acne.[15] Psychiatric morbidity in acne can be as severe and serious as that arising from chronic conditions such as asthma and diabetes.[16]

Unlike psoriasis, the physical severity of acne does not always correlate with the severity of depression and even mild to moderate acne has been associated with depression and suicide.[2] Many patients experience a worsening of their symptoms during periods of stress and Cunliffe[5] suggests a link between the pituitary-adrenal axis involved in stress and androgenic stimulation of the pilosebaceous unit. It is clear that addressing the psychological aspects of each case is as important as choosing essential oils for their antibacterial and anti-inflammatory actions. Table 11.2 lists oils that meet these criteria in one or more areas. Finally, even though the researched antibacterial activity of essential oils against *P. acnes* is mainly limited to *Melaleuca alternifolia*, *Backhousia citriodora* and *Ocimum gratissimum*, other essential oils with broad antibacterial activity are still worthy of consideration and further research.

Mediums

The choice of medium used in topical applications will largely be determined by user preference. Compliance in any treatment regime is crucial as treatment is often long term and poor compliance has been linked with the failure of some conventional treatments. Lotions and gels are generally pleasant to use, being non-greasy and having a slightly drying effect, helping to counter hyperseborrhoeic skin. *Aloe vera* gel has been shown to enhance the anti-acne properties of *Ocimum gratissimum* oil.[27] In this particular study, the efficacy of the essential oil based products increased in line with the increased content of *Aloe vera* gel, with 2% *Ocimum* oil in 50% aloe gel aqueous dilution proving to be the best formulation.

The inclusion of hydrosols in the water phase when preparing gels, creams and lotions adds to the anti-inflammatory and antibacterial activity of the final product. *Hamamelis virginiana* (witch hazel) hydrosol is widely used in skin-care products for its anti-inflammatory and wound-healing activity.[28,29] It is essential that only true hydrosol be used rather than any alcohol-based witch hazel, which may increase the risk of irritation. Hydrosols can be used neat for daily skin cleansing or used as a cool compress on inflamed lesions. Ointments are best avoided, as they can be comedogenic.

In one double-blind, placebo-controlled, randomised cross-over study[30] linoleic acid was topically applied to comedones in patients with mild acne. Results showed a 25% reduction in comedone size over a one-month period, compared with no change in the placebo-treated group. It was suggested that topical linoleic acid might be useful in the treatment of acne. Drawing upon these research findings, the topical application of vegetable oils with lipid profiles that are rich in linoleic acid (e.g. *Carthamus tinctorius* and *Helianthus annuus*) offers two possible benefits for acneic skin. First, by seeping into hypercornified ducts this may help them to normalise, increase desquamation of the stratum corneum and thus prevent comedo formation and the inflammatory sequelae. Second, it is entirely plausible that the potential supplementation of linoleic acid will occur, following skin metabolism of triglycerides from the oils, thereby reducing comedone size.

Light exfoliation assists in the shedding of cells from the stratum corneum, including cells from the pilosebaceous duct. It is essential that exfoliation is not done excessively nor with abrasive agents as overstimulation of the epidermis may lead to an aggravation of the hypercornification of the pilosebaceous duct[31] and further inflammatory changes. Additional vegetable oils such as *Corylus avellana* (hazelnut) and *Simmondsia chinensis* (jojoba) wax can be used as natural exfoliants. Jojoba is of particular use in reducing inflammation.[32] Table 11.3 offers sample formulations for the treatment of mild acne.

Table 11.3 Sample formulations for mild acne.

Essential oil spot treatment	*Hydrosol cleanser*
Essential oils: • *Melaleuca alternifolia* 50% • *Lavandula angustifolia* 20% • *Pogostemon cablin* 20% • *Matricaria recutita* 10%. Apply neat to each lesion morning and evening using a cotton bud.	Hydrosols: • *Lavandula angustifolia* 40% • *Hamamelis virginiana* 40% • *Thymus vulgaris* 20%. Use as cleanser morning and evening, or apply as cold compress to inflamed lesions, leaving in place for 10 minutes.
Weekly exfoliating mask for face and body	
Essential oils: • *Pelargonium graveolens* 0.25 ml • *Cistus ladaniferus* 0.25 ml • *Chamaemelum nobile* 0.25 ml • *Melaleuca alternifolia* 0.25 ml.	Vegetable/carrier oils: • *Simmondsia chinensis* 10 ml • *Helianthus annuus* 20 ml. Hydrosol: • *Mentha piperita* 150 ml.
Mix everything into 200 g of green clay. Apply for 10 minutes once a week.	

Rosacea and perioral dermatitis

Although most common in middle age, rosacea occurs in people over the age of 30 with the highest prevalence among the fair-skinned and those of Celtic and northern and eastern European descent.[33] It is a chronic inflammatory condition, characterised by erythema, telangiectasia and recurrent papulopustules and the cause remains unknown. The mites *Demodex folliculorum* and *D. brevis*, found in the follicular infundibulum and sebaceous glands respectively, have been identified as cofactors in the pathogenesis of rosacea[34] and, although not the sole cause, increased populations of mites may play a role in provoking inflammatory or allergic reactions.[34,35] This view is supported by reports of the prevalence and density of mites being statistically significant in those cases progressing to the papulopustular stage.[34]

The clinical picture sometimes includes lymphoedema of the cheeks, nose, forehead and chin. Chronic sebaceous hyperplasia of the nose leads to an irreversible hypertrophy (rhinophyma) usually affecting men. The lack of comedones distinguishes rosacea from late-onset acne vulgaris. The disease is chronic, persistent and in some cases there may be periods of remission, followed by relapse. Sebum secretion is normal, but, histologically, sebaceous gland hyperplasia, dilated dermal vasculature and an inflammatory cell infiltrate are seen.[36]

Perioral dermatitis presents with papules and pustules around the mouth, chin and nose. There are several similarities between rosacea and perioral dermatitis: the skin feels tight, dryness is marked, moisturisers and cosmetics readily cause burning or stinging sensations and both are aggravated by topical corticosteroids. The similar clinical pattern of these conditions has led some to maintain that perioral dermatitis is a variant of rosacea.[37] In both cases exact causes are unknown but suggestions include the possible role of cosmetic preparations and overuse of moisturisers, perhaps by an occlusive mechanism in conjunction with proliferation of skin flora.[35] Kobayashi and Tagami[38] suggest that as the perioral region has the poorest stratum corneum barrier function and highest skin surface temperature of anywhere on the face, this may lead to hypersensitivity reactions in the area. They also identified differences in transepidermal water loss (TEWL) values in different facial regions, with the perioral region showing the highest. Furthermore, the stratum corneum of the nasolabial fold showed a low hydration state probably related to skin lipid levels.

Aromatherapeutic options

In both conditions no cure exists and treatments aim to suppress the distressing signs and symptoms. Main principles include keeping the skin cool, avoiding vasodilation and ensuring that nothing be done to provoke irritation. As overzealous use of occlusive moisturisers may be a causative factor, lotions offer the right moisture-balancing medium as well as providing a soothing, cooling effect on the skin. Along with lotions, gels are also recommended, as they are refreshing and cooling and the incorporation of vegetable oils in their preparation helps to counterbalance their drying tendency.

Exfoliation and any drying agents are to be avoided, including all alcohol-based products. Essential oils must be used with care, as adverse reactions to all

Table 11.4 Endogenous and exogenous rosacea triggers. Avoidance can play a major role in the management of flare-ups.

Weather	Sunlight, cold, humidity, strong winds.
Food and drink	Dairy products, hydrogenated fats, citrus fruits, chocolate, spicy food, tomatoes, bananas, alcohol, hot drinks, coffee and tea, refined sugars.
Emotional	Stress, anxiety, anger.
Temperature	Hot humid environments, e.g. saunas, steam rooms, hot baths.
Exercise	Although gentle exercise is beneficial, overheating and profuse sweating is best avoided.
Medication	Topical corticosteroids, vasodilators.
Cosmetics	Hairsprays, alcohol-based products, fragrances, occlusive moisturisers.

externally applied products are a real possibility considering the heightened sensitivity of rosaceous skin. Suitable anti-inflammatory oils are given in Table 11.2. In addition, oils traditionally considered to have astringent effects are appropriate, such as *Cupressus sempervirens* (cypress), *Citrus aurantium var. amara* flos. (neroli), and *Cistus ladaniferus* (rock rose). (Note the distinction between synthetic alcohol-based astringents, which work by stripping the skin of its oils and are thus contraindicated in rosacea treatment, and the reputed astringent effect of essential oils.)

Hydrosols offer excellent cooling, refreshing properties and can be included in the formulation of lotions as well as being used individually in cool compresses and atomiser sprays to control flushing. Suitable hydrosols include *Anthemis nobilis* (Roman chamomile), *Citrus aurantium* flos. (neroli), *Cistus ladaniferus* (rock rose), *Lavandula angustifolia* (lavender), *Rosa damascena* (rose) and *Pelargonium graveolens* (geranium).

Initially testing a small area of affected skin with any preparation is advisable to assess individual tolerance, and clients should be advised to discontinue use immediately if flare occurs. The nature of rosacea with its unknown aetiology and somewhat unpredictable reactions to a host of triggers can easily result in the provocation of unpleasant flare and irritation. There are a number of recognised triggers for rosacea and these are given in Table 11.4. Working with the client to identify their individual trigger profile helps in developing strategies to avoid these factors to control flare-ups.

Once individual triggers have been identified, as well as avoidance, simple measures can be adopted such as wearing sunscreen, using only water-based hypo-allergenic cosmetics and cooling the skin with hydrosol sprays and compresses, all of which can make a substantial contribution to controlling the disorder.

Hair

A range of disorders affect the hair and scalp throughout the human lifespan, from 'cradle cap' in infants to dandruff and poorly understood disorders such as alopecia areata along with the common but often upsetting disorder, androgenic alopecia (male pattern baldness). Comorbidity with major psychiatric illness is recognised in disorders such as alopecia areata and research has identified that patients with stress-reactive alopecia may have higher depression scores than the general population.[2]

General care

Using aromatherapy to maintain scalp and hair health is simple and effective. For conditions involving dryness, irritation and flaking, oily scalp soaks are indicated but user compliance may be difficult to maintain.

In light of recent studies that have identified the influence played by hair follicles on the penetration of topically applied substances,[39] high absorption rates can be assumed when formulating for scalp preparations. The phenomenon of active and inactive hair follicles is known to influence the extent of absorption, with active follicles being those where hair growth and sebum production is detected and where absorption occurs.[40] On a healthy scalp, usually more than 70% of hair follicles are active at any one time, but in conditions involving sebaceous gland and follicular destruction, such as scarring alopecia, permeation rates will be reduced.

Alopecia

The hair follicle is an invaginated structure of the dermis and epidermis and has been described as having one of the most complex functions of all bodily structures.[41] It is required to produce a multicellular hair shaft on the skin surface over a lengthy period while preserving in the dermis an 'epithelial finger' that produces the shaft. Hair growth is a complex, cyclically driven biological process, co-ordinated by and dependent upon a variety of exogenous stimuli and endogenous signals. Unlike in some mammals, hair loss and growth is not seasonal but occurs randomly and is a continual process.[35,36] The three phases of hair follicle development are as follows.

- *Anagen:* which is the growing phase and approximately 80–95% of scalp hairs are in anagen, with 50 to 100 follicles switching to catagen daily. This phase lasts between two and eight years.
- *Catagen:* is the transitional or resting phase, which lasts two to three weeks and it signals the end of anagen. The hair follicle shrinks in length as the lower part loosens from the connective tissue papilla and the dermal papilla moves upwards. At any one time, 5–20% of scalp hairs are in catagen.
- *Telogen:* is where activity stops; this is sometimes described as the resting or shedding phase and around 5% of scalp hairs are in telogen at any one time. It lasts around two to three months. After telogen, the cycle is complete and the hair goes back into the anagen phase.

Most hair-loss disorders are due to changes in these cycles but the under-standing of their causes remains incomplete. Classification of hair loss can be based upon distribution and scarring (*see* Tables 11.5 and 11.6). It has been suggested that the sebaceous gland may play an important role in ensuring the

Table 11.5 Classification of hair loss.

Non-scarring	Causes and appearance
Diffuse	
Androgenic alopecia (males) Androgenetic alopecia (females)	Male pattern baldness occurs in genetically predisposed individuals and is due to the shortening of successive anagen cycles. Androgen-sensitive follicles are distributed on the top of the head while those on the sides and back of the scalp are androgen-independent, which accounts for the characteristic pattern of hair loss in men. In contrast, women with diffuse alopecia tend to retain a normal hairline without recession, but experience pronounced central thinning.
Telogen effluvium	Hair follicles are synchronised into terminating anagen, entering telogen, and shedding at once. It occurs post-partum, following high fever, emotional stress and some cytotoxic drugs. The hair follicle is not diseased and there is no inflammation.
Trichotillomania, traction, trauma, cosmetic alopecia	Obsessive pulling or rubbing the hair results in hair loss, which recovers once the behaviour stops. Traction from hair styles, excessive straightening and bleaching all damage hair, leading to loss. The scalp may be inflamed.
Localised	
Alopecia areata	A common condition, which starts with sharply defined, non-inflamed spreading bald patches. Itching, tenderness or burning precedes hair loss in some cases. Alopecia totalis (complete scalp involvement) or universalis (whole body hair loss) are rare. Spontaneous re-growth is likely if the condition is localised.
Tinea capitis	Common in children, usually caused by anthropophilic fungi. Zoophilic infection produces a more severe inflammatory, boggy swelling known as a kerion which requires medical care. Scarring may result in severe cases.
Psoriasis	Temporary hair loss can occur if adherent plaques on the scalp are roughly removed.

Scarring	
Localised/diffuse	These involve either destruction of the hair follicle or scarring of the reticular dermis and hair loss is permanent.
Irradiation, burns	Chemical or thermal burns scar the scalp, causing hair loss.
Herpes zoster	Shingles of the first trigeminal dermatome may cause scarring of the scalp.
Lichen planus Discoid lupus erythematosus	When these conditions affect the scalp, erythema, scaling and follicular changes are seen.
Pseudopelade	A term used to describe the end-stage of an idiopathic destructive inflammatory process of the scalp without any apparent co-existing skin disease.

Table 11.6 Systemic causes of hair loss.

Thyroid disease.
Iron deficiency.
Systemic lupus erythematosus.
Malnutrition or crash dieting.
Secondary syphilis.

shaft exits the skin; destruction of the gland is implicated in the pathogenesis of scarring alopecias.[41]

Aromatherapy treatment

To date there has only been one randomised controlled trial investigating the efficacy of aromatherapy in the treatment of alopecia.[42] Eighty-four patients with alopecia areata (non-androgenic) were randomised into two groups. The active group self-massaged an essential oil mixture of *Thymus vulgaris* (thyme), *Lavandula angustifolia* (lavender), *Rosmarinus officinalis* (rosemary) and *Cedrus atlantica* (cedarwood) blended into a jojoba–grapeseed mix into the scalp each night for a period of seven months. The control group followed the same regimen using only the carrier oils. There was a statistically significant improvement in the aromatherapy group. Although the study has received some criticism[43] (centring on the fact that in half of adult patients with recent onset alopecia, spontaneous remission occurs within the first year), the study illustrates that, for some patients involved, aromatherapy was successful and this success could not be solely attributed to the benefits of massage alone.

Although further evidence from clinical trials for the efficacy of aromatherapy in this area is lacking, regular scalp massage using oils with a traditional place in hair care is appropriate and those in Table 11.7 offer a reliable option.

Seborrheic dermatitis of the scalp and dandruff

These conditions are frequently discussed together and it has been suggested that dandruff is a generic term for scalp flaking irrespective of cause;[44] they have similar aetiology and variable severity.[1] Here, dandruff will be used to refer to mild seborrheic dermatitis of the scalp.

Table 11.7 Vegetable and essential oils traditionally used in hair care.

Vegetable oils	Essential oils
Cocos nucifera	Cedrus atlantica, C. deodara
Simmondsia chinensis	Cupressus sempervirens
Calophyllum inophyllum	Citrus aurantium fol.
Juglans regia	Rosmarinus officinalis
Triticum vulgare	Cananga odorata var. genuina

Seborrheic dermatitis is a common, chronic inflammatory condition characterised by itching and the appearance of fine scaling and redness occurring in the seborrheic areas, most commonly the scalp, scalp margins, nasolabial folds, ears and eyebrows. Dandruff and seborrheic dermatitis represent more than superficial disorders of the stratum corneum: they involve hyperproliferation of the epidermis, disruption of intercellular and intracellular lipids and parakeratosis. Although the name implies that seborrhoea is involved, studies have shown that sebum excretion rates are not necessarily different from those in unaffected skin.[45] Despite the fact that a direct causative link has yet to be identified with sebum secretion and the condition, it does seem that some relationship exists. It is common in adolescence when sebaceous glands are most active and the distribution of lesions mirrors the distribution of sebaceous glands. Further, the prevalence is highest among men, suggesting an androgenic influence on the pilosebaceous unit.

Sebaceous gland secretions are distinct from the intercellular lipids of the stratum corneum, the depletion of which has been shown to be a characteristic feature of dandruff.[46] Work by Harding et al.[46] identified reduced levels of long-chain ceramides in dandruff, which are absent in sebum, a finding in line with typical dry skin. It was speculated that a seasonal decline in ceramide levels in the winter might help to explain the seasonal prevalence of dandruff. Although the cause of reduced lipids in scalp skin is not yet identified, the role of the commensal yeast *Malassezia* warrants attention.

The lipophilic yeasts of the genus *Malassezia* were formerly classified as *Pityrosporum* species[47] and the genus has recently been revised to include 10 species.[1] The distribution of *Malassezia* species in resident skin flora relates to sebaceous gland density, with the scalp, face, chest and back having the highest numbers. The peak age for normal carriage or disease by *Malassezia* is the early twenties, coinciding with high rates of sebaceous gland activity.[48]

In individuals with dandruff or seborrheic dermatitis, *Malassezia* found on the scalp have been reported to make up a high proportion of scalp microflora. *Malassezia* has an absolute requirement for fatty acids for growth thus actively metabolising and potentially depleting scalp lipids.[46] They consume the very specific saturated fatty acids necessary for their proliferation, leaving behind the unsaturated fatty acids. It has been shown that the *Malassezia* cause reversible changes in sebum composition, with a return to normal triglycerides and fatty acids occurring when scalp microflora are removed with an antifungal shampoo.[1] The presence of altered sebaceous secretions in the stratum corneum breaks down the skin barrier function, resulting in inflammation, irritation and flaking.

It has also been suggested that the inflammatory reaction of seborrheic dermatitis may be due to an abnormal reaction to the yeasts or to the penetration of *Malassezia*-derived toxins.[44,46] The work of Harding et al.[46] suggests an intrinsic predisposition to dandruff, with susceptible individuals having inherently reduced stratum corneum lipid levels and a readily perturbed permeability barrier, which makes them more prone to the adverse effects of microbial activity in scalp skin, as well as exogenous factors.

Treatment of dandruff

Although there is currently no consensus about the exact cause of seborrheic dermatitis and dandruff, it is noteworthy that, in recent years, effective allopathic treatment has switched from focusing on anti-inflammatory agents to the greater use of antifungals.[1] The in vitro activity of *Melaleuca alternifolia* (tea tree) oil against *Malassezia* species has been compared favourably with that of the antifungals ketoconazole, econazole and miconazole[49] and could be considered in formulations for both antifungal and anti-inflammatory activity.[24,49,50] Oregano oil (*Origanum vulgare ssp. hirtum*)[51] has good activity against *Malassezia sp.* but the high phenol content makes it problematic for long-term use on the scalp. Table 11.8 lists oils that either have proven antifungal activity against a range of organisms, if not specifically *Malassezia,* or which are worth considering for their anti-inflammatory, antipruritic activity.

In conjunction with targeting microbial activity on the scalp, inflammation along with the perturbed barrier function can be corrected by topical application of vegetable oils such as *Simmondsia chinensis* (jojoba) liquid wax and *Helianthus annus* (sunflower)[54] and macerated *Calendula officinalis* (calendula).[55] *Calophyllum inophyllum* (tamanu) has a long traditional use in hair and skin care and, although not everyone likes the aroma, small amounts can be included in formulations for its anti-inflammatory and emollient effects.[56]

It is common for those with dandruff and seborrheic dermatitis to avoid washing their hair, in the belief that washing will aggravate the dryness. This needs discouraging as washing minimises the accumulation of scale, which can exacerbate inflammation. Daily shampooing is advisable using a mild non-perfumed shampoo base into which a total of 5% essential oils from Table 11.8 can be added. Where possible, clients should be instructed to apply an oily scalp soak at night, covering with a shower cap if preferred. Shampooing it off in the morning is best done by massaging shampoo into the scalp before wetting the hair for ease of oil removal.

Although oil-based formulations are ideal to counter dryness and scaling, gels make an appropriate medium for occasional use as they tend to be better accepted. A pragmatic approach is often needed, as compliance over a sustained time period will only be achieved if formulations are aesthetically pleasing. If this means a gel is most likely to be used and an oily soak rejected, negotiating with the client the realistic use for each while stressing the therapeutic benefit should achieve a successful outcome. It must be recognised that using gels without the

Table 11.8 Essential oils with antifungal and/or anti-inflammatory activity, suitable for inclusion in anti-dandruff treatments.

Cedrus deodara[19]
Commiphora myrrha[20]
Cymbopogon martinii[21,53]
Lavandula angustifolia[25,52]
Matricaria recutita, Chamomilla recutita[20,22]
Melaleuca alternifolia[49,52,53]
Pelargonium graveolens[53]
Pogostemon cablin[53]
Santalum album[20,53]

Table 11.9 Sample formulations for seborrheic dermatitis and dandruff.

Nightly scalp soak

Essential oils:	Vegetable oils:
Melaleuca alternifolia 1 ml	*Calophyllum inophyllum* 8.5 ml
Lavandula angustifolia 0.5 ml	*Simmondsia chinensis* 90 ml
Cymbopogon martinii 0.5 ml	
Pogostemon cablin 0.5 ml	

Massage thoroughly into the scalp for at least five minutes, leaving on overnight. If necessary cover with a shower cap. To wash out, massage shampoo into the scalp before getting the hair wet. This formula should be used for two weeks, together with the shampoo formula.

Shampoo

Essential oils:
Thymus vulgaris 15%
Melaleuca alternifolia 60%
Lavandula angustifolia 25%

Add 5% of this formula to a mild, non-perfumed shampoo base and use daily.
Can be used regularly as prophylactic.

Hydrosol after-shampoo spray

Pelargonium graveolens 50%
Rosmarinus officinalis 50%

After shampooing, spray liberally over the scalp and if possible leave to dry naturally.
Can be used regularly as prophylactic.

support of oily soaks will have a drying effect on an already dry scalp and will exacerbate the condition.

Table 11.9 lists some examples of sample formulations for seborrheic dermatitis and dandruff.

Case example

A 50-year-old male presented with chronic dandruff and itchy scalp. Over the years several anti-dandruff shampoos had been used with varying degrees of efficacy. The scalp was red and he had noticed recent increased hair loss. As the scalp was extremely dry, nightly oily scalp soaks were prescribed.

Formula 1

Vegetable oils	Essential oils
Triticum vulgare 3.5 ml	*Syzygium aromaticum* gem. 0.1 ml
Simmondsia chinensis 20 ml	*Pelargonium graveolens* 0.4 ml
	Cedrus atlantica 1 ml

This was massaged into the scalp and left overnight, then shampooed off in the morning using a mild, herbal-based shampoo formulated for frequent use. After 10 days the redness and flakiness appeared less on inspection but itchiness was still present so the formula was changed.

Formula 2

Vegetable oils	Essential oils
Triticum vulgare 3 ml	*Melaleuca alternifolia* 1 ml
Simmondsia chinensis 15 ml	*Pelargonium graveolens* 0.5 ml
Calophyllum inophyllum 5 ml	*Matricaria recutita* 0.5 ml

The same regime was followed for a further 14 days by which time the itchiness had gone. The aroma was not well liked and to encourage compliance an alternative formula was prescribed.

Formula 3

Vegetable oils	Essential oils
Helianthus annuus 5 ml	*Melaleuca alternifolia* 0.75 ml
Simmondsia chinensis 16 ml	*Pelargonium graveolens* 0.25 ml
Calophyllum inophyllum 2.5 ml	*Pogostemon cablin* 0.5 ml

This formula proved aesthetically acceptable and was used three times a week for a further month, by which time all flakiness, itching and irritation had gone.

He continued to use this formula once a week and over a period of several months reported a marked improvement in scalp health and no return of symptoms.

The benefits of honey

The value of honey in cosmetics has been recorded across centuries of traditional use and its therapeutic potential in the management of seborrheic dermatitis and dandruff has been investigated.[57] Thirty patients with chronic seborrheic dermatitis of the scalp, face and chest were asked to apply diluted crude honey (90% honey diluted in warm water) every other day for four weeks to the lesions with gentle rubbing for two to three minutes. The mixture was left for three hours before rinsing with warm water. The patients were followed daily for itching, scaling and hair loss and the lesions were examined. All patients showed marked improvements, itching was relieved and scaling disappeared within one week and lesions completely within a fortnight. In addition, patients showed subjective improvement in hair loss.

Patients showing improvements were then included in a six-month prophylactic phase where half continued the weekly honey treatment while the other half served as a control. None of the patients treated with honey relapsed while the non-treated patients experienced a relapse of the lesions two to four months after stopping treatment. It is valid to suggest that honey offers a suitable medium for essential oil-based prophylactic care of dandruff and seborrheic dermatitis if clients can be persuaded to adopt a regular regime.

Cradle cap

Infantile seborrheic dermatitis usually affects the scalp and is commonly known as cradle cap. It presents as patchy, yellow, greasy scales over the scalp area and can extend to the face, behind the ears and neck creases. It is not itchy and usually appears within the first few weeks after birth and clears within a few months. The causes are not clearly defined, but are likely to involve *Malassezia*.

Treatment is aimed at softening and removing the accumulated scales with gentle vegetable oil massage prior to shampooing.

Nail disorders

The nail is made up of a nail bed, nail matrix and a nail plate and consists of a dense plate of hardened keratin between 0.3 and 0.5 mm thick (*see* Figure 1.4 in Chapter 1). Fingernails grow at 0.1 mm per day; the toenails grow more slowly, taking over a year to replace a large toenail. Primary skin disease, trauma, infections and some systemic diseases can alter nail structure, leaving visible signs. Table 11.10 gives an overview of nail involvement in common skin disorders (also *see* Table 11.11).

Treatment of nails with aromatherapy

General advice for maintaining healthy nails includes avoiding exposing them to harsh chemicals, trauma and water by wearing cotton-lined vinyl gloves when required. Regular moisturising with ointments, especially following immersion in water helps to prevent dry and splitting nails. Weekly nail soaks promote nail

Table 11.10 Clinical signs on the nail of common dermatoses.

Dermatoses	Nail changes
Alopecia areata	Shallow pitting, uniform surface stippling.
Eczema	Coarse pitting, transverse ridging, dystrophy.
Lichen planus	Thin nail plate, longitudinal grooving and ridging, complete nail loss, adhesion of proximal nail fold to nail bed (pterygium).
Psoriasis	Pitting, thickening, irregular separation of nail from nail bed (onycholysis) as scale accumulates, brown or yellow discolouration. Pitting distinguishes it from fungal infection.

Table 11.11 Nail infections.

Infection	Cause and presentation
Acute paronychia	An abscess usually caused by staphylococci. The onset is rapid and presents with a painful, red swelling of the proximal and lateral nail fold. Draining the abscess provides immediate relief.
Chronic paronychia	Presents with tenderness and mild swelling of the lateral and proximal nail folds which become boggy and swollen. *Candida albicans* and gram-negative bacteria are involved but are probably opportunistic colonisers. Several nails will be involved and it occurs in those whose hands are repeatedly wet. The nail plate becomes discoloured and rippled but not thickened as in *Tinea unguium*.
Onychomycosis (*Tinea unguium*)	*Tinea rubrum* and *T. mentagrophytes* are responsible for most fungal nail infections. Trauma predisposes the nail to infection and distal subungual infection, spreading proximally is the most common pattern of nail invasion. Fungal growth in the plate causes the nail to separate from the bed, crumble and turn yellow.

Table 11.12 Essential oils
active against nail-infective
fungi.

Cinnamomum zeylanicum cort.[60]
Foeniculum vulgare[61]
Melaleuca alternifolia[58–60,62]
Ocimum gratissimum[63,64]
Thymus vulgaris[60]

---

integrity and strength and can be incorporated into regular home manicure and pedicure sessions.

As the nail plate prevents penetration of essential oils into the nail bed and the matrix, which is covered by the proximal nail fold, chronic fungal nail diseases are notoriously difficult to treat topically. For a topical antifungal to be effective, it must be capable of penetrating the hardened keratin and staying in situ in sufficient concentration long enough to destroy the causative organism. Essential oils subjected to the rigours of randomised clinical trials in this area are few and far between but limited evidence for some oils does exist.

Twice-daily neat application of *Melaleuca alternifolia* (tea tree) oil compared favourably with 1% clotrimazole in one trial, with both patient groups showing similar improvements after six months.[58] Syed *et al.*[59] administered 2% butenafine hydrochloride and 5% *Melaleuca alternifolia* cream in a randomised placebo-controlled trial, where the placebo cream contained *Melaleuca alternifolia*. Results showed an 80% cure rate in the active group and no relapse after one year. It was concluded that the combination of tea tree and butenafine hydrochloride offered a safe, effective alternative to systemic administration of antifungals.

Table 11.12 identifies essential oils with proven activity against nail-infective fungi which can be incorporated into nail treatments. Application over the long term – at least three months – is required for full mycological cure.

References

1 Ro BI, Dawson TL. The role of sebaceous gland activity and scalp microfloral metabolism in the etiology of seborrheic dermatitis and dandruff. *J Investigative Dermatol SP*. 2005; **10**(3): 194–7.

2 Gupta MA. Psychiatric comorbidity in dermatological disorders. In: Walker C, Papadopoulos L, editors. *Psychodermatology*. Cambridge: Cambridge University Press; 2005. p. 29–43.

3 Brown SK, Shalita AR. Acne vulgaris. *Lancet*. 1998; **351**: 1871–6.

4 Morganti P, Randazzo SD, Giardina A *et al.* Effect of phosphatidylcholine linoleic acid-rich and glycolic acid in acne vulgaris. *J Appl Cosmetol*. 1997; **15**: 21–32.

5 Cunliffe B. Diseases of the skin and their treatment – acne. *Pharm J*. 2001; **267**: 749–52.

6 Zouboulis CC. Acne and sebaceous gland function. *Clin Dermatol*. 2004; **22**: 360–6.

7 Carson CF, Riley TV. Susceptibility of *Propionibacterium acnes* to the essential oil of *Melaleuca alternifolia*. *Lett Appl Microbiol*. 1994; **19**(1): 24–5.

8 Bassett IB, Pannowitz DL, Barneston RS. A comparative study of tea tree oil versus benzoylperoxide in the treatment of acne. *Med J Aust*. 1990; **153**: 455–8.

9 Raman A, Weir U, Bloomfield SF. Antimicrobial effects of tea tree oil, and its major components on *Staphylococcus aureus, Staphylococcus epidermidis* and *Propionibacterium acnes*. *Lett Appl Microbiol*. 1995; **21**(4): 242–5.

10 Khalil Z, Pearce AL, Satkunanathan N. Regulation of wheal and flare by tea tree oil: complementary human and rodent studies. *J Invest Dermatol*. 2004; **123**: 683–90.

11 Koh KJ, Pearce AL, Marshman G *et al*. Tea tree oil reduces histamine-induced skin inflammation. *Br J Dermatol*. 2002; **147**: 1212–17.

12 Hayes AJ, Markovic B. Toxicity of Australian essential oil *Backhousia citriodora* (lemon myrtle). Part 1. Antimicrobial activity and in vitro cytotoxicity. *Food Chem Toxicol*. 2002; **40**: 535–43.

13 Opdyke DLJ. Inhibition of sensitisation reactions induced by certain aldehydes. *Food Cosmet Toxicol*. 1976; **14**: 197–8.

14 Orafidiya LO, Agbani EO, Oyedele AO *et al*. Preliminary clinical tests on topical preparations of *Ocimum gratissimum* Linn. leaf essential oil for the treatment of acne vulgaris. *Clin Drug Invest*. 2002; **22**(5): 313–19.

15 Lasek RJ, Chren M. Acne vulgaris and the quality of life of adult dermatology patients. *Arch Dermatol*. 1998; **134**: 454–8.

16 Mallon E, Newton JN, Klassen A *et al*. The quality of life in acne: a comparison with general medical conditions using generic questionnaires. *Br J Dermatol*. 1999; **140**: 672–6.

17 Rossi T, Melegari M, Bianchi A *et al*. Sedative, anti-inflammatory and anti-diuretic effects induced in rats by essential oils of varieties of *Anthemis nobilis*: a comparative study. *Pharmacol Res Commun*. 1988; **20**(Suppl. 5): 71–4.

18 Melegari M, Albasini A, Pecorari G *et al*. Chemical characteristics and pharmacological properties of the essential oils of *Anthemis nobilis*. *Fitoterapia*. 1989; **59**(6): 449–55.

19 Shinde UA, Kulkarni KR, Phadke AS *et al*. Mast cell stabilising and lipoxygenase inhibitory activity of *Cedrus deodara* (Roxb.) Loud. Wood oil. *Ind J Exp Biol*. 1999; **37**: 258–61.

20 Baylac S, Racine P. Inhibition of 5-lipoxygenase by essential oils and other natural fragrant extracts. *Int J Aromatherapy*. 2003; **13**(2/3): 138–42.

21 Krishnamoorthy G, Kavimani S, Loganathan C. Anti-inflammatory activity of the essential oil of *Cymbopogon martini*. *Ind J Pharm Sci*. 1998; **60**(2): 114–16.

22 Miller TM, Wittstock U, Lindequist U *et al*. Effects of some components of the essential oil of chamomile, *Chamomilla recutita*, on histamine release from rat mast cells. *Planta Med*. 1996; **62**(1): 60–1.

23 Khalil Z, Pearce AL, Satkunanathan N. Regulation of wheal and flare by tea tree oil: complementary human and rodent studies. *J Invest Dermatol*. 2004; **23**: 683–90.

24 Koh KJ, Pearce AL, Marshman G *et al*. Tea tree oil reduces histamine-induced skin inflammation. *Br J Dermatol*. 2002; **147**: 1212–17.

25 Kim H-M, Cho S-H. Lavender oil inhibits immediate-type allergic reaction in mice and rats. *J Pharm Pharmacol*. 1999; **51**(2): 221–6.

26 Maruyama N, Sekimoto Y, Ishibashi H *et al*. Suppression of neutrophils accumulation in mice by cutaneous application of geranium essential oil. *J Inflammation*. 2005; **2**(1): www.journal-inflammation.com/content/2/1/1 (accessed 04.11.05).

27 Orafidiya LO, Agbani EO, Oyedele AO *et al*. The effect of *Aloe vera* gel on the anti-acne properties of the essential oil of *Ocimum gratissimum* Linn leaf – a preliminary clinical investigation. *Int J Aromatherapy*. 2004; **14**: 15–21.

28 Korting HC, Schafer-Korting M, Hart H *et al*. Anti-inflammatory activity of *Hamamelis* distillate applied topically to the skin. Influence of vehicle and dose. *Eur J Clin Pharmacol*. 1993; **44**: 315–18.

29 Korting HC, Schafer-Korting M, Klovekorn W *et al*. Comparative efficacy of *Hamamelis* distillate and hydrocortisone cream in atopic eczema. *Eur J Clin Pharmacol*. 1995; **48**: 461–5.

30 Letawe C, Boone M, Pierard GE. Digital image analysis of the effect of topically applied linoleic acid on acne microcomedones. *Clin Exp Dermatol.* 1998; **23**: 56–8.

31 Pugliese PT. *Physiology of the Skin.* Illinois: Allured Publishing; 1996.

32 Habashy RR. Abdel-Naim AB. Khalifa AE *et al.* Anti-inflammatory effects of jojoba liquid wax in experimental models. *Pharmacol Res.* 2004; **51**(2): 95–105.

33 Gupta AK, Chaudhry MM. Rosacea and its management: an overview. *JEADV.* 2005; **19**: 273–85.

34 Georgala S, Katoulis AC, Kylafis GD *et al.* Increased density of *Demodex folliculorum* and evidence of delayed hypersensitivity reaction in subjects with papulopustular rosacea. *JEADV.* 2001; **15**: 441–4.

35 Habif TP. *Clinical Dermatology.* 4th ed. Edinburgh: Mosby; 2004.

36 Gawkrodger DJ. *Dermatology, An Illustrated Colour Text.* 3rd ed. Edinburgh: Churchill Livingstone; 2002.

37 Dirschka T, Tronnier H. Epithelial barrier function and atopic diathesis in rosacea and perioral dermatitis. *Br J Dermatol.* 2004; **150**: 1136–41.

38 Kobayashi H, Tagami H. Distinct locational differences observable in biophysical functions of the facial skin: with special emphasis on the poor functional properties of the SC of the perioral region. *Int J Cosmet Sci.* 2004; **26**(2): 91–101.

39 Biju SS, Ahuja A, Khar RK. Tea tree oil concentration in follicular casts after topical delivery: determination by high-performance thin layer chromatography using a perfused bovine udder model. *J Pharm Sci.* 2005; **94**(2): 240–5.

40 Teichmann A, Jacobi U, Ossadnik M *et al.* Differential stripping: determination of the amount of topically applied substances penetrated into the hair follicles. *J Investig Dematol.* 2005; **125**(2): 264–9.

41 Stenn KS. Hair follicle biology, the sebaceous gland and scarring alopecias. *Arch Dermatol.* 1999; **135**: 973–4.

42 Hay IC, Jamieson M, Ormerod AD. Randomized trial of aromatherapy. *Arch Dermatol.* 1998; **134**: 1349–52.

43 Kalish RS. Randomized trial of aromatherapy: successful treatment for alopecia areata. *Arch Dermatol.* 1999; **135**: 602–3.

44 Gupta AK, Bluhm R. Seborrheic dermatitis. *J Europ Acad Dermatol Venereol.* 2004; **18**(1): 13–26.

45 Burton JL, Pye RJ. Seborrhoea is not a feature of seborrhoeic dermatitis. *Br Med J (Clin Res Ed).* 1983; **286**(6372): 1169–70.

46 Harding CR, Moore AE, Rogers JS. Dandruff: a condition characterised by decreased levels of intercellular lipids in scalp stratum corneum and impaired barrier function. *Arch Dermatol Res.* 2002; **294**: 221–30.

47 Gupta AK. Nicol K, Batra R. Role of antifungal agents in the treatment of seborrheic dermatitis. *Am J Clin Dermatol.* 2004; **5**(6): 417–22.

48 Inamadar AC, Palit A. The genus *Malassezia* and human disease. *Indian J Dermatol Venereol Leprol.* 2003; **69**(4): 265–70.

49 Hammer KA, Carson CF, Riley TV. In vitro activities of ketoconazole, econazole, miconazole and *Melaleuca alternifolia* (tea tree) oil against *Malassezia* species. *Antimicrob Agents Chemother.* 2000; **44**(2): 467–9.

50 Caldefie-Chezet F, Guerry M, Chalchat JC *et al.* Anti-inflammatory effects of *Melaleuca alternifolia* essential oil on human polymorphonuclear neutrophils and monocytes. *Free Radical Res.* 2004; **38**(8): 805–11.

51 Adam K, Sivropoulou A, Kokkini S *et al.* Antifungal activities of *Origanum vulgare* subsp. *hirtum, Mentha spicata, Lavandula angustifolia* and *Salvia fruticosa* essential oils against human pathogenic fungi. *J Agric Food Chem.* 1998; **46**: 1739–45.

52 Cassella S, Cassella J, Smith I. Synergistic antifungal activity of tea tree (*Melaleuca alternifolia*) and lavender (*Lavandula angustifolia)* essential oils against dermatophytes infection. *Int J Aromatherapy.* 2002; **12**(1): 2–15.

53 Hammer KA, Carson CF, Riley TV. Antimicrobial activity of essential oils and other plant extracts. *J of Appl Microbiol.* 1999; **86**: 985–90.

54 Loden M, Andersson AC. Effect of topically applied lipids on surfactant-irritated skin. *Br J Dermatol.* 1996; **134**: 215–20.

55 Lavagna SM, Secci D, Chimenti P *et al.* Efficacy of hypericum and calendula oils in the epithelial reconstruction of surgical wounds in childbirth with caesarean section. *Il Farmaco.* 2001; **56**: 451–3.

56 Dweck AC, Meadows T. Tamanu (*Calophyllum inophyllum*) – the African, Asian, Polynesian and Pacific panacea. *Int J Cosm Sci.* 2002; **24**: 341–8.

57 Al-Waili NS. Therapeutic and prophylactic effects of crude honey on chronic seborrheic dermatitis and dandruff. *Eur J Med Res.* 2001; **6**(7): 306–8.

58 Buck DS, Nidorf DM, Addino JG. Comparison of two topical preparations for the treatment of onychomycosis: *Melaleuca alternifolia* (tea tree) oil and clotrimazole. *J Fam Pract.* 1994; **38**(6): 601–5.

59 Syed TA, Qureshi ZA, Ali SM *et al.* Treatment of toenail onychomycosis with 2% butenafine and 5% *Melaleuca alternifolia* (tea tree) oil in cream. *Trop Med Int Health.* 1999; **4**(4): 284–7.

60 Inouye S, Uchida K, Yamaguchi H. *In vitro* and *in vivo* anti-*Trichophyton* activity of essential oils by vapour contact. *Mycoses.* 2001; **44**: 99–107.

61 Patra M, Shahi SK, Midgely G *et al.* Utilization of essential oil as natural antifungal against nail-infective fungi. *Flav Frag J.* 2002; **17**: 91–4.

62 Hammer KA, Carson CF, Riley TV. *In vitro* activity of *Melaleuca alternifolia* (tea tree) oil against dermatophytes and other filamentous fungi. *J Antimicrob Chemother.* 2002; **50**: 195–9.

63 Silva MRR, Oliveira JG, Fernandes OFL *et al.* Antifungal activity of *Ocimum gratissimum* towards dermatophytes. *Mycoses.* 2005; **48**: 172–5.

64 Amvam Zollo PH, Tchoumbougnang F, Menut C *et al.* Aromatic plants of tropical Africa. Part XXXII. Chemical composition and antifungal activity of thirteen essential oils from aromatic plants of Cameroon. *Flav Fragr J.* 1998; **13**: 107–14.

Glossary

Absolute	Material obtained from plants by enfleurage or solvent extraction.
Acanthosis	Excessive thickening of the spinous layer of the epidermis (as seen in psoriasis).
Acaricide	An agent that destroys mites.
Acute exposure	Contact with a substance that occurs once or for only a short time (up to 14 days).
Adsorption	Accumulation, commonly of a gas, on the surface of a solid, forming a thin film.
Adulteration	The addition of materials to a whole genuine essential oil which alters its original composition or odour.
Anaphylaxis	Extreme sensitivity to foreign protein or other substances, induced by the introduction of one or more of these substances into system and characterised by acute systemic reactions.
Angiogenesis	The development of blood vessels from an existing vasculature.
Annular	Ring-shaped.
Antiphlogistic	An agent that reduces inflammation.
Aqueous	Involving water.
Aromatic	Having an aroma or fragrance. Chemistry – organic compound containing one or more six-carbon rings in which the electrons are found to be delocalised, characteristic of the benzene series.
Astringent	Constriction of tissues which arrests secretion or bleeding.
Atopic	Predisposition to allergic reactions.
Biodegradation	Decomposition or breakdown of a substance through the action of micro-organisms or other natural physical processes such as sunlight.
Carbuncle	An infection of a group of hair follicles, accompanied by intense inflammation and resulting in an abscess.
Carcinogen	A substance that causes cancer.
Cicatrisant	An agent that promotes the formation of scar tissue.
Circumscribed	With a definite outline.
Cis and trans stereoisomers	This involves a double bond, usually C=C, that does not allow *free rotation* of the attached atoms or groups (unlike a C-C single bond), e.g. *cis*-but-2-ene and *trans*-but-2-ene. The *cis* isomer has the methyl groups on the same side of the bond while the *trans* isomer has them on opposite sides.
Comedone	A blackhead or whitehead caused by dilation of a hair follicle filled with keratin debris, bacteria and sebum.

Commensals	Micro-organisms which normally live on the body without causing harm to the host.
Conglobate	Clumped together to form rounded masses.
Covalent bond	Linkage of two atoms by the sharing of two electrons.
Crust	Dried secretion from an oozing, moist primary skin lesion.
Cyst	An abnormal swelling which may contain keratin, sebum, synovial fluid or mucus.
Dermatophyte	Fungus which invades and infects the skin.
Desquamation	The shedding of the outer layer of the skin in the form of scales.
Diffusion	A passive process in which there is a greater movement of molecules or ions from a region of high concentration to a region of low concentration until equilibrium is reached.
Dose	The amount of a substance to which a person is exposed over some time. Dose is a measurement of exposure.
Double bond	Some atoms share two pairs of electrons forming a double bond (i.e. two covalent bonds).
Emollient	An agent that softens or soothes the skin, preventing water loss.
Erosion	The surface of the skin exposed when the full thickness of the epidermis is removed.
Erythema	Reddening of the skin, resulting from vasodilation.
Excoriation	Linear damage to the epidermis and the upper dermis caused by scratching.
Extensor	Outside skin surface of a joint.
Exudation	Weeping of a fluid from tissues.
Fissure	A painful, deep, linear crack in the surface of the skin.
Flexor	The inner skin surface at a joint.
Fumigant	Air disinfectant.
Furuncle	An infection localised in a hair follicle.
Haemostatic	An agent that stops bleeding.
Hapten	Molecule of low molecular weight that elicits an immune response only when attached to a large carrier such as a protein; the carrier may not elicit a response by itself.
Hazard	A source of potential harm from past, current or future exposures.
Hydrocarbon	An organic chemical compound that is comprised of only carbon (C) and hydrogen (H) atoms.
Hyperkeratinisation	Excessive deposition of keratin in cellular tissue.
Hyperkeratosis	Thickening of the stratum corneum.
Hyperosmia	Hypersensitivity to odours.
Hyperseborrhoea	Excess sebum secretion.
Immunostimulant	Stimulates immune system.
Infundibulum	Top of a duct shaped like a funnel.
Intertrigo	An inflammatory and infected area of opposing surfaces such as beneath a pendulous breast.
In vitro	In an artificial environment outside a living organism or body.

In vivo	Within a living organism or body.
Keratin	A water-insoluble protein which forms the bulk of the stratum corneum, nails and hair.
Keratolytic	An agent which counteracts the excessive production of keratin.
Koebner's phenonemon	Development of lesions (for example of psoriasis) along areas of trauma.
Langerhans cells	Antigen-fixing and antigen-processing cells in the mid-epidermis.
Lichenification	Dry, leathery, thickened skin.
Maceration	Softening of the tissues.
Macule	A non-palpable lesion up to 1–2 cm in diameter.
Melanin	The pigment which gives colour to the skin.
Melanocytes	Epidermal cells which produce pigment granules.
Metabolism	The conversion or breakdown of a substance from one form to another by a living organism.
Mutagen	A substance that causes mutations (genetic damage).
Neonatal	First four weeks after birth.
Nodule	Localised malformations of the skin or mucous membranes.
Onycholysis	Separation of the nail from the nail bed.
Papule	An elevated solid lesion having a diameter less than 5 mm.
Parakeratosis	Retention of nuclei in the cells of the stratum corneum, as in psoriasis.
Paronychia	An inflammation of the nail folds.
Partition	Where two immiscible phases are placed in contact with each other, one containing a solute soluble in both phases, the solute will distribute itself so that when equilibrium is reached no further net transfer of solute will occur.
Patch	A non-palpable lesion larger than 2 cm in diameter.
Perifollicular	Around the hair follicles.
Pilosebaceous	Relating to a hair follicle or its sebaceous gland.
Pityriasis	Scaling of the skin.
Plaque	A flat-topped, palpable, superficial lesion, greater than 0.5 cm in diameter.
ppm	Parts per million.
Pruritus	Itching.
Pustule	A lesion filled with pus. Often associated with hair follicles.
Risk	The probability that something will cause injury or harm.
Rubefacient	Dilates capillaries on skin, reddening the skin.
Saturated compound	Term given to organic molecules which contain no multiple bonds (i.e. double or triple bonds).
Scale	An accumulation of stratum corneum cells which have separated from the remainder of the epidermis. Usually white or pale yellow but can be yellow-brown when thick.
Sebaceous glands	Glands within the skin which secrete sebum.
Sebum	A fatty fluid which lubricates the hair and spreads over the adjacent skin.

Sedative	Allays activity and excitement, calms, relaxes, reduces anxiety.
Striae atrophicae	Stretch marks.
Surfactant	Agent that lowers the surface tension of a liquid, e.g. soaps and detergents.
Tachyphylaxis	Regarding the skin – tolerance the skin develops to a topically applied drug or chemical with repeated applications.
Telangiectasia	Chronic dilation of groups of dermal capillaries making them more visible as seen in rosacea.
Teratogen	A substance that causes defects in the development of the foetus between conception and birth.
Topical anaesthetic	An agent that causes the loss of sensation from the skin or external mucous membranes when applied directly to that area.
Ulcer	Loss of an area of epidermis extending into the dermis.
Unsaturated compound	Term given to organic molecules which contain multiple bonds, i.e. double and triple bonds.
Vesicle	A small blister. A fluid-filled lesion less than 5 mm in diameter.
Vulnerary	An agent used to assist wound healing.
Wheal	A transitory compressible papule of dermal oedema, usually indicating urticaria.
Xerosis	Dry skin.

Appendix

Botanical names of essential oils and hydrosols

Botanical name with naming botanist	Synonym	Family
Achillea millefolium L.	yarrow	Asteraceae
Ammi copticum L.	ajowan	Apiaceae
Angelica archangelica L.	angelica	Apiaceae
Aniba rosaeodora Ducke	rosewood	Lauraceae
Anthemis nobile L.	Roman chamomile	Asteraceae
Apium graveolens L.	celery	Apiaceae
Backhousia citriodora F. Muell.	lemon myrtle	Myrtaceae
Boswellia carterii Birdw.	frankincense	Burseraceae
Boswellia thurifera Roxb. ex Flem	frankincense	Burseraceae
Callitris intratropica R.T. Baker & H.G. Sm.	blue cypress	Cupressaceae
Cananga odorata (Lam.) Hook. F. & Thomson	cananga	Annonaceae
Cananga odorata var. genuina	ylang ylang	Annonaceae
Carum carvi L.	caraway	Apiaceae
Carum copticum L.	ajowan	Apiaceae
Cedrus atlantica Manetti	cedarwood	Pinaceae
Cedrus deodara (Roxb. ex Lambert) G. Don	cedarwood	Pinaceae
Chamaemelum nobile L.	Roman chamomile	Asteraceae
Chamomilla chamomilla Rydb.	German chamomile	Asteraceae
Chamomilla recutita (L.) Rauschert	German chamomile	Asteraceae
Cinnamomum camphora L.	ravintsara	Lauraceae
Cinnamomum camphora L. var. *linaloolifera*	ho wood	Lauraceae
Cinnamomum zeylanicum fol. Blume	cinnamon leaf	Lauraceae
Cistus ladaniferus L.	rock rose	Cistaceae
Citrus aurantifolia Swingle	lime	Rutaceae
Citrus aurantium flos. L.	neroli	Rutaceae
Citrus aurantium L.	bitter orange	Rutaceae
Citrus aurantium ssp. amara fol. L.	petitgrain	Rutaceae
Citrus bergamia Risso	bergamot	Rutaceae
Citrus limon (L.) Burm. f.	lemon	Rutaceae
Citrus paradisi MacFad.	grapefruit	Rutaceae
Citrus reticulata Blanco	mandarin; tangerine	Rutaceae
Citrus reticulata var. mandarin fol.	petitgrain mandarin	Rutaceae

Citrus sinensis Osbeck	orange	Rutaceae
Commiphora myrrha var. molmol Engl.	myrrh	Burseraceae
Coriandrum sativum L.	coriander	Apiaceae
Cuminum cyminum L.	cumin	Apiaceae
Cupressus sempervirens L.	cypress	Cupressaceae
Curcuma longa L.	turmeric	Zingiberaceae
Cymbopogon citratus Stapf	lemongrass	Poaceae
Cymbopogon flexuosus Stapf	East Indian lemongrass	Poaceae
Cymbopogon martini Stapf	palmarosa	Poaceae
Cymbopogon nardus L.	citronella	Poaceae
Daucus carota L.	carrot	Apiaceae
Eucalyptus citriodora Hook.	lemon scented eucalyptus	Myrtaceae
Eucalyptus polybractea R.T. Baker ct cryptone	blue mallee eucalyptus	Myrtaceae
Eugenia caryophyllata Thunb.	clove	Myrtaceae
Foeniculum vulgare P. Mill.	fennel	Apiaceae
Helichrysum italicum (Roth) G. Don	immortelle; everlasting	Asteraceae
Hyssopus officinalis L.	hyssop	Lamiaceae
Illicium verum Hook. f.	star anise	Illiciaceae
Inula helenium L.	elecampane	Asteraceae
Jasminum grandiflorum L.	jasmine	Oleaceae
Laurus nobilis L.	bay	Lauraceae
Lavandula angustifolia Mill.	lavender	Lamiaceae
Lavandula latifolia Medik.	spike lavender	Lamiaceae
Lavandula latifolia spica	spike lavender	Lamiaceae
Lavandula officinalis Chaix	lavender	Lamiaceae
Leptospermum scoparium J.R. Forst & G. Forst.	manuka	Myrtaceae
Lippia citriodora H.B. & K.	lemon verbena	Verbenaceae
Litsea cubeba (Lour.) Pers.	may chang	Lauraceae
Matricaria recutita L.	German chamomile	Asteraceae
Melaleuca alternifolia Cheel	tea tree	Myrtaceae
Melaleuca cajuputi Roxb.	cajeput	Myrtaceae
Melaleuca ericifolia Sm.	rosalina	Myrtaceae
Melaleuca leucadendron L.	niaouli	Myrtaceae
Melaleuca quinquenervia (Cav.) S.T. Blake	niaouli	Myrtaceae
Melaleuca viridiflora Gaertn.	niaouli	Myrtaceae
Melissa officinalis L.	lemon balm	Lamiaceae
Mentha arvensis L.	cornmint	Lamiaceae
Mentha piperita L.	peppermint	Lamiaceae
Mentha pulegium L.	pennyroyal	Lamiaceae
Mentha spicata L.	spearmint	Lamiaceae
Myrtus communis L.	myrtle	Myrtaceae
Ocimum basilicum L.	sweet basil	Lamiaceae

Ocimum gratissimum L.	clove basil; African basil	Lamiaceae
Origanum compactum Benth.	oregano	Lamiaceae
Origanum majorana L.	sweet marjoram	Lamiaceae
Origanum onites L.	oregano (Turkish)	Lamiaceae
Origanum vulgare L.	oregano	Lamiaceae
Origanum vulgare ssp. hirtum Kuntze	oregano (Greek)	Lamiaceae
Pelargonium asperum Willd.	geranium	Geraniaceae
Pelargonium graveolens L'Her.	geranium	Geraniaceae
Petroselinum crispum (Mill.) A.W. Hill	parsley	Apiaceae
Picea mariana (P. Mill.) B.S.P.	black spruce	Pinaceae
Pinus sylvestris L.	Scots pine	Pinaceae
Piper nigrum L.	black pepper	Piperaceae
Pogostemon cablin (Blanco) Benth.	patchouli	Lamiaceae
Pogostemon patchouli Bell	patchouli	Lamiaceae
Ravensara aromatica Sonn.	ravintsara	Lauraceae
Rosa centifolia L.	rose	Rosaceae
Rosa damascena Mill.	rose	Rosaceae
Rosmarinus officinalis ct camphor	rosemary ct camphor	Lamiaceae
Rosmarinus officinalis L.	rosemary	Lamiaceae
Rosmarinus officinalis L. ct verbenone	rosemary ct verbenone	Lamiaceae
Rosmarinus pyramidalis L.	upright rosemary	Lamiaceae
Salvia lavandulifolia Vahl	Spanish sage	Lamiaceae
Salvia officinalis L.	common sage	Lamiaceae
Salvia sclarea L.	clary sage	Lamiaceae
Santalum album L.	sandalwood	Santalaceae
Satureja hortensis L.	summer savory	Lamiaceae
Satureja montana L.	winter savory	Lamiaceae
Saussurea lappa C.B. Clarke	costus	Asteraceae
Syzygium aromaticum (L.) Merr. & L.M. Perry	clove	Myrtaceae
Tanacetum vulgare L.	tansy	Asteraceae
Thuja occidentalis L.	cedar leaf; thuja	Cupressaceae
Thymus capitatus L.	thyme	Lamiaceae
Thymus vulgaris ct carvacrol	thyme ct carvacrol	Lamiaceae
Thymus vulgaris ct linalol	thyme ct linalol	Lamiaceae
Thymus vulgaris ct thymol	thyme ct thymol	Lamiaceae
Thymus vulgaris L.	common thyme	Lamiaceae
Trachyspermum ammi L.	ajowan	Apiaceae
Valeriana officinalis L.	valerian	Valerianaceae
Vetiveria zizanioides (L.) Nash ex Small	vetiver	Poaceae

Vegetable/fixed/infused oils

Botanical name	Synonym
Azadirachta indica	neem
Borago officinalis	borage
Butyrospermum paradoxa	shea butter; karité butter
Calendula officinalis	calendula; marigold
Calophyllum inophyllum	tamanu
Carthamus tinctorius	safflower
Cocos nucifera	coconut
Corylus avellana	hazelnut
Helianthus annuus	sunflower seed
Hypericum perforatum	St John's wort
Juglans regia	walnut
Oenothera biennis	evening primrose
Olea europaea	olive
Persea americana	avocado
Persea gratissima	avocado
Prunus dulcis	sweet almond
Rosa mosqueta	rosehip seed
Rosa rubiginosa	rosehip seed
Simmondsia chinensis	jojoba
Simmondsia sinensis	jojoba
Theobroma cacao	cocoa butter
Vitellaria paradoxa	shea butter; karité butter
Vitis vinifera	grape seed

Some voluntary organisations and support groups

Acne Support Group
PO Box 9
Newquay
Cornwall
TR9 6WG
Tel: 0870 8702263
www.stopspots.org

Hairline International – The Alopecia Patients' Society
Lyons Court
1668 High Street
Knowle
West Midlands
B93 0LY
Tel: 01564 775281
www.hairlineinternational.co.uk

Herpes Viruses Association
41 North Road
London
N7 9DP
Tel: 0845 1232305
www.herpes.org.uk

National Eczema Society
Hill House
Highgate Hill
London
N19 5NA
Tel: 020 7281 3553
www.eczema.org

Patch test requirements (Finn chambers)
Bio-Diagnostics Ltd
Upton Industrial Estate
Rectory Road
Upton-upon-Severn
Worcestershire
Tel: 01684 592262

Psoriasis Association
Milton House
7 Milton Street
Northampton
NN2 7JG
Tel: 0845 6760076
www.psoriasis-association.org.uk

Scar Information Service
PO Box 2003
Hull
HU3 4DJ
Tel: 0845 1200022
www.scarinfo.org

Sun Know How Campaign
Health Education Authority
Hamilton House
Mabledon Place
London
WC1H 9TX
Tel: 0800 665544

Index

Page numbers in *italic* refer to tables or figures.